The Royal Doctors
1485–1714

The Royal Doctors 1485-1714

Medical Personnel at the Tudor and Stuart Courts

Elizabeth Lane Furdell

University of Rochester Press

University of Rochester Press
668 Mt. Hope Avenue
Rochester, New York, 14620, USA
and at P.O. Box 9, Woodbridge, Suffolk IP12 3DF, UK

Library of Congress Cataloging-in-Publication Data

Furdell, Elizabeth Lane.
The royal doctors, 1485–1714 : medical personnel at the Tudor and Stuart courts / Elizabeth Lane Furdell.
p. cm.
Includes bibliographical references and index.
ISBN 1-58046-051-8 (alk. paper)
1. Physicians—England—History—16th century. 2. Physicians—England—History—17th century. 3. Medicine—England—History—16th century. 4. Medicine—England—History—17th century. I. Title.
R487.F87 2001
610'.945'09031—dc21 00-078308
CIP

British Library Cataloguing-in-Publication Data

A catalogue record for this book is available from the British Library

This publication is printed on acid-free paper
Printed in the United States of America
Designed and typeset by Isis-1 Corporation

For Theo

Contents

Acknowledgments

A book of this sort, which has taken over a decade to research, organize, and write, owes its existence to the generosity of institutions and individuals alike. The librarians and archivists at the British Library, especially Rachel Stockdale in the Department of Manuscripts, and at the Royal College of Physicians of London, the Royal College of Surgeons, the Public Record Office, and the Wellcome Institute helped me in countless ways, as did my fellow residents at Crosby Hall in London, former haven for female academics sponsored by the British Federation of University Women. I am particularly grateful to Barbara Tuck and Alisa Craddock, respectively research librarian and interlibrary loan specialist at the University of North Florida (UNF). Elizabeth Simmons, UNF graduate assistant, scoured microfilmed state papers of the Commonwealth to locate interregnum court apothecaries and Caroline McCants, my informal research assistant, pursued miscellaneous leads for me at the University of Florida. I wish to acknowledge the support of the University of North Florida for a sabbatical leave in 1997–98 and a summer research grant in 1999. I express my appreciation also for the perspicacity of Timothy Madigan, Editorial Director at the University of Rochester Press, and to Louise Goldberg, Managing Editor, for helping me bring the project to completion as I originally envisioned it.

Several scholars on both sides of the Atlantic provided information and interpretation that shaped my work. J. C. Sainty (K. C. B.) and R. O. Bucholz have compiled and published the names of officials of the royal household for the period after the Restoration. Sir John also graciously provided me with some of the names of the pre-1660 medical staff that he accumulated for a project now abandoned. Lady Sheila de Bellaigue, Registrar of the Royal Archives at Windsor Castle, furnished me with indispensable information culled from the Establishment Books. I thank Geoffrey Davenport, Registrar at the Royal College of Physicians of London, for permission to quote from the College's unpublished Annals, and Dee Cook, Archivist to the Society of Apothecaries, for her help in tracking the lost state apothecaries of the Interregnum. I owe a debt of gratitude to Harold Cook, Barrett Beer, Anita Guerrini, Robert Frank, Pat Rogers, Donald Pierce, Sharon Arnoult, Mordechai Feingold, and my dear friend, Robert Remini, for suggestions and cautions along the way. Fellow members of the electronic network H-Albion have been generous with their bibliographic and interpretive tips. Most importantly, special thanks for their encouragement and love go to my sons, James and Andrew Furdell, and to my husband and colleague, Theophilus Prousis.

Portions of chapter 7 relating to Dr. James Welwood are fashioned from part of my biography, *James Welwood: Physician to the Glorious Revolution*

(Conshohocken, Penn.: Combined Publishing, 1998), and from "The Surprising Dr. Welwood: Physician and Polemicist," *Journal of the Royal Society of Medicine* 87 (1994): 682–84. Comments on the unique Clippingdale manuscript have their basis in "The Life and Work of Samuel Dodd Clippingdale, Physician and Antiquarian," *Journal of the Royal Society of Medicine* 82 (1989): 758–60. Information I gathered on Drs. Bate, Boorde, Harris, and Welwood will appear in entries written by me for the *New Dictionary of National Biography*, forthcoming from Oxford University Press in 2004. An earlier version of my treatment of Queen Anne's doctors appeared as "Medical Personnel in the Court of Queen Anne," *The Historian* 68 (1986): 412–429. Additional material on royal physicians Walter Bayley, Robert Jacob, and surgeon William Clowes came from a paper, "Tudor Medical Travellers," presented at the 1993 Sixteenth-Century Studies Conference in Atlanta. Panel commentator Ellen Macek provided me with cogent advice for my work in medical history that I have tried to follow.

Most but not all spellings have been modernized for clarity in this work. Dates are Old Style, based on the Julian Calendar, in use in England until 1752, except that I have calculated the New Year as beginning in January rather than March. Providing monetary equivalents is always tricky, especially over a span of 250 years, and estimates from economic historians vary wildly, but multiplying amounts by one hundred will give a rough approximation of today's value. Until the mid-twentieth century, pounds (£) were made up of twenty shillings (s.) and each shilling of twelve pence (d.).

Introduction

Dr. John Arbuthnot, Augustan Age wit and physician to Queen Anne, opined that biography was one of the new terrors of death.[1] Imagine, then, the dread wrought by prosopography, the composite biography of people with something in common. Such a collection of people was the medical staff of the Tudor and Stuart kings and queens of England, who ministered to the health needs of the monarchs from 1485 to 1714. Using the term "royal doctor" broadly to include both officially designated medical personnel and ad hoc iatric consultants, over three hundred men and a handful of women practiced medicine at the highest levels during the twelve distinct regimes of the Tudor-Stuart centuries, chosen from among their peers to receive appointment to the sovereign, to members of the royal family, and to the household.[2] Their separate stories, examined in chapters chronologically arranged according to reign, offer a unique perspective on the fractured state of medicine in early modern England superimposed on a fractious nation-state. The details of their lives illuminate the transitional nature of political and medical science, both fluctuating between medieval and modern impulses, and the varied ways in which practitioners coped with dangerous inconsistencies in both domains. The royal doctors were likewise important as a group, intimately involved with the fundamental well-being of the nation: responsible for the fitness of its dynasts and through the government prompting changes within the profession of medicine. As an anointed monarch, the ruler claimed both inherent sacred gifts that enabled him to cure the sick and exalted prerogatives that gave him mastery over all the medical world. This theme of mutual effect—of individuals and institutions on one another—unfolds throughout the saga of the royal doctors.

Kings could confer with whomever they wished about health problems, but formal assignments, permanent or temporary, were public concerns that had significant ramifications for all involved. While no single pattern for obtaining royal appointments can be traced from the careers of these medicos, several factors made their appointments more likely, if not certain. Royal doctors often knew the monarch before his accession to the throne in a professional, military, or social capacity. Tudor and Stuart kings and princes frequently had direct association with the army and navy, some commanding campaigns and laying sieges; their serjeant-surgeons accompanied them into combat. Henry VII acquired the services of the surgeon William Altofte after admiring his prowess on the battlefield where the founding Tudor won his crown. Richard Wiseman, surgeon to troops in the Royalist army, so impressed Charles, Prince of Wales, with his useful skills that the prince asked for Wiseman's personal service. Wiseman accompanied him throughout the ordeal of Civil War and exile to become the royal surgeon to a restored Charles II. Edward VI continued the aulic placements of those who had taken care of him as Prince of Wales, and other sovereigns did the same, some bringing medical men from abroad. Upon his accession to the throne of England in 1603, James I brought his favorite Scottish court physician with him from Edinburgh; Charles I's queen, Henrietta Maria, had her doctor, Le Sieur Chartier, accompany her from France; and William of Orange employed Dutch practitioners in his household after the so-called "Glorious Revolution."

Preeminence in a London-based practice or renown in the medical profession might seem to be *sine qua non* for royal favor, but occasionally a little-respected quack would sneak through the screening process. Henry VIII's principal doctor, Thomas Linacre, and surgeon, Thomas Vicary, were at the top of their respective fields. William Clowes the Elder, experienced in military medicine, gained prominence in London in 1575 and the attention of Elizabethan courtiers as surgeon to St. Bartholomew's Hospital. As physician to Henri IV of France, Theodore de Mayerne attracted the attention of James I and, after the French king's death, was summoned to the English court. His spirited defense of chemical remedies propelled him into the forefront of the English medical scene, providing him with a large clientele and substantial influence within the Royal College of Physicians. Dr. Walter Harris, physician-in-ordinary to William and Mary, lectured and published extensively, most notably on acute diseases in infants. At the other end of the spectrum, William Read, a London tailor and creator of miraculous eyedrops, received special favor from near-sighted Queen Anne as her royal oculist.

Politics and religious preference could influence royal patronage of healers as well. Catholic Queen Mary I favored like-minded doctors such as the Italian physician Caesar Dalmaris, whom she naturalized and provided with a tax immunity, and her French-born apothecary, John de Soda I. Sir William Paddy, an early Stuart physician, staunchly defended his collegiate friend, William Laud, when the latter's High Church policies as Charles I's Archbishop of Canterbury elicited Parliamentary enmity. Before becoming the physician of William and Mary in 1691, Dr. James Welwood wrote Whiggish tracts in London and launched a newspaper unfailingly supportive of the Williamite faction. However, several medical appointees, including Dalmaris, transcended politics to serve successive, and very different, households. Remarkably, George Bate was physician to Charles I, beheaded in 1649, Oliver Cromwell, Lord Protector and chief regicide, and Charles II, son of the executed king.

Familial and fraternal connections often proved decisive in landing a coveted royal office. William Clowes, Sr., passed along serjeant-surgeoncy to William Clowes, Jr.; members of the Lister family from Yorkshire doctored Elizabeth I and James I; several generations of Chases served the Stuarts as court apothecaries; Queen Anne's apothecary, Daniel Malthus, arranged for his nephew to receive a preferment to succeed him; and Theodore de Vaux, physician to Charles II, was the godson of Dr. Mayerne. Knowing an illustrious peer might help one garner a key post. The Duke of Norfolk recommended the services of Andrew Boorde to Henry VIII, but Thomas Cromwell devised a different function for the itinerant doctor as a reporter on foreign reactions to the king's divorce. Many of Elizabeth I's key medical appointees were members of the Leicester circle, men of science patronized by Elizabeth's favorite, Robert Dudley, Earl of Leicester. Before becoming James I's personal physician in Scotland in 1616, Dr. George Eglisham enjoyed the patronage of the Marquis of Hamilton. Ambrose Dickins "inherited" his job as serjeant surgeon to Queen Anne in 1710 after serving as apprentice to Charles Bernard, Anne's surgeon for seven years, and marrying Bernard's daughter.

There seems to have been something akin to an "old boys' network" at Oxford and Cambridge through which mentors and their protégés in the sciences established lifelong connections with one another through their colleges. Medical scholars created informal intellectual communities that could easily be transferred, by necessity since there were few academic vacancies, to practice in London and at court; elder royal doctors probably recommended their collegiate associates or students to the monarch or the Lord Chamberlain. For instance, at Merton College, Oxford, in the 1640s and 1650s when William Harvey and Jonathan Goddard were wardens, Charles Scarburgh and Edmund Dickenson were their pupils; at Christchurch, Oxford, in the 1660s medical don Thomas Willis took on Richard Lower as his assistant. After the Stuart Restoration, when Francis Glisson, a graduate of Caius College, was Regius Professor of Physic at Cambridge, his deputy was Robert Brady, Master of Caius. These men were the royal doctors of their respective generations. Historian Robert G. Frank, Jr. points out that patterns of university association colored the membership of the Royal Society, which was dominated by Oxonians, and the College of Physicians in London, which was distinctly Cantabrigian.[3] Those physicians who studied at continental universities developed comparable circles of friendship and reference, probably made even closer by their shared British roots. Elizabethan royal doctors John James and William Paddy were at Leiden at about the same time in the 1580s, as were their Stuart aulic counterparts, Christian Harrell and Thomas Burnet, a hundred years later. Two physicians to the Dual Monarchs, John Hutton and Thomas Lawrence, received their M.D.s from Padua a generation apart, but worked together ministering to the forces of King William; James Welwood and David Hamilton graduated from Reims in the mid-1680s. Barber-surgeons and apothecaries also had their institutions of apprenticeship and guild membership with which to create bonds and alliances that were valuable professionally.

When an ambitious doctor lacked the reputation or affiliations to acquire a post at court, monetary inducements to various superior officials might do the trick. Those with leverage could then recommend the applicant to the Lord Chamberlain or his deputy, who ruled the roost. James I himself rhetorically inquired of his Chamberlain, Robert Carr: "Do not all court graces and place come through your office as Chamberlain, and rewards through [the] treasurer? Do not you two, as it were, hedge in all the court with a manner of necessity to depend upon you?"[4] Besides patrimony and patronage, advancement in the

Tudor and Stuart households always entailed purchase. Bribery was endemic to the preferment process, especially since aspirants expected movement from royal court office to a well-paying position in the administration. Incentives to indispensable friends in high places did not necessarily stop at the conclusion of a successful campaign; moreover, substantial offerings to kings and their councillors were continually expected from medical officeholders. As a result, many medical hopefuls spent beyond their means to procure and retain appointments. Several of the royal doctors almost impoverished themselves in the quest to be physician-in-ordinary, serjeant-surgeon, or chief apothecary, necessitating agitation for increased wages as compensation for their considerable outlay, wages they did not always receive during times of war, revolution, or kingly insolvency.

Luck and auspicious endeavors provide a final explanation for certain royal appointments. John James, the earliest English medical graduate of the University of Leiden, initially came to the attention of Queen Elizabeth when he represented St. Ives in the Parliament of 1585; by 1595 he was physician to her household. John Hinton helped Charles I's queen escape from England during the Civil War and settle safely in France; in gratitude her son, Charles II, made Hinton physician-in-ordinary and knighted him. After Scotsman Robert Morison was wounded in the Civil War, he fled to France where he became a superintendent of the Duke of Orleans's gardens at Blois and met Prince Charles in exile; summoned to England in 1660, Morison became Charles II's senior physician and king's botanist. Flora and fauna featured in two other appointments. Queen Elizabeth designated John Ryche, a member of the Grocers' Company, her royal apothecary upon the recommendation of William Turner, the "Father of English Botany," who saw and admired Ryche's garden. The last of the Stuart monarchs, Queen Anne, consulted Hans Sloane after he made a name for himself collecting specimens in Jamaica in the late 1680s as physician to the Duke of Albemarle; his collection eventually spawned the British Museum. As a concluding example, Queen Anne first encountered the quotable John Arbuthnot at the races. Her consort, Prince George of Denmark, became suddenly sick at Epsom and, after Arbuthnot revived George, the queen rewarded the doctor with a place at court. Arbuthnot's luck continued, as he was able to advance in the ordered list of physicians' ranks when another appointee fell ill. Arbuthnot, a close friend of Tory publicist Jonathan Swift, became Anne's favorite physician and may have impelled her shift away from the Whigs to their rivals, the Tories.

Doctors faced enormous challenges in the Tudor-Stuart centuries from diseases that swept through all classes of people and respected no rank. Plague, sweating sickness, typhus, scurvy, and leprosy infested England periodically during the Tudor-Stuart era. Epidemics of fever and smallpox consumed London throughout the sixteenth and seventeenth centuries. In 1659 smallpox carried off fifteen hundred souls; standard treatments included powdered root of pestilence-wort (butter-burr) dissolved in wine. Understandably, amulets were also popular.[5] Ten thousand Londoners died of plague in 1636; nearly seventy thousand succumbed in 1665, the capital's greatest disaster. London burials exceeded baptisms until late in the eighteenth century.[6] Ague (malaria) was endemic to marshy environments like the east coast of Great Britain and laid its victims low with intermittent fevers.[7] However, an "ordinary" ague raged all over England in the summer of 1612. Syphilis, labeled the "French pox" in England (and the "English disease" in France), ran rampant, a congenital form affecting the royal family and ruining its chances for ease of succession. Childbirth was a woman's greatest fear, and for good reason. Those who lived through it survived to bear a child every year for ten to fifteen years. Infant mortality rates were ghastly, highest among aristocratic families that employed wet nurses.[8] Almost half of all children died at birth or in infancy, and those who survived to toddlerhood were carried off by infectious diseases like smallpox; rickets spread through England in the early years of the seventeenth century.[9] Such was the state of the nation's health.

On top of the stresses and strains of caring for persons of the utmost importance to the realm during decades of decimation, the royal doctors had to cope with political and religious upheavals that led to regicide and revolution, as well as with sharp theoretical and jurisdictional divisions in English medicine.[10] Jealous competitors for governmental favor might point out iatric mistakes, made out of ignorance, incompetence, or even malice; royal physician Walter Harris blamed the death of Queen Mary II on his rival, Richard Lower. Attending to the illness of a king often required a constant presence at court, sometimes without lodgings there, or traveling long distances to rural palaces when called, taking away the opportunity to care for and derive income from other patients. Yet there was no dearth of applicants for official medical positions. Just as there were multiple ways to obtain royal employment, there appear to have been a number of reasons for seeking work with the sovereign. Prestige no doubt tempted many, though not all, skilled practitioners to compete for royal favor. The title physician-in-ordinary, sergeant surgeon, or royal apothecary carried with it immediate elevation to the upper echelons of the profession, including leadership of one's colleagues in occupational organizations. Being sergeant-surgeon meant automatically becoming Master of the Barber Surgeons.[11]

Royal doctors received handsome, often lifelong annuities, and the crown favored them with the chance to buy or lease lands and estates. The drawbacks involved slowness of payment, especially to the royal apothecaries for their supplies, but even then the promise of payment enabled the medical appointees to establish lines of credit in lieu of cash. The drawbacks seemed minor in comparison to such perquisites as the opportunity to work with and care for an elite clientele, to travel abroad or within Britain as part of the royal entourage, to function perhaps in a political or diplomatic capacity, and to pass on appointments to sons or other favored protégés by grants of reversion. Records of the Privy Seal testify to allowances for food, certain items of clothing, and lodging while attending the monarch, as well as other rewards in bonuses, lands, and houses. Henry VIII's physician, Thomas Linacre, received a canonry, three prebendaries, and five rectories from a grateful monarch; John Chambre, who succeeded Linacre at the Henrician court, came to hold several "livings" in England plus an archdeaconry in Ireland. Moreover, a gracious sovereign could bestow a knighthood, as well as armorial ensigns and other emoluments.[12]

The centuries of Tudor-Stuart rule began with the victory of Henry Tudor over Richard III at Bosworth Field in 1485 and the establishment of a new dynasty. Historians acknowledge that, when put into long-range perspective, Henry VII's reign marks a turning point in English history.[13] By 1714 the Tudors and their Scottish cousin-successors, the Stuarts, had exhausted their bloodlines; distant relatives from Germany arrived to fill the vacancy. In between these bookend years, England experienced a harrowing metamorphosis provoked by Henry VIII's momentous break in the 1530s with the Roman Catholic Church. From then on, religious division colored all aspects of life, exacerbating political difference and accelerating political transformation. Foreign relations on both sides of the Channel were reconfigured to reflect England's Protestant orientation. During the seventeenth century, domestic tensions deepened, resulting in the Civil War, regicide, and in 1688 the Glorious Revolution, a relocation of the center of governmental power in Parliament. Throughout this turmoil, any official with aulic duties needed to be adroit at withstanding the chaotic, potentially dangerous gyrations of public life.

To complicate matters, English medicine itself underwent significant alteration in the pivotal 230 years of the Tudors and the Stuarts. Disputes over medical theory created one source of tension within the community of physicians as followers of newer, experimental approaches to diagnosis and treatment clashed with supporters of the traditional teachings of Galen, the Greek court physician to second-century Roman emperor Marcus Aurelius. The medical curricula at Oxford and Cambridge, the only universities in Britain conferring degrees in medicine during the period, adhered to Galenic precepts and the humoral explanation for illness. According to Galen, four "humors" or bodily fluids govern the body: blood, phlegm, yellow bile, and black bile. Personality is also affected by the humors. People with too much blood are sanguine, or ardent and hopeful; those with an excess of phlegm are phlegmatic, or dull and apathetic; melancholiacs, the depressed and unhappy among us, suffer from immoderate black bile; and the peevish and cross are understandably bilious, burdened with superfluous yellow bile.

Classical Galenism embraced the notion of balance and moderation, postulating that human beings are a balance of warm, cold, dry, and moist. Thomas Elyot popularized a Renaissance version of Galenism in Britain in his 1534 book, *The Castel of Helth*, the earliest manual in the vernacular that warned the layman not to make his own diagnosis, but explained how to maintain humoral balance.[14] Stability strengthened good health; conversely, a surfeit or deficit of any of the humors caused sickness and had to be rectified. An overabundance of blood caused fever, but bleeding a patient of that surplus could restore wellness. Purging with laxatives, vomitories, and emmenagogues eliminated other redundant humors, while certain prescriptives relieved humoral shortages. Medications or other recipes promised restoration and rejuvenation, albeit they were usually taken by a patient denied fresh air or sunlight.

Even food was considered medicinal if prepared properly, reflecting the ancient conviction that internal medicine was a specialized construct of dietetics and that preparing food was akin to preparing medicines. Cooking must display the Galenic ideal of balance: wet, dry, cold, and hot; a tempered diet should contain food from each category. Beans, for instance, were deemed cold, so they should be supplemented with hot spices to counteract them. Febrile patients should eat predominantly cold foods. Accordingly, a royal physician advised the monarch on his diet, and discussed victuals with the steward, the head server, and the master cook.[15] John Archer, an advertising empiric who treated Charles II, categorized hare as "a melancholy meat, and therefore not good for those who have dry bodies."[16] Auxiliary to these theories was the idea that each person had a unique constitution and therefore needed to be treated individually; particular treatments in one case might not be good for someone else. Furthermore, since disease could deviate over time as the physiology of the patient changed, treatment needed to be varied according to the current state of the illness. Galen's theories went virtually unchallenged until the mid-sixteenth century; in fact, the Renaissance passion for classical learning only bolstered the prestige of Galenic medicine, thus inhibiting much scientific investigation and experimentation.

The faculties at continental universities like Salerno and Leiden taught something else, inspired by the teachings of the Swiss chemist Paracelsus (1493–1541). Paracelsus, nom de plume of Theophrastus Bombastus von Hohenheim, ridiculed Galenism and its four humors and insisted that other factors caused illness, factors that could be arrested with chemical medicines. Since specific cures would check specific diseases, only intensive laboratory experimentation could unlock the secrets of sickness. Paracelsus upset the medical profession with his unorthodox ideas, monumental ego, and insistence on writing in German rather than "popish" Latin. He was exiled from his post at the University of Basel and led an itinerant life, practicing medicine, writing books, and studying diseases of miners. Paracelsus moved back and forth between magic and science. Nevertheless, his consequence was as conspicuous as his defiance, in ways parallel to Martin Luther's contempt for the Roman Catholic Church, but even more thorough, given Paracelsus' consistent disdain for all authority.[17] One by-product of Paracelsianism was symptom observation and greater participation by the physician in the care afforded to the patient. Myriad diseases, his followers held, revealed themselves through fairly constant symptoms easily recognized by the patient and easily diagnosed by any observer. Once diagnosed, exact countermeasures could be prescribed rather than the protean regimen required by Galenists. Those English doctors who trained abroad learned the precepts of Paracelsus and took them to heart. Thomas Sydenham, the "English Hippocrates," studied at Montpellier and developed a taxonomy of syndromes. He also claimed that the body has its own powerful means of dealing with disease, and that the recuperative energy possessed by everyone ought not to be interfered with.[18] By the middle of the seventeenth century, about half of the Fellows in the Royal College of Physicians were graduates of continental universities. Only then, with empiricism the fashion in London, did Oxford and Cambridge substantially alter their curricula. A few English monarchs, notably James I and William III, deliberately engaged advocates of the new medicine, but others seemed oblivious to the ideological struggle within the profession.

This leads to the other line of fracture in Tudor-Stuart medicine—professional jurisdiction. Galen had written that surgery was only a method of treatment; hence, a separation of physicians from surgeons existed in imperial Rome. Although this division was not observed in medieval Italian universities, the medical faculty-physicians at Paris did subscribe to the division, perhaps out of professional self-defensiveness.[19] Moreover, there was a strong ecclesiastical impulse for the scission. Discrete, functional categories within the medical community developed from an edict in 1163 issued by the Council of Tours under Pope Alexander III that members of the clergy could not participate in operations involving the shedding of blood.[20] Since medieval physicians were almost always priests, they were forbidden from practicing surgery; hence, another vocational group—first barbers, then surgeons—must perform that function along with the administration of purgatives, the setting of bones, and the extraction of teeth. Moreover, university-trained doctors were neither cooks nor brewers; they were "second philosophers."[21] Accordingly, someone else had to mix the recipes and make the elixirs prescribed by physicians for the sick. The apothecaries had their origins among the Norman spicers and pepperers who preserved food or disguised its taste, so their gradual evolution into herbal mixers filled a need and made sense. However, the apothecaries had social precedence over barber-surgeons because their guild ranked higher in the English civic order.[22]

The appointed positions of physician, surgeon, and apothecary to the English monarch date from medieval times. William the Conqueror (r. 1066–87) was attended by a fellow Norman, the physician-bishop Gilbert Maminot, who also represented the king on church business in Rome.[23] However, Edward II (r. 1307–27) was the king of England who initiated the appointment of a medical staff for the court; his son and successor, Edward III (r. 1327–77), employed four doctors and surgeons. Primary tasks for royal physician-priests included saying grace at meals, recommending and tasting the monarch's food, and witnessing the royal testament. They prescribed medicines within the household and kept the court free from infected persons. Later, the king's physicians also certified the bills of the court apothecaries. The Ordinances for the Royal Household in 1604 regulated the fees paid to physicians. Dr. John Craig, who had accompanied James I from Scotland as his "principal mediciner," collected £160 for daily attendance plus the "bouche of the court:" one loaf and a gallon of ale in the morning, another meal in the afternoon, plus supplies of wine, torches, and coal.[24] Bouche could be a moneymaking perquisite; Dr. William Harvey, the king's physician in 1640, exchanged his board for an allowance of £200 a year.[25] Being ranked annoyed the royal healers, but the sovereign specified ordinal status for each appointee to the Person, thereby dictating levels of standing and salary within the medical corps.

Monarchs themselves deliberately influenced the evolution of the medical profession. In 1518 Henry VIII chartered the Royal College of Physicians of London in response to urging from his physician, Thomas Linacre, who became its inaugural President; Henry's serjeant-surgeon, Thomas Vicary, likewise persuaded the king to commission the united Barber-Surgeons' Company in 1540.[26] That same year, the king created Regius Professorships in Medicine at Oxford and Cambridge, the first endowed chairs of medicine in England.[27] James I agreed to incorporate the Apothecaries' Society in 1614 after that group separated from the Grocers' Company, and Charles II established the Royal Society in 1662. Significantly, it was the Royal College of Physicians that came to dominate and regulate Tudor-Stuart iatric practices, taking over from bishops the function of licensing doctors in the capital. Just as significant was the deliberate pruning of College authority by the government of William III and his forceful encouragement of the physicians' more pragmatic challengers, the surgeons and apothecaries, in providing for the military needs of his regime.

Much of the activity of the Fellows of the College involved investigating unlicensed practitioners in London and prosecuting them. One can understand the jealousy with which physicians guarded their privileges. A medical degree took fourteen years to obtain at Oxford, with bachelor's and master's of arts degrees as prerequisites to commencing the study of medicine. However, the College created some of its own problems by keeping the number of licensed physicians preposterously small in a burgeoning metropolis. At the beginning of the seventeenth century, for instance, fewer than fifty men belonged to the College, serving a populace of around two hundred and fifty thousand; by the middle of the century the number of Fellows had doubled, but so had the population. In 1700 the paucity of physicians reached scandalous proportions: one College member for 1300 serious cases of illness per day.[28] Impoverished, London-born patients received care free of charge at three local hospitals, but the middle class needed doctors, too. Since London was woefully short of physicians, the bourgeoisie sought out others who could, for smaller fees, fix what ailed them. A blossoming "medical marketplace" emerged from the demand for more doctors and a supply of new health-care entrepreneurs. Large numbers of enterprising people advertised their medical goods and services to the public in printed handbills and newspapers.[29] Consequently, while the ratio of bona fide physicians to Londoners remained at about 1:5,000 throughout the seventeenth century, the ratio of all medical practitioners to citizens was

1:400.[30]

An Act of 1540 defined medicine to encompass surgery, but most physicians did not perform operations or make medicines, preferring the tradition of working consistently with the same surgeon and apothecary.[31] Ironically, by collaborating with those whom they regarded as mere tradesmen, physicians inadvertently gave credence to those tradesmen's skills. Moreover, during the worst epidemics in the city, doctors often left town, abdicating their responsibilities and their clients to others.[32] Barber-surgeons, apothecaries, and unlicensed "irregulars" steadfastly tended to the needs of ordinary Londoners. Even some monarchs endorsed unlicensed medical men and women, and by appointing the occasional charlatan they undermined the professional monopoly of the Fellows.[33]

Henry VII appointed Benedict Frietre as the inaugural Tudor royal physician in 1485, allocating him £40 per annum and giving him keepership of Prince Arthur's wardrobe the following year. Thus begins the litany of Tudor-Stuart medical staff, a group challenged with the enormous assignment of keeping crowned heads and regal bodies healthy. Elizabeth I introduced the title physician-in-ordinary when she nominated Robert Huicke as the premier medical man in her service; physician-to-the-household was a separate job, as was physician extraordinary. Besides a handful of physicians, there were also serjeant-surgeons, principal surgeons, surgeons-in-ordinary and to the household, court herbalists and botanical physicians, chemical physicians and apothecaries, midwives, oculists for the royal eyes, and aurists who syringed the royal ears. The king's barber could pull teeth, the only surgical procedure permitted him after 1540, but there was no official "operator for the teeth" until 1727.[34] Serjeant-surgeoncy dates back to the fifteenth century, when the crown rewarded service with a gift of land or other honors. William Hobbes became the archetypal serjeant-surgeon; in 1461 he was alloted "forty marks with wine, wax, and requisites."[35] The wax referred to a perquisite connected with the duty of embalming members of the royal family. Besides salary, each serjeant-surgeon merited bouche of the court. Richard Wiseman, Charles II's principal surgeon, received £80 per annum and a special pension of £150 for services to the king in exile during the Interregnum.[36] The serjeant-surgeon ranked below the king's physician, but above the surgeon-in-ordinary. Early duties included being present at the torture or maiming of state prisoners. The serjeant-surgeon screened applicants hoping to be touched by the monarch for the "King's Evil," a ritual believed to cure scrofula. Surgeons followed the king onto the field of battle; as late as 1743 John Ranby accompanied George II at Dettingen. For their wartime service they received special compensation of £10 per quarter plus the right to prisoners and plunder.[37] James I's surgeon, Christopher Frederick, treated him for a broken collarbone and hemorrhoids, but when therapies failed, the serjeant-surgeon was responsible for embalming the princely corpse. From 1560 to 1891, two serjeant-surgeons served the household, aided occasionally by a third who received no remuneration.[38] The Barber-Surgeons'

Company recognized the importance of the office in its 1540 rules, requiring that the serjeant-surgeon be seated next to the past Master of the Company and urging that he be made Master as soon as possible.

The office of court apothecary has an unbroken history from the thirteenth-century reign of King John. Two court apothecaries attended the first Tudor king and his queen; they received £10 yearly plus seven houses and lands for their services. Henry VII engaged a serjeant of the King's Confectionary, the man responsible for sweetmeats. Henry VIII liked his desserts so much that he summoned confectioner Richard Babham, who was also the court apothecary, to his coronation and brought Babham along in 1520 to his meeting with Francis I of France at the Field of the Cloth of Gold. Tudor royal apothecaries were entitled, like the other iatric personnel, to bouche of the court. Their employment could be very lucrative as long as they kept scrupulous accounts of the materials they bought, for which they were reimbursed. In addition to medicines, the court apothecaries made perfumes, gargles, and candies of anise seed and sweet fennel; they also supplied sugar for the king's hounds and rhubarb in horehound water for the king's hawks. The apothecaries prepared the monarch's bath with herbs and musk and, following the royal ablutions, took care of the wooden bath tub itself. The court apothecary also furnished the king's council members with disposable, perfumed urinals for use during meetings. Later apothecaries inspected drugs sold in London and some grew rare specimens of plants brought from the New World.[39]

Some royal doctors proved notable in nonmedical matters. William Butts, Henry VIII's physician, advocated radical Protestantism while ministering to the king. Queen Elizabeth I had Robert Jacob negotiate a possible marriage between Lady Mary Hastings and Ivan the Terrible, Tsar of Russia. John Knight, serjeant-surgeon to the Stuarts and a staunch Cavalier, worked in the secret service in 1648.[40] Charles II drafted Alexander Fraizer for political matters and William III facilitated his invasion of England in 1688 with an espionage squadron that utilized his physician and cryptographer, Dr. John Hutton. King William's co-ruler, Queen Mary II, invited her polymath-physician, James Welwood, to write a history of England.

All of these appointments are hard to trace in the years before 1660, because no sources systematically record court medical personnel and precision is rarely attainable. Nonetheless, since the medical staff were compensated at the exchequer and not by one of the household paymasters, their salaries are usually recorded in the exchequer books. Scattered information can also be gleaned from the printed *Calendars of the Patent Rolls* for the years 1485–1509 and 1547–78, the *Calendars of Close Rolls*, and the *Letters and Papers of Henry VIII*, edited by J. S. Brewer, R. H. Brodie, and J. Gairdner, for the years 1509–47. In 1526 Henry VIII issued the Eltham Ordinances, providing for a streamlined royal household and tightened accounting procedures, but uncovering the medical corps is still hit-and-miss. After 1578 evidence of many appointments can be unearthed in the *Calendars of State Papers, Domestic*. Authenticating periods of service is even more problematical, since the relevant exchequer books are not included in the calendars and since not everyone got paid before leaving office. After 1660, when medical openings were filled by the Lord Chamberlain's warrant they were in most cases embodied in Letters Patent under the Great Seal.[41] Royal medical personnel in the northern kingdom of Scotland, not the same persons who served the Stuart dynasty after its accession to the throne in England, have been specified by the Scottish Record Office. Local appointments could be made when necessary to meet the requirements of the court.

Previous attempts to compile information for the whole Tudor-Stuart period resulted in lists that often contained those who only bragged about their connections to kings and queens.[42] Biographical data on unrenowned doctors are sketchy and sometimes apocryphal, and searching is complicated by a lack of standardized spelling during the period, even of surnames. For instance, John Macelo, physician to James I and author of a book on iatrochemical theory, might be discovered as Maccolo or McKulio; James Moleyns, surgeon before and after the Restoration, appears in records as Mullins and Molines. I have relied on several biographical sources of professional information on medicos: Munk's *Roll of the Royal College of Physicians*; Young's *Annals of the Barber-Surgeons of London*; histories of the Apothecaries' Society; collections on alumni from Oxford, Cambridge, and prominent continental universities; and the *Dictionary of National Biography*. Apart from these institutional histories, there now exists a wealth of newer scholarship by trained academics reluctant to accept a narrow, elite focus for medicine; this new scholarship explores the social history of medicine and the role of the suffering patient rather than the doctor.[43]

The "royal doctors," however, were by definition elite, as were their patients. Therefore, my work revives a more traditional concentration on the medical establishment in London, which, given the absence of even a comprehensive listing of the Tudor-Stuart physicians, surgeons, and apothecaries, is still essential to an understanding of the sovereign's household and its iatric personnel. Accordingly, I have explored the unpublished annals of the Royal College of Physicians, whose founding twenty Fellows were all successful medical consultants at the court of Henry VIII, and manuscripts at the Royal College of Surgeons and the Wellcome Institute for the History of Medicine. Luckily, though the private diaries and letters of sixteenth- and seventeenth-century doctors seldom survive, many medical men and a few women published extensively, if not always about medicine.[44] I have examined the mountain of their printed materials and any unpublished manuscript evidence including scattered letters and recipes in the British Library in order to illuminate individual lives and to reveal a collective portrait. For those truly obscure ministers to sick monarchs, as Peter Ackroyd has advised biographers, one must simply invent more freely.[45]

Notes

1. Robert Carruthers, ed., *The Poetical Works of Alexander Pope*, 4 vols. (London: Ingram, 1953) 1: 3. The cause of Arbuthnot's consternation was a series of "deathbed lives" published by Edmund Curll to acknowledge notable deaths during the previous year. See J. LeNeve, *Lives and Characters of the Most Illustrious Persons Who Died in the Year* (London: S. Holt, 1712). The author thanks Pat Rogers for this information. A similar quotation, "biography lends to death a new terror," is attributed to another wit, Oscar Wilde.

2. Though not nominally "royal," I am including the Interregnum (1649–60) republican rule of Oliver Cromwell as a discrete period of medical interest since significant doctors attended him during the Commonwealth and the Protectorate.

3. Robert G. Frank, Jr., "Science, Medicine and the Universities of Early Modern England: Background and Sources, Part 2," *History of Science* 11 (1973): 263.

4. Neil Cuddy, "The Revival of the Entourage: The Bedchamber of James I," in *The English Court from the Wars of the Roses to the Civil War*, ed. David Starkey et al. (London: Longman, 1987), 213.

5. Christina Hole, *The English Housewife in the Seventeenth Century* (London: Chatto and Windus, 1953), 92; see also Lloyd G. Stevenson, "New Diseases of the Seventeenth Century," *Bulletin for the History of Medicine* 39 (1965): 1–21.

6. Charles Creighton, *A History of Epidemics in Britain* 2 vols., (Cambridge: Cambridge University Press, 1891) 1: 532–33; Roy Porter, *London* (Cambridge, Mass.: Harvard University Press, 1996), 42.

7. Malaria, referred to as ague by Chaucer in 1386, had a prolonged incubation in England where summer and autumn infections caused an outbreak each spring. L. W. Hackett, *Malaria in Europe* (London: Oxford University Press, 1937), 31, 61; Henry A. Skinner, *The Origin of Medical Terms* (Baltimore: Johns Hopkins University Press, 1961), 84.

8. Dorothy McLaren, "Fertility, Infant Mortality, and Breast Feeding in the Seventeenth Century," *Medical History* 22 (1978): 380. Roger Schofield and E. A. Wrigley note a sharp rise in child mortality rates between the late sixteenth and early seventeenth centuries. See their "Infant and Child Mortality in England in the Late Tudor and Early Stuart period," in *Health, Medicine and Mortality in the Sixteenth Century*, ed. Charles Webster (Cambridge: Cambridge University Press, 1979), 95.

9. Schofield and Wrigley calculate that 34% of English children died under the age of ten; "Infant Mortality," 61. Lady Anne Fanshawe, wife of Sir Richard Fanshawe, Charles II's ambassador to Portugal, wrote:

> Harrison, my second son, Richard my third, Henry my fourth, and Richard my fifth are all dead; my second lies buried in the Protestant churchyard in Paris; my eldest daughter Anne lies buried in Yorkshire where she died; Elizabeth lies in Madrid where she died of a feve at ten days old; my next daughter of her name lies buried in Kent and my daughter Mary lies in my father's vault in Hertford with my first son, Henry.

See Anne Harrison Fanshawe, *Memoirs of Lady Fanshawe*, ed. N. H. Nicolas (London: Henry Colburn, 1829).

10. Hugh Trevor-Roper calls the European sixteenth and seventeenth centuries an age, like our own, in which medicine was degraded by international politics that combined absolute power with ideological war; see his essay, "Medicine in Politics," *American Scholar* 51 (Winter 1982): 34.

11. "Serjeant Surgeons of England and Their Office," *British Medical Journal* (1900) 1: 583.

12. Knighthood was conferred on countless royal doctors, such as William Butts, another physician to Henry VIII; Gideon de Laune, James I's apothecary, adopted as his coat of arms a gold lion pennant with a fleur-de-lis. Samuel Dodd Clippingdale, Medical Court Roll, 2 vols., 1: xiv, Library of the Royal College of Surgeons, London (LRCS). Clippingdale sent his unpublished historical

scrapbook to the Royal College of Surgeons in 1922; the Library of the Royal College of Physicians has a photocopy.

13. For a discussion of the multiple reasons to consider 1485 as the beginning of a new period in English history, see Alexander Grant, *Henry VII* (London: Methuen, 1985).

14. There is no evidence that Elyot attended Henry VIII. See Stanford Lehmberg, *Sir Thomas Elyot: Tudor Humanist* (Austin: University of Texas Press, 1960); Pearl Hogrefe, *The Life and Times of Sir Thomas Elyot, Englishman* (Ames, Iowa: Iowa State University Press, 1967).

15. George Clark, *History of the Royal College of Physicians of London*, 2 vols. (Oxford: Clarendon Press, 1964–66), 1: 17–18.

16. John Archer, *Every Man His Own Doctor* (London: Peter Lillicrap, 1671), 34.

17. For more on the contention that Paracelsianism was far more radical than Lutheranism, see Hugh Trevor-Roper, "The Paracelsian Movement," in his *Renaissance Essays* (Chicago: University of Chicago Press, 1985), and Trevor-Roper, "The Court Physician and Paracelsianism," in *Medicine at the Courts of Europe* ed. Vivian Nutton (London: Routledge, 1990).

18. Sydenham, despite his influence on medicine and his friendship with the leading intellectuals of his day, never became a Fellow of the Royal College of Physicians of London (although he was a licentiate) and never enjoyed the favor of the Stuarts. He finally received an M.D. from Cambridge in 1676. See Kenneth Dewhurst, *Dr. Thomas Sydenham* (Berkeley: University of California Press, 1966).

19. Clark, *Royal College of Physicians*, 1: 17.

20. Although the separation of physicians and surgeons was nearly complete by the end of the twelfth century, Pope Innocent III issued another ordinance in 1215 reiterating the restriction for ecclesiastics. John Simon, *English Sanitary Institutions*, 2nd ed. (London: John Murray, 1897), 70.

21. The English universities helped standardize medical skills and collected medical texts, giving learned physicians elite status. However, Jews, women, and, after the reign of Henry VIII, non-Anglicans were deliberately excluded from university education in medicine.

22. See Margaret Pelling's revisionist challenge to institutional historians, in "Medical Practice in Early Modern England: Trade or Profession?," *The Professions in Early Modern England*, ed. Wilfrid Prest (London: Croom Helm, 1987), 90–128.

23. Gilbert also ministered to William's queen, Matilda, and was present at the king's death after a riding accident near Rouen in 1087. Faye Getz, *Medicine in the English Middle Ages* (Princeton: Princeton University Press, 1998), 25.

24. Leslie G. Matthews, *The Royal Apothecaries* (London: Wellcome Medical Library, 1967), 84. Bouche could sometimes include clothing and lodging while in attendance on the monarch.

25. D'Arcy Power, "The Serjeant Surgeons of England and Their Office," *St. Bartholomew's Hospital Journal* 8 (March 1901): 81. "Bouche" was eventually augmented with "diet," which included a specified number of dishes, five per day around 1600, twelve to sixteen per day when William Harvey tended King Charles I. Charles, by contrast, enjoyed twenty-eight dishes on a day when meat was eaten and awarded the right to his leftovers to the Groom of the Stool. Kevin Sharpe, "The Image of Virtue: The Court and Household of Charles I," in *The English Court from the Wars of the Roses to the Civil War*, ed. David Starkey et al. (London: Longman, 1987), 235.

26. An earlier attempt by Gilbert Kymer, in 1423, to join university physicians and London surgeons in a Conjoint College of Physicians and Surgeons aimed at regulating medical practice. The group heard one case, then dissolved, probably due to internal squabbling. Getz, *Medicine in the English Middle Ages*, 70.

27. Phyllis Allen, "Medical Education in Seventeenth-Century England," *Journal of the History of Medicine and Allied Sciences* 1 (1946): 117. See also A. Chaplin, "A History of Medical Education in the Universities of Oxford and Cambridge 1500–1850," *Proceedings of the Royal Society of Medicine* 13 (1920): 83–107.

28. Roy Porter reckons the population of London at under 50,000 in 1500, and 180,000 in 1600. Rattansi estimates 225,000 Londoners in 1600–1620, 500,000 by 1660. Owing to the lack of a census, historians differ over the population of London during the Tudor-Stuart era, but most concur on the scarcity of licensed physicians. An exception is Margaret Pelling, who argues that if

one takes into account all medical practitioners, "a high ratio of practitioners to population emerges . . . at least 1:400." Porter, *London*, 42; Pyrali Rattansi, "The Helmontian-Galenist Controversy in Restoration England," *Ambix* 12 (1964): 6–7; Roger A. Hambridge, "Empiricomany or an Infatuation in Favour of Empiricism or Quackery," in *Literature, Science and Medicine*, ed. Serge Soupel and Roger A, Hambridge (Los Angeles: UCLA, 1982), 64; Pelling, "Medical Practice in Early Modern England," 100.

29. Elizabeth Lane Furdell, " 'Every Man His Own Doctor:' Medical Publishers and Booksellers in the Augustan Age," unpublished paper read at the DeBartolo Conference on "Revolutions in Print," Tampa FL, 1999. I have determined that the political or religious affiliation of publishers had little bearing on the sorts of medical pieces published; everyone, even Fellows of the College of Physicians, wanted to make money by selling medical information to the public. See also Anne Digby, *Making a Medical Living* (Cambridge: Cambridge University Press, 1994).

30. Harold Cook, "Good Advice and Little Medicine: The Professional Authority of Early Modern English Physicians," *Journal of British Studies* 33 (1994): 4 n; Margaret Pelling and Charles Webster, "Medical Practitioners," in *Health, Medicine and Mortality in the Sixteenth Century*, ed. Charles Webster (Cambridge: Cambridge University Press, 1979), 188.

31. The Act was a manifestation of the break with Rome and the priest-physician custom. By defining medicine to include surgery, which priests could not perform, Parliament further distanced itself from the authority of the Catholic Church.

32. During the plague epidemic of 1665, so few Fellows were at the College that their treasure chest containing gold plate and coin was stolen. Annals of the Royal College of Physicians of London, vol. 4, f. 89a, Library of the Royal College of Physicians, London (LRCP). The author thanks the College for permission to cite the unpublished records.

33. For more on the rise and fall of the College, see Harold J. Cook, *The Decline of the Old Medical Regime in Stuart London* (Ithaca, N.Y.: Cornell University Press, 1986. Charlatans usually remained in the same location; mountebanks traveled from city to city with a stage, often a servant, and sometimes a monkey to entertain potential customers. Leslie G. Matthews, "Italian Charlatans in England," *Pharmaceutical Historian* 9/2 (1979): 2.

34. Charles II's queen, Henrietta Maria, used Dr. Theodore Mayerne's recommended dentifrice: a mixture of pumice stone, cuttlefish bones, powdered coral, pearl, and deer horn. Godfrey Bidloo functioned as William III's dentist in Holland in 1697 when the king's teeth were loose and painful; Bidloo advised a mouthwash of tincture of myrrh and fair water. Dr. John Radcliffe advocated that two grains of opium be put on a sore tooth and that "gum arabic and dragonwort" be used for bleeding teeth. See J. Dobson, "The Royal Dentists," *Annals of the Royal College of Surgeons* 46 (1970): 277–91.

35. Quoted in "Doctors at Court: The Medical Household," *British Medical Journal* (1953) 1: 1217–18.

36. "Serjeant Surgeons of England," 583.

37. If the plunder exceeded £20, one-third went to the king, but the surgeon received two "buttes of sack" yearly from the royal cellars in which to drown his sorrows. See Henry R. Thompson, "Serjeant Surgeons to Their Majesties," *Annals of the Royal College of Surgeons* 26 (1960): 1–23.

38. See "Serjeant Surgeons to the King," *British Medical Journal* (1925) 1: 224.

39. Leslie Matthews, "Royal Apothecaries of the Tudor Period," *Medical History* 8 (1964): 170–80.

40. Knight was sufficiently pragmatic to accept the job of serjeant-surgeon to Oliver Cromwell and after the Stuart Restoration was Surgeon General to the Royal Forces. See E. M Calvert and R. T. C. Calvert, *Serjeant Surgeon John Knight* (London: W. Heinemann, 1939).

41. J. C. Sainty and R. O. Bucholz, *Officials of the Royal Household 1660–1837 Part I: Department of the Lord Chamberlain and Associated Offices* (London: Institute of Historical Research, 1997). I thank Sir John Sainty for a typescript of some pre-Restoration household officials.

42. Harold J. Cook warns about the dangers of pretended "royal" physicians in *Decline of the Old Medical Regime*, Appendix 3.

43. Roy Porter's prodigious output of such works includes *Disease, Medicine and Society in England 1550–1860* (London: Macmillan, 1987); Porter, ed., *The Popularization of Medicine 1650–1850* (New York: Routledge, 1992); and the volume edited with Dorothy Porter, *Doctors, Politics and Society* (Amsterdam: Rodopi, 1993). In addition, *The Social History of Medicine*, a journal published by the Oxford University Press, regularly explores this avenue of scholarly pursuit.

44. Although the majority of the royal doctors were men, a number of women served the Tudor-Stuart monarchs and developed some repute, among them Elizabeth I's herbalist Margaret Kennix and the Jacobean organizer of midwives, Alice Dennis . For more, see Lynette Hunter and Sarah Hutton, eds., *Women, Science and Medicine 1500–1700* (Stroud, England: Sutton, 1997).

45. Peter Ackroyd, "Biography: The Short Form," *New York Times Book Review*, January 10, 1999, 4. "In biography," he writes, " the devices and tricks of historical narrative are so abundant that it is much easier to disguise lack of knowledge or loss of comprehension."

Chapter 1

Henrician Doctors and the Founding of the Royal College of Physicians (1485–1547)

Henry VII established the Tudor dynasty by conquest, defeating and killing Richard III on the field of battle in 1485, effectively putting an end to the aristocratic struggle known as the Wars of the Roses.[1] A Lancastrian claimant to the throne himself, Henry Tudor then married Elizabeth of York, joining the two rival houses and bolstering his right and that of his descendants to the crown. In striking contrast to his predecessors, Henry VII kept his throne and was able to introduce control by the king of the kingdom's affairs. Some historians credit him with laying the groundwork for a later revolution in government.[2] At the same time, Henry VII maintained many of the traditions of prior royal households, including the appointment of outstanding medical personnel.[3] However, England was frankly underdeveloped in most areas of medical progress compared to continental Europe; in other kingdoms, such as Sicily, Castile, and Aragon, rulers had already established institutions with disciplinary powers over physicians and surgeons. During the period of aristocratic infighting that had afflicted England for three lifetimes, kings had lacked the authority and power to act in a similar fashion.

What changed with the arrival of the Tudors was the actual strength of the English monarchy itself. Sir George Clark has argued that only a strong sovereign could set up medical control independent of the universities, and that under Henry VII the chances for regulation of medical affairs were greater than ever before.[4] The king, familiar with medical provision in France and the Low Countries, demonstrated his intention to improve the English medical scene in his will, which contained detailed stipulations for the foundation of three large hospitals, in London, York, and Coventry. He modeled his bequest on the statutes of the famous Santa Maria Nuova in Florence.[5]

However, the very power of the first Tudor kings precipitated political crisis with which all English subjects, especially those at court, had to deal. If any new administration, not to mention a new dynasty, brings the unknown, the government of Henry VII surely made its share of unsettling innovations; that of his successor shattered established tradition and practice. Henry VIII married six times, broke with the Roman Catholic Church, and set up an independent national church with himself as its head. Matters of dogma were harder to settle, and for generations religious differences divided England and made foreign relations with continental states problematical. In the wake of the split from Rome, ecclesiastical property was confiscated by the crown for profit; many activities formerly the province of the church became the responsibility of the state. Henry VIII, no doctrinal Protestant, used the reformers to get his way and then abandoned them when they were too troublesome. Four of the king's most indispensable men, all Thomases, suffered for their successes in his name; two were priests—Cardinal Thomas Wolsey, and Archbishop Thomas Cranmer—and two were lawyers—Sir Thomas More and Thomas Cromwell.[6] In sum, Tudor might enabled the state to grow, but the monarch would not scruple to use individuals as pawns for that end. Medical men at court were not exempt from that fate.

The royal household formed the basis of the court, and people eagerly angled for a place on the permanent establishment of this household. Such a place brought with it free board and lodging, as well as the opportunity for influence. During the Tudor era, rulers carried on the medieval peripatetic tradition of moving their entourage around with them from palace to palace on progresses, but that convention hardly deterred applicants. The household was composed of two distinct groupings: the Lord Steward's complex, comprised of domestic offices like the laundry and the bakery, and the department of the Lord Chamberlain, made up of specialized agencies including the medical corps. Since factions within the household posed a problem for the new king, Henry VII strengthened monarchical dominion over the household by restricting direct access to him. He created a Privy Chamber past whose door few could pass into the royal presence. Among those who were admitted to discharge their functions were the king's medical personnel.[7]

Two physicians joined the household staff of Henry VII during the early months of the new dynasty's existence—Benedict Frietre and Walter Lemster. Henry Tudor brought Frietre, already his physician, along with him to do battle at Bosworth Field in 1485. After his victory there over Richard III, Henry VII made Frietre, alternately spelled Frutze or Fentre, his first royal physician following the royal coronation.[8] It was to be a lifetime commission with assurances that Parliament would not alter the physician's salary or responsibilities. A servant in Henry's household for many years prior to 1485, Frietre also received another £30 for service to the king while abroad.[9] Walter Lemster (Leinster, Lymster), born in 1444, earned a medical degree from Cambridge in 1465. He was designated a royal doctor in 1486 and probably also attended Elizabeth, Duchess of Norfolk. At Lemstar's death in 1487, he bequeathed her a ring that she had earlier given to him.[10] Both Frietre and Lemster had to handle medical affairs in the castle during an epidemic of the sweating sickness, probably a form of influenza with pulmonary complications, that gripped the kingdom in 1486. Many felt that the "sweats" were God's scourge on those without the right religion or piety; some whispered that sickness accompanied the Tudor usurper; still others argued that the disease emanated from corrupt air.[11]

The royal doctors also had to deal with Henry VII's gout. In the fifteenth century, with classical Galenism as yet unchallenged, gout was categorized by physicians as a "catarrh" thought to be caused by a liquid secretion from the diseased part. It flowed downward from the brain through the base of the skull to various organs, the classic product of humoral pathology. Moving from one part of the body to another, gout brought distress and pain from the extremities to the head. Physicians stipulated that gout was a male condition, and one associated with rank.[12] Renaissance humanists cautioned that extravagant living brought on malevolent afflictions, echoing Hippocrates' opinion that gout arose from sexual excess. The usual treatment in the Tudor period was a sort of purgative, but medieval authors who had other ideas were often consulted. Gilbertus Anglicus recommended an herbal ointment made of puppy boiled with cucumber, rue, and juniper.[13] A later physician called for a hot drink made of boiled "biritite and new milk" to which brown sugar had been added.[14] Henry VII particularly complained of his goutish ailments in the final years of his life.

Shortly before Easter 1507, the king suffered a devastating attack of "quinsies," a peritonsillar abscess, and for nearly a week had been unable to swallow; he was left so feeble he thought he might die.[15] He recovered slowly and spent much of the summer and fall hunting, seeming to grow stronger and enjoying the sport with his son. In February 1508 he was ill again, suffering from consumption or phthisis, a progressive wasting disease, though his doctors told him it was gout again. One medical historian contends that the Tudors had a hereditary disposition to tuberculosis associated with asthma that began with Henry VII.[16] A few weeks after the February attack, the king was so incapacitated that his mother, Margaret Beaufort, moved with her servants into Richmond Palace to watch over him; one year later he died, on his deathbed making "the Lady Margaret," as she was popularly known, his chief executrix.[17]

Early royal surgeons are harder to trace than physicians, but the office goes back to the fifteenth century.[18] The crown regularly rewarded those who provided medical services, such as the surgeons who operated on royal patients when monks were forbidden to do so, with grants of land or other honors without land. The first serjeant-surgeon was William Hobbes, paid "forty marks with wine, wax, and requisites" in 1461; "serjeant" comes from the Latin "serviens," by definition an aulic official.[19] As royal surgeon to Richard, Duke of York (father of Edward IV), Edward IV, and Richard III, it is not surprising that he did not continue in that capacity under the Tudors. Hobbes died in 1488 and his tomb inscription reiterates his loyalty to the House of York. In his will he left a silver cup to the Barbers' Company, which contained a group of surgeons and whose livery he wore, but nothing to the Fellowship of Surgeons, a separate but intertwined entity too small to seek incorporation.[20] Whatever qualms Hobbes may have felt about an autonomous organization of surgeons mirrored that of the fifteenth-century medical community at large.

A Barbers' Company with surgeons included predates Hobbes's appointment by nearly three generations, but barbers were far more numerous and actually senior to the surgeons in their civic guild or mystery, as it was then called. When beards went out of fashion in the mid-fifteenth century, shaving and haircutting became more lucrative and less demanding activities than surgery. Some surgeons formed their own association and the crown recognized the two groups as distinct crafts, each with its special grant of arms.[21] Henry VII specifically acknowledged the services of the unincorporated surgeons in 1492 by awarding them a device depicting the patron saints of surgeons, Cosmas and Damian. For its part, the Barbers' Company in 1499 obtained affirmation of its charter under Edward IV, perhaps as a manifestation of its own strength. Nonetheless, as surgeons acquired the use of various sophisticated techniques based on battlefield experiences in war, their reputations improved and broadened; London surgeons, whether of the Company or the Fellowship, strove to initiate and implement high professional standards. Besides performing amputations, cutting out tumors, and setting bones, surgeons treated patients for syphilis, a disease that would affect even the divinely chosen.[22] Eventually, coexistence between the Barbers' Company and the Fellowship of Surgeons led to coalescence. Although the medieval differentiation between physicians and surgeons persisted in the minds of the university-educated doctors, in reality by the time of Henry VII the distinctions had less lasting power in a compact urban center like London, where ideas and manuscripts circulated regularly and easily.[23]

The principal surgeon of Henry VII was William Altofte from Warwickshire, probably the personal surgeon of Henry's father-in-law, Thomas Stanley, at Bosworth Field. Though a nominal Yorkist, Lord Stanley's desertion of Richard III there contributed to the Tudor victory, and Altofte's battlefield ability persuaded the triumphant Henry to make Altofte his royal surgeon for life, an appointment Altofte held throughout the reign of the first Tudor king and into that of the second. His annuity was forty marks "out of the petty serjeantry in the counties of Bedford and Buckingham and £10. 11s. 1d. out of the issues of those counties."[24] In fact, as late as 1520, Altofte was still being paid his wages. He expired in 1521, leaving considerable property, and was buried in the chancel of St. Peter's, Manchester.[25] The first Tudor monarch demonstrated a real interest in medical matters with his project for the Savoy hospital in the parish of St. Clement Danes. Although the hospital was not completed in his lifetime, Henry VII demonstrated compassion for the poor and the sick by its commissioning. The king made many inquiries about the administration and planning of foreign hospitals and sought the advice of the master of the hospital in Florence in planning a cruciform structure with a chapel at the crossing for London, so that patients in each of the wards could view the altar. Henry also planned similar hospitals for Coventry and York.

The occasional woman received recompense for medical services performed in the court of Henry VII, usually in the capacity of midwife. Alice Massey was Elizabeth of York's midwife, for which she was paid a salary of £10 per year for life. Sadly, the Tudors proved to be a rather sickly dynasty.[26] Elizabeth bore eight children, but only three outlived her and reached maturity: the future Henry VIII, Margaret, later Queen of Scotland, and Mary, later Queen of France. Elizabeth died on her thirty-eighth birthday, February 11, 1503, after delivering Princess Katherine, shortly before the infant also succumbed. Because Tudor physicians regarded pregnancy and childbirth as natural events best not interfered with, midwives and wise women handled obstetrical responsibilities. Percival Willughby, author of a classic seventeenth-century discourse on midwifery, urged that most cases be left to the safe conduct of "the invisible midwife, Dame Nature."[27] Besides, male exclusion from childbirth on moral grounds persisted even to Willughby's day; he recounted that in 1657 he was obliged to crawl into a darkened room on his hands and knees when called to a pregnant patient.[28]

Two apothecaries, John Grice and John Pykenham, provided wares and services to Henry VII and his queen. Grice received £10 yearly for life plus the cost of supplies, £20 for 1502.[29] He also acquired seven grants for London houses and lands between 1497 and 1500. Grice supervised the preparation of the household's sweetmeats as serjeant of the King's Confectionary; Elizabeth gave his assistant in spicery, Leonard Twycross, sixteen shillings for a wedding gown. John Pykenham secured his appointment three days after Grice, probably receiving a lower rank, but garnering the same annual earnings for life.[30] The records are sketchy, but Pykenham may have moved up on the protocol scale when Grice died in 1505; the vacancy thus created may have been filled by Thomas Pierson, the first apothecary mentioned in the July 1509 book of payments and therefore likely first in rank at that time.[31] Richard Babham moved in later that year and stayed to become Henry VIII's "apothecary for life."[32]

The Tudors cemented the family's hold on the English throne by marrying Henry VII's children into the royal houses of Spain, Scotland, and France. After ten years of negotiations for a Spanish alliance, Arthur, Prince of Wales, wed Catherine of Aragon, daughter of Ferdinand and Isabella, in November 1501 at St. Paul's Cathedral. Catherine brought personnel to serve her needs in England including her French-born apothecary, John de Soda (de Soto). He soon came into the service of five-year-old Princess Mary Rose, the younger of Henry VII's daughters.[33] After Arthur passed away unexpectedly in April 1502, Catherine stayed on in England, betrothed to Arthur's brother and heir presumptive, Prince Henry. De Soda remained with Catherine through Henry VII's funeral, her own coronation as the new queen, and a state trip with Henry VIII to the continent in 1520 to meet Francis I.[34] De Soda's loyalty to Catherine proved stronger than that of her husband; de Soda maintained his service to her until her death from cancer in January 1536. He then became the household apothecary to Catherine's daughter, Mary, from 1536 to 1547.[35]

Those were dangerous years for the Spanish Tudor, as Mary is sometimes called. Declared a bastard in 1533 by Parliament in its eagerness to make the offspring of Anne Boleyn the king's legitimate heirs, Mary, formerly Princess of Wales, was a devout Roman Catholic whose household was ordered disbanded.

However, in 1536 after her mother's death and Anne Boleyn's beheading, Henry VIII offered her a new court and finances if she would admit that her parents' marriage had been incestuous. Mary yielded to the king's demands, but suffered enormous regret at her actions and became seriously ill. De Soda ministered to her while she resided away from court. De Soda lived long enough to see her reinstated in the succession, but retired in 1547. His son and replacement as Mary's apothecary, also named John, witnessed the day when she became queen of England.

Another bridge between the reigns of the two Henrys, Thomas Linacre, ranks among England's most illustrious physicians. He is credited with persuading Henry VIII to assent to the Medical Act of 1512 and to issue letters patent in 1518 setting up a body to supervise the practice of medicine in London. Born in Canterbury in 1460, Linacre mastered Greek under Cornelius Vitelli at All Souls College, Oxford, where he became a Fellow in 1484; a true Renaissance man, he was also accomplished in Latin, grammar, and theology.[36] Like other Renaissance successes, Linacre benefited from patronage, advancing thanks to Henry VII's policy of preferment based on merit. Linacre traveled to Italy with England's ambassador to Rome, Cambridge scholar William de Selling, probably a relative of his, but stayed on in Florence to study with the Italian classical scholar, Angelo Poliziano. While in Florence, Linacre met and befriended two sons of Lorenzo de Medici, also students of Poliziano; one of them later became Pope Leo X. He sojourned in Rome, where he was influenced to study medicine by the scholar Ermolao Barbaro, and in Venice, where he stayed with Aldus Manutius, founder of the Aldine Press. In 1496 Linacre received his medical degree at Padua, among the most prestigious institutions of higher learning in Europe, and had his degree incorporated (accepted and assimilated) at Oxford and Cambridge by 1499.[37] He had fashioned impressive credentials and connections.

Linacre ensconced himself at Oxford as a lecturer on medical subjects and on Greek. The Dutch humanist Erasmus came to the university in 1499 to study Greek with him. Linacre was appalled by the poor quality of medical education in England and undertook the renewal of Galenic medicine. The Renaissance medical humanism that Linacre championed sought to cleanse medicine of complicated and unwarranted additions and to restore the classical foundation of humoral therapy, especially the work of Hippocrates and his great interpreter, Galen.[38] Seeing himself as a true progressive who sought to enlighten the darkness of medievalism, Linacre translated Galen's treatises on hygiene and medical treatment from Greek into Latin. Like most physicians of his day, he was also a cleric (albeit a late-blooming one, ordained in 1509), and supplemented his medical income with prebendaries at Easton-in-Gordano and South Newbold.[39] Linacre held several other ecclesiastical benefices, but in accordance with the custom of the period he did not take up residence in those places; instead, he sold the livings to other clergymen and amassed considerable wealth.

In 1501, Henry VII summoned Linacre to court to become tutor and physician to Prince Arthur; Linacre also instructed Princess Mary in Italian. Although the Prince of Wales died of consumption not long afterward, Linacre maintained high visibility as physician to the elite. Erasmus, a frequent visitor to England, called him in when he fell sick in 1506; Linacre tended Sir Thomas More, Bishop Cuthbert Tunstall, and the fiery reformer Hugh Latimer. His remedy for "gravel" called for a poultice of camomile flowers and parsley boiled in linen.[40] Never relaxed and always busy with his profession, Linacre became court physician to Henry VIII in 1509 at £50 per annum. Henry's chief minister and a patient of Linacre, Cardinal Wolsey, procured yet another living for the doctor as precentor (choir director) of Wells Cathedral, but Linacre lived in London.

Linacre's organizational accomplishments began with the Medical Act of 1512, the first parliamentary enactment about medical affairs. The preamble to the Act complained about the disreputable hacks selling bogus medical cures throughout the realm, and then ordered, for anyone other than Oxford or Cambridge M.D.s who wished to perform as a doctor within a seven-mile radius of the City, a compulsory examination by the Bishop of London, who was to be advised by four physicians and surgeons.[41] Outside of the metropolis, the bishop of the appropriate diocese should examine the applicant with expert help. Failure to observe this requirement resulted in a fine of £5 for every month, half of which was to go to the king and half to any informer.[42] Competency testing was important, as Henry VIII wished to raise medical standards; seventy-two surgeons passed the examination and were licensed in 1514.[43] The universities still could grant physicians licenses to practice locally with their diplomas, but examinations were required of even the degreed beyond those bailiwicks. The medical system was placed under ecclesiastical control because no other institution had a national administration capable of conducting the examinations, but it is likely that Linacre's great friends, John Colet, Dean of St. Paul's, and Thomas More, then under-sheriff in London, spearheaded the action in Parliament.[44]

Perhaps in response to a sense of emergency as plague drove the court from London and devastated Oxford, Linacre next persuaded Henry VIII to found the Royal College of Physicians in September 1518. The College charter was modeled after those of comparable institutions in Italian cities, and was presented to the king by "seven weighty men," including three royal physicians—John Chambre, Ferdinand de Victoria, and Thomas Linacre.[45] The College had the same geographic jurisdiction as set up in the Medical Act of 1512; its creation clearly abrogated the licensing power of the bishop. In 1523 the licensing capacity of the College was broadened to include all of England, but the absence of any enforcement machinery made national control nebulous.[46] Nonetheless, the College matured into much more than a local association and for the first time extended recognized professional status for medical practitioners. The charter protected the Fellows from "common artificers [such] as smiths, weavers, and women" and from those who could not "discern the cunning from the uncunning"; later legal enhancements exempted members from civic responsibilities such as serving as constables, ostensibly to safeguard their noble and indispensable patients.[47]

The College's statutes were enacted by the members themselves, and included a provision making royal physicians *ex officio* members regardless of their nationality or university.[48] Linacre became its President and its meetings were held at his house in Knightrider Street near St. Paul's. Linacre retained the presidency until his death "from the stone" in 1524, although he had retired from medical practice in 1520 to devote himself to literary work, especially to a Latin translation of Galen. Linacre's last royal appointment in 1523 was that of tutor to five-year-old Princess Mary, later Mary I. Just before his death he founded three Linacre lectureships in medicine, two at Oxford and one at Cambridge. He was buried in St. Paul's Cathedral.[49]

Listed first in the letters patent founding the College, John Chambre or Chambers, like Linacre, combined medicine with the priesthood. A native of Northumberland, Chambre came to Merton College, Oxford, for the undergraduate and graduate arts courses, and then enrolled at Padua for the M.D. He became physician to the king upon his return to England. With Linacre as President of the College, Chambre served as one of the College's censors, officers responsible for inquiring about all medical practices in the kingdom and for burning impure medicines used by unlicensed practitioners.[50] He held the post of canon of Windsor from 1509 until his death, plus prebendaries in Sarum and Lincoln, and in 1524 was appointed Archdeacon of Bedford. Later that year he succeeded Linacre as the king's principal physician. Unlike Linacre, however, Chambre had to wrestle with Henry VIII's decision to establish a national church in England and split from the Roman Catholic fold; in 1536 he subscribed to the Articles of Faith and was rewarded for his loyalty to the king with the deanship of the collegiate chapel of St. Stephen's in Westminster. Additional ecclesiastical perquisites by 1540 included the post of treasurer of the cathedral of Bath and Wells, preferments in one Irish and three English dioceses, and the headship of his alma mater, Merton College. Dr. Chambre used his substantial fortune to build new cloisters for the collegiate chapel.[51]

Chambre cared for Anne Boleyn in her confinement and delivery of the Princess Elizabeth, as well as attending the disastrous labor of Henry's third wife, Jane Seymour. Although the king got the son he desperately wanted, Queen Jane died in October 1537 after a reported Caesarean section led to a fatal infection. George Owen, another Henrician physician, probably performed the operation, along with William Butts and Chambre. Fittingly, perhaps, in view of the virtual death sentence to which Jane was doomed, Chambre signed himself "priest" on the letter announcing the seriousness of her condition.[52] With Dr. Butts, he also attested to the non-consummation bulletin prepared for Henry's divorce from wife number four, the German princess Anne of Cleves. The king told the doctors that "he found her body disordered and indisposed to excite and provoke any lust in him."[53] Despite his manifold aulic responsibilities, Chambre had time for outside consultations, and probably was physician to Margaret, Countess of Richmond. He outlived the king by two years, dying in 1549. Chambre's recipes—along with those of three of Henry VIII's other doctors, William Butts, Walter Cromar, and Augustin de Angustinus—formed a pharmacopoeia of over 230 prescriptions for Henry VIII. Containing directions for plasters for various parts of the body, lotions, balms, and ointments, the recipe album includes an enema for pain that seems more like a genteel beverage: rosewater, white wine, ginger, and violet leaves. One prescription for imbalanced humors called for a mixture of leaves of centgrene and nightshade, roses, pomegranates, sumac, hepocistides, and the barks of barberry and sloe.[54] The king himself, something of an amateur apothecary, may have contributed over one hundred recipes for plasters and ointments to the collection.[55]

The third royal doctor whose name appeared on the petition for a College of Physicians was Ferdinand de Victoria, a Spaniard whose medical degree came "from beyond the seas," but which was eventually incorporated at Oxford in 1520.[56] De Victoria and his wife, a "gentlewoman" among the attendants to Henry VIII's first consort, Catherine of Aragon, came to England prior to 1515; royal favor to him included a 1519 license "to export yearly 500 woollen cloths."[57] De Victoria was a censor along with Chambre for the College, but the gathering storm over the king's desire for a divorce from the queen enveloped the physician. In 1527 Henry VIII initiated a secret suit with the purpose of getting his marriage to Catherine declared invalid.[58] Catherine sent de Victoria to inform her nephew, Holy Roman Emperor Charles V, of her plight, effectively ending the doctor's English connections. He died in 1529, before Catherine's ultimate humiliation and the break with Rome. Catherine also employed Peter Farnando (sometimes Vernando) as queen's physician around the time that the Princess Mary was born, paying him a yearly wage of £66 13s. 4d. and arranging a warrant for him to transport his wife from Spain to England in 1518; no payments to him appear after that year.[59]

Edward Wotton was appointed to take de Victoria's place on the royal medical staff in 1528.[60] Born in Oxfordshire around 1492, the son of the university beadle, Wotton graduated from Magdalen College in 1513 and became a Fellow there in 1516. Under the influence of John Claymond, President of Magdalen and author of an exegesis on Pliny's *Natural History*, Wotton moved to Corpus Christi College, where he became its first Reader in Greek. He procured a leave from the College, traveling for several years in Italy perfecting his skills and obtaining a medical degree from Padua, incorporated in 1526 at Oxford. Wotton was instrumental in getting the complete works of Galen published in their original Greek. He also studied natural history and wrote a ten-book summary of the subject, published in a splendid folio in Paris in 1552, the first such work written by an Englishman. *De Differentiis Animalium*, dedicated to Edward VI, covers the whole range of the animal world and is a useful compendium of traditional lore. A large part of the work is devoted to medicinal uses of insects, especially parasites, as potent drugs.[61] Wotton became a Fellow of the College of Physicians in 1528 and served as its President from 1541 to 1543. He died in 1555, leaving a large family.

The doctors besides Chambre who created medications for Henry VIII's use—Cromar, Angustinus, and Butts—deserve consideration. About Walter Cromar the least is known including the source of his medical degree. He was active in the College of Physicians as a Fellow in 1530, an elect in 1541, and a censor in 1544. Cromar, who died in 1547, worked closely with a court apothecary, Thomas Ashe, in tending to the needs of persons at court.[62] Augustin de Angustinus, a Venetian, tended Cardinal Wolsey from about 1523. When away from England, Angustinus (occasionally referred to as Dr. Ang) wrote regularly to London for supplies of leeches.[63] When Wolsey fell mortally ill in January 1530, Angustinus beseeched Thomas Cromwell, a protégé of the Cardinal, to send along Dr. Butts, Dr. Cromar, and a stock of hungry annelids. He also requested that Balthasar Guersie, a fellow Italian and surgeon to Catherine of Aragon, be dispatched to apply the leeches. Another of his patients was Sir Thomas Elyot, author in 1534 of the Galenic *Castel of Helth*, and himself an Oxford M.D. Elyot referred with gratitude to the medical treatment Angustinus afforded him.[64] Dr. Angustinus joined the College of Physicians in 1536 and became one of its censors in 1543.[65]

William Butts, M.D., parlayed his medical relationship with the king into a position as a strong influence for radical Protestantism within the Henrician court.[66] A native of Norfolk, Butts took all of his arts and medical degrees by 1518 at Gonville College, Cambridge, and he became a Fellow of the College of Physicians and the king's domestic physician, just as Henry's "Great Matter," the divorce from Catherine of Aragon, was heating up. Although a friend of Wolsey, Butts was from the outset favorable to religious reform and was one of the first physicians to make a distinguished lay, rather than clerical, career. He patronized Hugh Latimer when the future Bishop of Worcester was a mere preacher with a social conscience and brought him to court after Wolsey died. Knowing that Anne Boleyn protected foreign evangelicals and supported the "new" religion, Dr. Butts interceded with her to sustain Nicolas Bourbon, who had been imprisoned in France for speaking out against the Pope. He asked that she obtain his release from prison and subsidize his living expenses once he had safely arrived in England. Bourbon later wrote poems of gratitude to Anne, Henry, and Dr. Butts.[67]

Dr. Butts cared for the medical needs of the most important men and women of the palace. Besides Butts's personal attendance on the king, who called Linacre his first physician and Butts his second, he ministered to Anne Boleyn and her brother, George. After the Boleyns' executions in the spring of 1536, Butts doctored the new queen, Jane Seymour, the Duke of Norfolk, and Henry's bastard son, Henry Fitzroy, Earl of Richmond. Butts' salary was £100 per year plus forty marks and an additional £20 for attending Richmond, who died of tuberculosis in July 1536.[68] Dr. Butts received a suit of blue and green damask for taking care of Princess Mary, liveries for his servants, and cloth for his apothecary, probably Philip Greenacre. The king knighted Butts, who was only the second English physician to be so honored, and placed Butts's wife Margaret in Princess Mary's service as a gentlewoman. As Sir William, he acquired royal augmentation, a caduceus for his family crest, and real estate.

As a consequence of Henry VIII's momentous break from Rome, the government confiscated church properties, particularly monastic lands and buildings. These holdings could be kept by the crown, sold to the highest bidder, or dispensed by the king at bargain prices to his favorites. The dissolution of the monasteries had a profound impact on medicine since clergy often cared for the sick, especially in the provinces. Some have argued that the English Reformation created an immediate problem for poor patients, but it was surely beneficial to several of the royal doctors.[69] King Henry secured abbey lands for Dr. Butts after the dissolution of the monasteries and Butts lived for a time at the Chapterhouse of the Whitefriars monastery. Evidently, Butts tried to convert the monks of Sion to acknowledge Henry's supremacy over the Church of England, but they demurred. Butts also enjoyed the income from the manor of Thornage in Norfolk.[70]

Henry VIII disclosed to Dr. Butts the most intimate details of his failed marriage to Anne of Cleves. He sought out his physician and explained that his failure to have intercourse with the queen was not due to impotence on his part. The king boasted that he had experienced nocturnal emissions twice during their wedding night and that he was surely able to perform the sex act with others. Dr. Butts testified at the July 1540 annulment hearing in the House of Lords that since the king had wet dreams while married to Anne, intercourse had not taken place.[71] Dr. Butts is well-known for defending Thomas Cranmer, Archbishop of Canterbury, when the reforming cleric's fortunes were at a low ebb in 1543 and for interceding on his behalf in 1544, when hopeful religious conservatives tried to commit Cranmer to the Tower. He also successfully championed the candidacy of the erudite but radical Cambridge scholar, John Cheke, to become Prince Edward's and Princess Elizabeth's tutor. In his later years Queen Katherine Parr, Henry's sixth wife, was a close friend and religious ally. William Butts died of malaria, a "double quaternary fever," in November 1545 and was buried in Fulham church with an epitaph that begins: "Of what worth is medicine, honour, royal favour, the love of the people, when cruel death comes? Piety which is built on Christ the Founder alone helps us. It alone in death avails: all other things pass away."[72] Butts's wife was interred beside him two years later. One of his three sons, Edmund, continued the Protestant tradition established by Dr. Butts, supporting Anne Askew, a repudiator of the Catholic doctrine of transubstantiation, who was burned at the stake in 1546.[73]

Occasionally a doctor not on the regular medical staff was called in to attend to the king during a particular illness. Robert Yaxley, a physician among the first six elects listed in the College of Physicians' charter, received payment in 1518 for medical services rendered to the household.[74] Anthony

Brasavola, Italian-born author of a commentary on and huge index to the works of Galen and physician to Francis I, attended Henry VIII when in France. Professor of medicine at Ferrara from 1536 until his death in 1555, he was also doctor to Popes Paul III, Leo X, Clement VII, and Julius III, but it was to the king of England that Brasavola respectfully dedicated his 1541 commentary on Hippocrates' *Aphorisms*. Praising Henry's intellectual achievements and his support of medical scholarship, Brasavola may have deliberately sought to cultivate Tudor friendship for his own patrons in Ferrara. Medical publications could easily become tools of princely diplomacy.[75] Brasavola is also remembered for arguing that syphilis, like any entity, could change over generations. His categorizing impulses led him to label new variations within the "French Disease." Brasavola pointed to sequential symptoms: loss of hair, teeth, and nails, blindness, and gonorrhea. Permutations within these symptoms led him to list varieties of the great pox.[76] Another Henrician irregular was Thomas Bille, an English M.D. from Pavia and physician at St. Bartholomew's Hospital, who had received his arts degrees from Cambridge. Dr. Bille received £100 for attending Henry in the last year of his reign.[77]

William Bullein, described as a nurse-surgeon who cared for the king, wrote an early herbal and other works on pleurisy and the sweating sickness.[78] If Bullein had a medical degree, he likely obtained it abroad after 1554, as he was never admitted to the College of Physicians. Bullein's book on the "sweat" addressed the terrible epidemic of 1517 that decimated London and its environs. It struck its victims "with a great sweating and stinking, with redness of the face and of all the body, and a continual thirst, with a great heat and headache."[79] The "sweat" terrified with its swiftness; a pimply rash led to collapse and death, often with no time to make a will or call a priest. Tens of thousands succumbed in that summer; survivors whispered prayers and downed preventive medicines. Henry VIII sent his own recipe to friends and relatives. Despite his concoction, the king's household did not escape the contagion, and after several secretaries and pages perished, Henry fled to the countryside, stopping at several palaces, each further away from the capital. In the spring of 1518 the sickness resurfaced, even more virulent than before. Those who lived in households visited by the disease had to carry white rods to announce their proximity to infection.

Of all Henry VIII's irregular doctors, the most famous was Andrew Boorde, peripatetic scholar and author of cheery, sensible writings on health, who came to the attention of Henry VIII around 1530 through the Duke of Norfolk. Boorde pronounced the king fleshy with large arteries, possessed of ruddy cheeks and pale skin, "hair plenty and red, pulse great and full, digestion perfect, anger short, [and] sweat abundant."[80] Born in Sussex around 1490, Boorde entered the Carthusian Order at the London Charterhouse under the usual age but rose rapidly to be nominated Suffragan Bishop of Chichester. Falsely accused in 1517 of being "conversant with women," he was dismissed by papal bull from the post and his career in the church effectively ended. Boorde received a dispensation from his vows and went abroad to study medicine, visiting Orleans, Toulouse, Wittenburg, and Rome. Back in England by 1534, he took the Oath of Conformity, coaxed perhaps by a brief confinement in the London Charterhouse. Upon his release, he spent time in Hampshire with Thomas Cromwell, the king's new Secretary of State. Cromwell sent Boorde abroad to test elite opinion about Henry VIII's divorce and to corresponded with him about political matters.

Boorde dispatched rhubarb seeds from North Africa's Barbary States to Cromwell with directions for their cultivation, noting that the plant was greatly prized in Spain for curing excessive yellow bile. By 1536 Boorde was practicing medicine in Glasgow, informing Cromwell about the Scots, whom he did not like and who, he reported, did not like the English. After the dissolution of the monasteries, Boorde traveled again through Europe, ending in Jerusalem to see the Holy Sepulchre. He settled for a while in Montpellier, near his favorite university, where he penned his most important medical books: *The Dyetary* (dedicated to the Duke of Norfolk in 1542) and *The Breviarie of Health*. Boorde's *Dyetary* is a self-help book of remedies and preventives, which incorporated medical advice gleaned from his continental travels; the *Breviarie* is a book of useful home remedies, written in a confident style. Among his recommendations are green ginger for indigestion, garlic for intestinal worms, a mercury-based oil for running sores, and "olium costinum" for baldness.[81] He broached the problem of gout, a frequent complaint of Henry VIII, in both the *Dyetary* and the *Brevarie*, advocating spring and autumn bleeding and the wearing of dog-skin hosiery. Boorde prescribed daily applications to the aching joints of cabbage-wrapped, baked ox-dung and infusions of ash bark, a preferred recipe all over Europe for gout.[82] Boorde often presented a variety of internal and external treatments for sicknesses as did most of his Galenist colleagues, all hoping to produce a harmonious balance in their patients.

Another of Boorde's publications, *The First Book of the Introduction of Knowledge* (also printed in 1547), was illustrated with woodcuts and used rhyme, dialect, and other amusing techniques to provide delightful details about fashions, foods, costumes, weather, and business in dozens of continental regions from Norway to Greece.[83] The book contained numbers in various languages, monetary information, and key foreign phrases including the first printed specimen of the Gypsy language. Boorde dedicated the *Introduction* to the Princess Mary. Back in England by 1547 to supervise publication of his works, Boorde penned a tract, *The Book of Berdes*, which protested the unhygienic nature of facial hair. An anonymous critic in an answer to this disparagement accused Boorde of blaming his drunken stench on his own beard.[84] Boorde took up residence in Winchester, but his fame as an author did little to protect him from a charge made by John Ponet, later Bishop of Winchester, that Boorde kept prostitutes in his domicile. He was put into Fleet Prison in 1547 and, his old patrons dead or powerless, he never left it alive. Andrew Boorde died in 1549. His will was drawn up in jail on April 9, 1549, and probated on April 25.

No record exists about his burial, leaving future admirers of Boorde, often called "Merry Andrew," with an uncharacteristically muted ending to an otherwise spirited life.[85]

Henry VIII had enjoyed reasonably good health throughout his youth, but to assure continued vitality his doctors had kept busy through the years examining the royal urine, stools, and sputum. To keep his humoral balance in tune, they had bled and cupped him in accordance with the phases of the moon. Their therapies had gotten him through fevers and sinusitis in 1521, chronic headaches that began in 1528, painful attacks in the extremities beginning in 1532, a possible minor pulmonary embolism in 1537, and the flare-up of an old leg wound in 1541. Smitten with Katherine Howard, his youthful fifth wife, Henry began a special regimen in December 1540 aimed at increasing his activity and reducing his weight. He rose at dawn and after hearing Mass would ride for two hours; he was reported to be feeling better.[86] But after the leg wound ulcerated, the king stayed unhealthy, experiencing recurrent colds, swelling with obesity, and manifesting a choleric disposition; his doctors plied him with rhubarb and kept the concupiscent Katherine out of his presence.[87] From youthful fitness, in middleage Henry had expanded to obese proportions, the waistline of his armor measuring an astounding fifty-four inches.

What was wrong with the king? Historians have constructed various diagnoses for Henry VIII's ailments including malaria, gout, alcoholism, and syphilis. He had bladder trouble as early as 1528 and himself recommended a cure for tumor of the testicles.[88] Despite the king's popular reputation in his own day as a womanizer, the first suggestion that syphilis might be the culprit came from A. S. Currie in an 1888 article in *The Edinburgh Medical Journal*.[89] The king did have appalling leg ulcers, considered by his physicians to be a secondary symptom of syphilis; however, no evidence that Henry received any of the standard treatments for syphilis can be gleaned from the record.[90] More recently, Sir Arthur MacNalty has claimed that Henry may have suffered from osteomyelitis, in his case a chronic septic infection of the thigh bone, probably caused by a serious jousting accident in January 1536. On that occasion, the armored king was unhorsed by an opponent and fell underneath the mailed animal; he lay unconscious for two hours. MacNalty argued that the wound would have discharged pus and bits of necrosed bone, allowing the king the occasional periods of remission from pain that commentators noted.[91] Susan Maclean Kybett has argued persuasively that Henry VIII exhibited every sign of scurvy, which progressively debilitated him and produced violent changes of temper.[92] Whatever ailed him, his doctors could not help and he never regained his old vigor.

Three physicians presided over Henry VIII's final years and their service extended to his successors: George Owen, Thomas Wendy, and Robert Huicke. Worcester-born Owen, likely chief accoucheur to Jane Seymour, received his M.D. from Oxford in 1527 but did not become a Fellow of the College of Physicians until 1545. He prescribed for little Prince Edward and in gratitude

Henry VIII bestowed manors and abbey sites on Owen, including Inn Hall and St. Alban Hall, formerly the properties of Cardinal Wolsey. Owen resided at Godstow Abbey, another gift from the king. Henry left Owen £100 in his will, a document to which Owen was a witness. Owen served as Edward VI's doctor and received more houses and lands from the young king, such as the buildings and grounds of Durham College, Oxford, which he then sold. Owen purchased St. Giles', Oxford, in 1550. Despite the seesaw state of England's religious situation under Edward and his successor, Mary I, Owen managed to stay on as royal physician after Mary's accession in 1553. Mary held him in such esteem that she acceded to his request for an enlargement of the powers of the College of Physicians during her first year on the throne, the same year that Owen was the College President. Owen demonstrated his loyalty to the Roman Catholic Mary by reporting to her on the condition of Princess Elizabeth's health while she was at Woodstock. George Owen wrote about diet and ague, but evidently the knowledge did not help him; he succumbed to a fever in 1558.[93]

Thomas Wendy, William Butts's successor as a royal physician, also witnessed the king's testamentary signature and received a legacy of £100. Wendy took his arts degree at Gonville College, Cambridge, but unlike most of the later Henrician physicians, studied medicine abroad; his medical degree from Ferrara was incorporated at Cambridge in 1527. Like other physicians to the household, Wendy prospered thanks to royal largesse. Henry VIII granted Wendy a manor and rectory at Haslingfield in 1541. Dr. Wendy also benefited from serving as an ecclesiastical visitor to Oxford, Cambridge, and Eton in 1546 and 1548. The king confided in Dr. Wendy, complaining to him in 1546 of the heretical religious views of Queen Katherine Parr and threatening to have her arrested. Wendy had to console the distraught queen when she learned of her husband's displeasure.[94] Like Owen, Wendy was a pragmatist when it came to his employers, serving on the medical staff for Henry and each of the king's ruling offspring. He was Edward VI's physician with a £100 annuity from the time of the boy's accession in 1547.[95] Though Wendy attended the Protestant Edward on his deathbed six years later, Catholic Queen Mary continued him as her doctor. He served in Parliament during her reign, as M.P. for St. Alban's and Cambridge in 1555. Thomas Wendy died in 1560.

Robert Huicke, physician to Henry VIII and his final consort, Katherine Parr, was a third witness to the king's will. A Berkshire native, Huicke took his M.A. at Oxford but received his M.D. from Cambridge in 1538. He, too, devoted much energy to the College of Physicians, serving as censor, elect, consilarius, and President throughout the 1550s. Huicke was appointed physician to Edward VI at £50 per annum. Contemporary commentators remarked on Huicke's acrimonious divorce in the mid-1540s from his wife, Elizabeth, and the cruelty that he displayed towards her.[96] Despite that reputation, Princess Elizabeth employed Huicke as her physician while she lived at Hatfield House waiting for her turn on the throne; she made him her royal physician in 1558. As queen, she rewarded him for his service with a mansion in Middlesex, White Webbs House. Huicke participated in a disputation on the Physic Act at Cambridge in 1564 and at Oxford in 1566. The naturalist William Turner cited Huicke in *Spirituall Physick* (1555)—along with Drs. Wendy, Owen, and Wotton—as being desirous of "more accurate herbarism" in England.[97]

Besides his physicians, Henry VIII employed a number of surgeons at court during his nearly forty years on the throne, beginning with foreign-born John Veyrier, who appears to have been a holdover from the previous reign and was present at the funeral of Henry VII; he also attended the new king's coronation in June 1509. Referred to as "chief surgeon to the body, and to the heirs of his body," Veyrier received a grant of forty marks "during pleasure," and was naturalized in May 1513. He died around 1516.[98] At about the same time that Veyrier's name fades from the official papers of Henry VIII's government, Anthony Chabo's surfaces. Chabo, a native of Savoy, received a grant of denization (naturalization) in 1514 and in 1519 an annuity of £20 for life; the amount had increased to £40 by 1521. Like many Tudor servants, Chabo benefited from opportunity in the form of royal licenses. In January 1531 he secured a license to import 200 tuns of Gascon wine and Toulouse woad, a license renewed in December 1531 and August 1534; another license issued in September 1538 authorized Chabo to buy and export 400 tuns of beer, and his authorization to import Gascon wine was increased to 600 tuns in September 1539.[99]

Marcellus de la More, in aulic service from August 1510 and appointed serjeant-surgeon in 1513, accompanied the king on campaign in France. Henry VIII took the Flemish city of Tournai during that campaign and made Wolsey its bishop; de la More acquired a prebendary in Tournai, until then held by Erasmus, for his son Henry, but not without some difficulty.[100] First, a papal nominee claimed the benefice and the king would have to make proper provision for him or "no Englishman would have a quiet benefice in Tournay." Then, the Dean of Cambray claimed the right to the first vacancy. Finally, Erasmus resigned the post to Henry de la More, but he did so "notwithstanding I think him not in heart so good English that I should desire many such in Tournay Church."[101] As serjeant-surgeon, Marcellus de la More's first salary was only forty marks, but in 1516 he received a lifetime annuity of more than £26. He also enjoyed a grant "of the customs on his imports or exports for three years to the amount of £1000 on the bonds" of a merchant of Florence, John Calvancanti.[102] Master of the Barbers' Company, de la More was in constant attendance on the royal household and is listed among the daily liveries, those retainers receiving provisions. When Marcellus de la More passed away in 1530 he was succeeded as serjeant-surgeon by Thomas Vicary.

The occupational line between surgeons and barbers continued to blur because they often performed similar functions, and Vicary personified that indistinction.[103] Born in 1490, Vicary served his apprenticeship, sat for the bishop's surgical licensing exam, and became a freeman of the Barbers' Company; by 1525 he was third warden and frequently acted as license examiner for the mystery. Nonetheless, Henry VIII made Vicary his new serjeant-surgeon in 1530 when he cured the king's sore leg.[104] Although the crown list of surgeons' fees always placed Vicary first, his was not the highest salary. He was rewarded and recognized in other ways, especially for his plan to unite the barbers and surgeons into one super-guild. Vicary urged the amalgamation of the barbers and all surgeons' associations, a fusion to which the king agreed in 1540. Under the Act of Union, the new Barber-Surgeons' Company had full parliamentary authority. The statutes specified that surgeons were prohibited from practicing barbing or shaving; barbers could pull teeth but were not allowed to bleed or operate on patients. To encourage surgical education, each year the Company was allotted the bodies of four executed felons to dissect.[105] The reestablished partnership of these occupations lasted for two hundred years, but there would be no blending of the separate callings.[106]

However, the Act of Union made oblique reference to the danger of surgeons spreading infectious diseases by treating infected people in their houses, and it paved the way for another statute two years later sanctioning traditional male and female healers and herbalists. According to the provisions of this law, honest persons knowledgeable in natural medicine, who ministered out of charity to their neighbors, were protected from harassment by mercenary medicos. Henry himself sponsored altruistic medicine and in August 1543 he sent the Lord Mayor of London a remedy against plague to be disseminated to the people for their protection. The recipe, preserved in the Corporation of London Record Office, calls for herbs, elder and briar leaves, and ginger, mixed with white wine and drunk for nine days. The first spoonful would protect for twenty-four days, the whole regimen for a year. If a person became sick before the nine days had elapsed and "the botch doth appeere," then he was instructed to sop up what remained of the liquid, mix it with the leaves and mustard seed, and apply it as a plaster directly to the skin.[107] By his creation of a college for the physicians and a united company of barber-surgeons, as well as through his own amateur pharmacy, Henry VIII repeatedly demonstrated serious royal patronage of and interest in medicine. Moreover, he had the good judgment to listen to visionaries like Linacre and Vicary.

Hans Holbein executed a famous if fanciful cartoon of the granting of the new Barber-Surgeons' Company's charter by the king in 1541; in it, Henry hands the charter to Vicary to commemorate the event, while appropriate, imagined witnesses look on.[108] The Barber-Surgeons were grateful, making Vicary Master of the Company more times than anyone else. The king was also grateful to Vicary for the recommendation and gave him a twenty-one-year lease and right to the tithes of the dissolved abbey of Boxley in Kent. Vicary served as governor of St. Bartholomew's Hospital in 1548 and was later resident surgical governor there. He published his *Anatomie of the Body of Man* in 1548, the first English anatomy printed in the vernacular.[109] In 1598 William Bremer appended some recipes of his own and an essay on baths by William

Turner, and published it as *The English-Man's Treasure*, "gathered and set forth for the benefit and cure of the poorer sort of people."[110] *The English-Man's Treasure* referred to surgery as "the last instrument of medicine" and discusses bones, nerves, and muscles in ways that ordinary readers could understand. In a separate section, Vicary dealt with remedies for wounds, gunshots, and ulcers, and for seasick captains and soldiers who travel by water. He provided correctives for insomnia, toothache, red nose, and sore eyes. For bad breath he endorsed a mouthwash of water, vinegar, anise, mint, and cloves; extraction of the tooth was another option mentioned.

Besides his serjeant-surgeon, the king employed John Ayliffe and James Monforde as royal surgeons. Ayliffe joined the Barbers' Company in 1522, becoming Master in 1538, a time when the Company outstripped all other London mysteries with 185 members. He successfully treated the king for a fistula; Henry showed his gratitude with a royal surgical appointment (at £30 per annum, £10 more than Vicary received) and the gift of a manor in Wiltshire.[111] Ayliffe participated in London politics, as sheriff in 1548, as alderman from Dowgate ward the following year, and as the first alderman from Bridge Without in 1550. Ayliffe expected to become mayor when he translated to the Grocers' Company, but he died before the certainty of his election was established. He made a substantial fortune as a woolen merchant and Master of Bakewell Hall, location of the weekly cloth market; he left many endowments for diverse charities.[112] James Monforde also functioned as the king's surgeon toward the end of Henry VIII's reign. Twice warden of the united Barber-Surgeons, Monforde bequeathed a silver hammer to the Company, which is still used by its Masters.[113]

One foreign Henrician surgeon demonstrated a remarkable ability to adjust to the shifting political winds inherent in religious change, particularly impressive for an Italian who was often the target of xenophobic jealousy. Balthazar Guersie, mentioned previously as a surgical colleague of Dr. Angustinus, entered into the service of Catherine of Aragon, and shortly thereafter a London surgeon, Thomas Roos, took exception to the advancement of an outsider and attacked him. Roos had to post £100 as a guarantee that he would not molest Guersie again.[114] Probably for his own protection, Guersie was naturalized in 1522. Unlike most surgeons, Guersie pursued a medical degree, graduating from Cambridge with a bachelor's in medicine around 1530. His medical skills induced Henry VIII to bring him onto his surgical staff.

Guersie's religious conservatism proved important as well. Guersie participated in the attempt to thwart the radical Protestant advance and to reiterate the official "Catholic" Henrician creed. Beginning in 1539, a return to orthodoxy was orchestrated by Stephen Gardiner, Bishop of Winchester. With Gardiner's encouragement, Henry assented to the Act of the Six Articles, reasserting a number of traditional doctrines such as transubstantiation. Archbishop Cranmer opposed the Six Articles, particularly a clause relating to clerical marriage. In May 1543, the king issued a formal declaration that he had written himself, articulating the Creed, the seven sacraments, the ten commandments, and his own royal supremacy. Cranmer continued to promote the Reformation in his diocese and to nominate preachers at Canterbury familiar with the "New Learning." Cranmer's enemies, especially Gardiner, attacked him repeatedly in the Privy Council; Guersie even collected accusations against the archbishop, pitting him against the king's physician, Dr. Butts.[115] Despite repeated attempts to destroy Cranmer, the king would not condemn him for heresy. "By special grace," Cambridge awarded Guersie an M.D. in 1546, probably in appreciation for the service he had done Bishop Gardiner, Chancellor of the University. Given his Romanist orientation, Guersie was not welcome in the Protestant household of Edward VI, but with the accession of Catholic Mary I and her intercession on his behalf, he became a Fellow of the College of Physicians in 1556. Guersie died the following year.

One of the responsibilities for the royal surgeons was treating syphilis. In Henrician times, various New World medicinal plants like guaiacum wood from the Caribbean were used for syphilis. Because it was thought that impure blood caused the disease, surgeons administered blood cleansers like sassafras, sarsaparilla, and China root. Later, prolonged dosing with mercury became the standard remedy for syphilis when it was first recognized as a venereal disease. "Spend a night with Venus and lifetime with Mercury" warned an often-repeated quip.[116]

Besides his doctors and surgeons, Henry VIII required the services of three barbers during his reign: Edmund Harman, Nicholas Simpson, and John Pen. The king's barber, held in high esteem by the royal household, was one of only fifteen persons allowed to enter the Privy Chamber; the term of office was one month at a time. At the ready when the monarch rose from bed every morning, the king's barber trimmed and dressed the king's head and beard with the royal comb, scissors, and knives as required. According to ordinance, he should keep himself and his own apparel clean, be prudent in his conversation, and avoid the company "of vile persons or misguided women."[117]

Edmund Harman ranks as one of Henry's favorite household attendants. A Londoner born in 1509 and a protégé of Cardinal Wolsey, Harman was in service to the king by 1535. As the king's barber, he received fifty shillings a quarter plus bouche; Harman was allowed to convert the bouche into money. Besides his tonsorial duties, Harman held another office—common packer for exports—meaning that he was the king's revenue officer at the port of London. The king presented Harman with lands in Buckinghamshire, lands that had reverted to the crown upon the attainder of Henry Norris. Harman doubtless appreciated the extra income; he had sixteen children. Harman even finagled a place at court for his brother, John. Harman's outspoken Lutheran opinions later got him into trouble with the Tudor offspring, none of whom had need of his barbering services, but Henry VIII had no doubts about Harman's devotion. Harman accompanied the king on a military expedition to Boulogne in 1544, attended by four horsemen, six archers, and six privates.[118] Harman also witnessed the signing of the king's will. He died in 1577.

Finally, Henry VIII outlasted Richard Babham, his apothecary for life, and Babham's successor, Cuthbert Blackeden. Babham, as has been noted already, was in attendance at Henry VII's funeral and at the coronation of his heir. As the new king's serjeant of the Confectionary, he accompanied Henry VIII in June 1520 along with the rest of the court to the Field of the Cloth of Gold, the historic meeting near Calais of the kings of England and France. Devised by Wolsey to effect détente with France, the Field of the Cloth of Gold enabled Henry to impress Francis I with an expensive chivalric display. Amidst prodigious extravagance, including fountains running with wine, the puerile monarchs frolicked and partied. No doubt there was great demand for the confectionery skills of Richard Babham at such a celebration and Henry awarded him £10 per annum for life.[119] But the demonstration of royal friendship between the kings proved shallow; during the following summer Wolsey concluded a treaty against France with Charles V, Holy Roman Emperor and King of Spain.

Richard Babham supplied the entire court with medicines, but was not always able to collect amounts he was owed. Babham died in 1527, still owed over £8 by Wolsey; the debt still had not been paid at the time of Wolsey's death three years later. Thomas Pierson, like John de Soda, took care of the specific needs of Catherine of Aragon; unlike de Soda, however, Pierson was a native Englishman and member of the Grocers' Company. Pierson may have succeeded John Grice as Henry VII's apothecary; he certainly was in service by 1509 when he received twenty marks (over £13) in salary and more for supplies. Pierson applied for and was granted an exemption from serving on juries in 1516, perhaps because the crush of household business prevented it; that was the year of the Princess Mary's birth, an event requiring Pierson's attendance on Queen Catherine and her daughter.[120] Elected warden of the Grocers in 1530, Pierson died the following year.

Also a member of the Grocers' Company, Cuthbert Blackeden began his aulic service as a yeoman (or assistant) apothecary, entitled to bouche and a quarterly allotment.[121] He tendered bills of about £60 annually for medical supplies in the 1530s, invoices that give an indication of the varied nature of an apothecary's tasks. For perfuming the Princess Mary's gloves that year, Blackeden requested 4s. 10d. As an officeholder, Blackeden attended the coronation of Anne Boleyn in 1533; he was later given some of Jane Seymour's jewelry after her death.[122] Blackeden died in 1540.

Thomas Alsop, Henry VIII's best-known apothecary, took Blackeden's place as "gentleman apothecary," and remained in office through Edward VI's reign and most of Queen Mary's. Alsop was immortalized in Hans Holbein's illustration of the chartering of the Barber-Surgeons' Company. Standing on the king's far right, tall and handsome, Alsop wears a fur-edged robe and chain, indicative of his stature and wealth. The royal apothecary profited from the dissolution of the monasteries and bought eight tenements, lay residences on monastic lands, in St. Stephen's Walbrook for £285, including a large house that ironically had once belonged to St. Thomas of Acon Hospital. He owned property elsewhere in London, Deptford, and Greenwich. Alsop probably earned his salary and whatever emoluments accompanied it, for after 1540 the king's various ailments grew steadily worse. Alsop made fomentations, plasters, sponges, decoctions, gargles, dragées of anise seed and sweet fennel, and *aqua lactis virginis*, a dilution of benzoin tincture for scurvy. Alsop's use of benjamin would seem to support the notion that the king's physicians thought Henry suffered from scurvy.[123] At the exhortation of Queen Katherine Parr, the king began to wear reading glasses with gilt frames, probably provided by Alsop.[124] From August 1546 to January 1547, Alsop's bills totaled £127, an indication of the attention that the royal physicians and surgeons paid to the languishing king. When Henry VIII expired in January 1547, Alsop made perfumes and potpourri for the king's funeral and coffin. He was left one hundred marks in the royal will.[125] Alsop continued in service to Edward VI and Mary I until his death in 1557.

John Hemingway (Emmyngwey) became apprenticed to Blackeden in 1531 and followed him in court service as yeoman apothecary to Henry VIII in 1542, when Hemingway's salary was listed as forty marks per annum. One of his chief duties was preparation of the royal bath, a particularly important therapy for the king's swollen legs. Hemingway kept track of all the herbs, sponges, and aromatic scents used as well as the tub itself, a large wooden cask bound with chestnut hoops; he saw to its storage and supervised repairs when needed. During his thirty-year tenure with the Tudors, assisted by his son Edward, Hemingway kept meticulous accounts of medicines and perfumes that he made, especially a rosewater mixture with cloves and benjamin, and of the vanilla-smelling storax he used for sweetening the royal clothes. Like Alsop, he performed as apothecary to Edward VI, but not to Mary. Hemingway worked for Queen Elizabeth I from her accession, and she compensated him in 1562 with a lease on Santyngley Grange in Yorkshire for a disbursement of £30. Once again, attendance upon the Tudors proved to be very rewarding.

The last apothecary brought into the Henrician household was Patrick Reynolds, also a subscribing witness to Henry VIII's will and the recipient of one hundred marks. He received forty marks a year for service from his appointment in 1546. One of Reynolds' tasks was to distill the dozens of waters made from herbs and flowers used by the court. The names of fifty different waters that the king's apothecary prepared within a few weeks included roses, ground ivy, henbane, oak and walnut leaves, strawberries, and snails.[126] These were in addition to the existing inventory of twenty-four waters concocted during the previous year. Most of these waters would have been used for medications, but a few were used to flavor jellies and candies. Reynolds, like Alsop, continued as a royal apothecary after the death of Henry VIII, working for several years in the household of the new king, Edward VI. Despite the continuity of some Tudor medical personnel, however, 1547 signals the end of a complex and dramatic era in England.[127]

Notes

1. For more on the lengthy contention for power between the houses of Lancaster and York, see John Gillingham, *The Wars of the Roses* (Baton Rouge: Louisiana State University Press, 1981). The standard biography of Henry VII is S. B. Chrimes, *Henry VII* (Berkely: University of California Press, 1972).

2. The phrase "Tudor revolution in government" belongs to Geoffrey R. Elton; he applied the phrase to the administrative reforms initiated by Thomas Cromwell, Henry VIII's chief minister after Cardinal Wolsey and Thomas More. See Elton, *Reform and Reformation England* (London: Arnold, 1977).

3. Henry VII knighted Cambridge-educated physician Lewis Caerleon in 1488, probably for his assistance in intrigue against Richard III rather than in recognition of his service as physician to the king and family. Getz, *Medicine in the English Middle Ages*, 18.

4. Clark, *Royal College of Physicians* 1: 35.

5. The statutes, handsomely illustrated, are reproduced in Fritz Saxl and Rudolf Wittkower, *British Art and the Mediterranean* (New York: Oxford University Press, 1948). The original text is in the Bodleian Library, Oxford.

6. All save Wolsey were executed, and he died *en route* to face a treason charge. Mary I had Cranmer burned at the stake for heresy in 1556.

7. For more on the complicated structure of the household, see D. A. L. Morgan, "The House of Policy," in *The English Court from the Wars of the Roses to the Civil War*, ed. David Starkey et al. (London: Longman, 1987), 32–33; and David Starkey, "Intimacy and Innovation: The Use of the Privy Chamber," in *The English Court*, 73–75. Scattered information about medical office holders under Henry VII may be gleaned from the *Calendar of the Patent Rolls Preserved in the Public Record Office: Henry VII* (1485–1509), 2 vols. (London: HMSO, 1914–16), hereafter *C.P.R.*; and from the *Calendar of the Close Rolls preserved in the Public Record Office* (1485–1500) (London: HMSO, 1955), hereafter *C.C.R.*

8. The appointment included keepership of Prince Arthur's wardrobe. See James Gairdner, *Henry the Seventh* (London: Macmillan, 1902). Medical appointments to the French royal household had to be bought, but carried important fringe benefits such as an aristocratic practice and social advancement: Laurence Brockliss and Colin Jones, *The Medical World of Early Modern France* (Oxford: Clarendon Press, 1997), 546.

9. C. H. Talbot and E. A. Hammond, *The Medical Practitioners in Medieval England: A Biographical Register* (London: Wellcome Medical Library, 1965), 24; Clippingdale, Medical Court Roll, 1: 17, LRCS.

10. Talbot and Hammond, *Medical Practitioners*, 369. The records of Henry VII's reign are very fragmentary. Sir John Sainty has been unable to confirm any physician appointments and Dr. Clippingdale could find no record of surgeons named during the reign.

11. Jon Arrizabalaga, John Henderson, and Roger French, *The Great Pox: The French Disease in Renaissance Europe* (New Haven, Conn.: Yale University Press, 1997), 265.

12. For an exhaustive history of gout, see Roy Porter and G. S. Rousseau, *Gout: The Patrician Malady* (New Haven, Conn.: Yale University Press, 1998).

13. Ibid., 27. For more on Gilbertus Anglicus (Gilbert Eagle), see Faye Marie Getz, *Healing and Society in Medieval England: A Middle English Translation of the Pharmaceutical Writings of Gilbertus Anglicus* (Madison: University of Wisconsin Press, 1991).

14. Skinner, *Medical Terms*, 195. The drink is William Butler's and can be found in the Sloane Manuscripts (hereafter SL MSS) 1087, British Library, London. Andrew Boorde, erstwhile doctor to Henry VIII, additionally recommended that goutish patients watch their diets after being purged. Thomas Sydenham published the classical account of gout at the end of the seventeenth century.

15. Eric N. Simons, *Henry VII: The First Tudor King* (London: Frederick Muller, 1968), 285.

16. Arthur MacNalty, *Henry VIII: A Difficult Patient* (London: C. Johnson, 1952), 25. MacNalty argues that Henry VII passed tuberculosis along to his son and heir, Arthur, and that Henry VIII, free himself from the active disease, had two sons who died from it—Edward VI and a natural son,

Henry, Duke of Richmond. See also Arthur MacNalty, *Elizabeth Tudor: The Lonely Queen* (New York: Frederick Ungar Publishing, 1961), 222–23.

17. The Queen Mother, afforded precedence over all the other royal women at Henry VII's funeral, died just two months later and was buried in her son's chapel at Westminster Abbey.

18. Neither Clippingdale nor Sainty and Bucholz have indexed any in their respective medical lists.

19. "Doctors at Court: The Medical Household," *British Medical Journal* (1953) 1: 1217–18; Thompson, "Serjeant Surgeons to Their Majesties," 2.

20. R. Theodore Beck, *The Cutting Edge: The Early History of the Surgeons of London* (London: Lund Humphries, 1974), 152–53.

21. Clark, *Royal College of Physicians* 1: 13.

22. According to one historian, syphilis came to Britain in 1497 when Neapolitan mercenaries of Perkin Warbeck, a phony claimant to the English throne, landed in Scotland and were garrisoned in Aberdeen: Rosemary O'Day, *The Tudor Age* (London: Longman, 1995), 6. However, the source of syphilis in Europe is a subject of much current controversy. See Roy Porter, ed., *Medicine: A History of Healing* (New York: Marlowe, 1997), 32.

23. R. S. Roberts, "Personnel and Practice of Medicine in Tudor Stuart England: Part 2:. London," *Medical History* 8 (1964): 219.

24. *C.P.R.* (1485–94) 1: 174; *C.C.R.* (1485–1500), 96.

25. Beck, *Cutting Edge*, 153; Altofte's will is reprinted on 167–68.

26. See Hector MacLennan, "A Gynecologist Looks at the Tudors," *Medical History* 11 (1967): 66–74.

27. Quoted in Irving S. Cutter and Henry R. Viets, *A Short History of Midwifery* (Philadelphia: Saunders, 1964), 39.

28. See Humphrey Arthure, "The Midwife," *Journal of Obstetrics and Gynecology of the British Commonwealth* 80 (1973): 1–9.

29. See N. H. Nicolas, *Privy Purse Expenses of Elizabeth of York* (New York: Barnes and Noble Reprint, 1972).

30. Matthews, *Royal Apothecaries*, 61.

31. Matthews, *Royal Apothecaries*, 62–63. Records of Henrician medical appointments after 1509 may be found scattered throughout J. S. Brewer, R. H. Brodie, and J. Gairdner, eds., *Letters and Papers, Foreign and Domestic, of the Reign of Henry VIII*, 2nd ed., 21 vols. (London: HMSO, 1862–1920), hereafter referred to as *L. & P.*

32. At least until his own death, that is. Babham died in 1527 and was succeeded by Cuthbert Blackeden.

33. Matthews, *Royal Apothecaries*, 70. In 1514 Mary was married, at age eighteen, to fifty-two-year-old Louis XII of France; he died the following year, leaving her free to wed a man of her own choosing. The other Tudor daughter, Margaret, married James IV of Scotland in 1503; through her, as Henry VII predicted, the greater would attract the lesser, when in 1603 Margaret's great-grandson James VI became James I of England.

34. De Soda received black cloth for the funeral, red cloth for the coronation, and livery for the celebrations at the Field of the Cloth of Gold (see below).

35. David Loades, *Mary Tudor* (Oxford: Blackwell, 1989), 352.

36. It was Dr. Samuel Johnson who called Linacre a Renaissance man; Fielding Garrison, famed medical historian, referred to him as a "Restorer of Learning." Johnson quoted in William Munk, *Roll of the Royal College of Physicians*, 2 vols. (London: Longman, Green and Roberts, 1861) 1: 12. See also John Pye, *Thomas Linacre: Scholar, Physician, Priest* (London: Catholic Truth Society, 1912).

37. For the influence of Padua on Renaissance England, see Jonathan Woolfson, *Padua and the Tudors: English Students in Italy, 1485–1603* (Cambridge: Cambridge University Press, 1999).

38. Vivian Nutton, "John Caius and the Linacre Tradition," *Medical History* 23 (1979): 374.

39. Linacre's ecclesiastical livings gave him leisure to enjoy the literary life. See Charles D. O'Malley, *English Medical Humanists* (Lawrence: University of Kansas Press, 1965).

40. William Macmichael, *Lives of British Physicians* (London: J. Murray, 1830), 5.

41. "Mr. Serjeant Surgeon John Knight," *British Medical Journal* (1940) 2: 129.

42. Clark, *College of Physicians* 1: 54–55. The bishop licensed midwives, although not because of the Act. Because midwives often had to baptize sickly or dying newborns, their religious reputations were more important than their medical prowess. Four or more women had to testify that the midwife-to-be had practical experience and manifest spiritual orthodoxy. J. H. Bloom and R. R. James, *Medical Practitioners 1529–1725* (Cambridge: Cambridge University Press, 1935), 11.

43. R. R. James, "Earliest List of Surgeons to Be Licensed by the Bishop of London," *Janus* 41 (1937): 255–60.

44. Clark, *College of Physicians* 1: 57.

45. The other petitioners were Cardinal Wolsey and physicians Nicholas Haswell, John Francis, and Robert Yaxley.

46. Licenses were not free: around the year 1600, £8 went to the College, £1 to its President, 13s. 4d. (thirteen shillings, four pence) to the treasurer, ten shillings for a certificate, and 6s. 8d. for the beadle. Total fees came to £10 10s. Eric Jameson, *The Natural History of Quackery* (London: C. C. Thomas, 1961), 28. The College had no control over graduates in medicine from Oxford or Cambridge as long as they stayed out of London.

47. Quoted in Joyce Youings, *Sixteenth-Century England* (New York: Penguin, 1984), 45. The 1540 Act freeing the Fellows from civic duties also strictly subordinated the apothecaries to a College committee. Clark, *College of Physicians* 1: 82–83.

48. Pelling and Webster, "Medical Practitioners," 169.

49. The standard biography of Linacre remains William Osler, *Thomas Linacre* (Cambridge: Cambridge University Press, 1908). For an assessment of Linacre's impact, see Francis Maddison, Margaret Pelling, and Charles Webster, *Essays on the Life and Work of Thomas Linacre* (Oxford: Clarendon Press, 1977); and Charles E. Raven, *English Naturalists from Neckam to Ray* (New York: Cambridge University Press, 1968), 36–38.

50. There were originally two, then four censors as the College tried to make its authority effective; the proliferation of apothecaries, some without shops, made enforcement difficult. Besides the President and censors, other officers of the College included a pro-president, two consiliarii (President's counselors), and a caduceator or beadle (guardian of the College's property). Clark, *College of Physicians* 1: 92–93.

51. Munk, *Roll* 1: 10.

52. Sidney Young, *The Annals of the Barber-Surgeons of London* (London: Blades, East and Blades, 1890), 85; MacLennan, "Gynecologist," 69. The first recorded Caesarean section in England in which both mother and child lived was in 1836: Skinner, *Medical Terms*, 84. Jack Dewhurst doubts that Queen Jane had a Caesarean section, since she survived for too long (two weeks) afterwards: Jack Dewhurst, *Royal Confinements: A Gynaecological History of Britain's Royal Family* (New York: St. Martin's Press, 1980), 7.

53. Quoted in Neville Williams, *Henry VIII and His Court* (New York: Macmillan, 1971), 176; Talbot and Hammond, *Medical Practitioners*, 132. For more on the sexual problems of Henry VIII and his fourth consort, see Retha M. Warnicke, *The Marrying of Anne of Cleves* (Cambridge: Cambridge University Press, 2000), 162–172.

54. SL MSS 1047, British Library. The book is water-damaged, but the handwriting is legible and identical throughout. Dr. Butts signed the prescriptions.

55. Blaxland Stubbs, "Royal Recipes for Plasters, Ointments and Other Medicaments," *Chemist and Druggist* 114 (1931): 792–94; Jameson, 36.

56. Munk, *Roll* 1: 14.

57. Talbot and Hammond, *Medical Practitioners*, 47.

58. Catherine had been married to Henry's deceased older brother, Arthur. Although a papal dispensation had been obtained for Henry to marry her in 1509, Henry argued that the Bible prohibited their union and that God had punished him by giving him no sons. Sir Hector MacLennan suggested that the royal couple's troubles may have stemmed, not from syphilis in the king, but from Catherine's Rh negative and Henry's Rh positive factors, and that simple replacement trans-

fusions might have saved the baby boys who died soon after birth; Sir Arthur MacNalty suggested that the problem was toxemia of pregnancy. See MacLennan, "Gynecologist," 68.

59. Beck, *Cutting Edge*, 169–70. Farnando died in June 1533 after identifying Margaret Bruges as his natural daughter and bequeathing to her all his goods; he is not listed in Munk.

60. Although the entry in *The Dictionary of National Biography* (DNB) casts doubt on whether Wotton was a physician-in-ordinary, it does call him physician to Thomas Howard, Duke of Norfolk, and to Margaret Pole, Countess of Salisbury.

61. The great naturalist, Conrad Gesner of Zurich, "corrected" some of Wotton's errors in the margins of the Wellcome Institute's copy of the treatise. Vivian Nutton, "Conrad Gesner and the English Naturalists," *Medical History* 29 (1985): 93–94. Charles Raven also dismisses Wotton as a man of books rather than an observer, a man who "has little claim to be called a naturalist." Raven, *English Naturalists*, 40–42.

62. Munk, *Roll* 1: 31; Matthews, *Royal Apothecaries*, 82. Ashe was owed money by the Earl of Northumberland and the Countess of Salisbury at their deaths.

63. Clippingdale, Medical Court Roll, 1: 23, LRCS. John Clement, though not a royal physician as Vivian Nutton maintained, did tend Wolsey in 1529 at the behest of Henry VIII. Clement, whose wife was a kinswoman of Sir Thomas More, presided over the College of Physicians in 1544. See Nutton, "John Caius and the Linacre Tradition," 379.

64. There is no evidence that Elyot ever attended Henry VIII in a professional capacity, but his own recommendations are fascinating: he suggests eating such "good metes" as partridge, pheasant, pigeon, and veal, but cautions that "quayle increases melancholye" and is of small nourishment. Elyot's *Castel of Helth* (London: Thomas Bertheleti, 1534), dedicated to Thomas Cromwell, popularized the humoral theory and urged care with food, cautioning readers not to consume old or putrid victuals. The most excellent milk, he said, is that of a woman. For more on Elyot, see Lehmberg, *Sir Thomas Elyot: Tudor Humanist*.

65. Munk concluded that Angustinus must have also served Henry VIII. Munk, *Roll* 1: 33–34.

66. Samuel Dodd Clippingdale reported that the doctor's name is Butt in the will and on the tombstone, but in Shakespeare's play, *Henry VIII*, it is Butts. The conceited and mercenary character of Dr. Butts became the prototype for a dramatic convention that exposed false learning and medical piety. See Clippingdale, "Sir William Butt, M.D.: A Local Link with Shakespeare," *West London Medical Journal* (July 1916); Philip C. Kolin, *Elizabethan Stage Doctor* (Salzburg: Institut für Englische Sprache und Literatur, 1975), 201.

67. Maria Dowling, "Anne Boleyn as Patron," in *Henry VIII: A European Court in England*, ed. David Starkey (London: Collins and Brown, 1991), 110.

68. Forty marks equalled a little over £26. One hundred marks, the sum the king left to his apothecaries, were worth about £67.

69. For more on the debate over the repercussions of the dissolution on medicine, see Youings, *Sixteenth-Century England*, 256–59; J. J. Scarisbrick, *Henry VIII* (Berkeley: University of California Press, 1970), 515–16; and Charles S. Webster, ed., *Health, Medicine and Mortality in the Sixteenth Century* (Cambridge: Cambridge University Press, 1979).

70. Young, *Annals*, 85.

71. Allison Weir, *The Six Wives of Henry VIII* (New York: Grove Weidenfeld, 1991), 421.

72. Munk, *Roll* 1: 29; Beck, *Cutting Edge*, 171. A copy of Hans Holbein's portrait of Dr. Butts is in the Isabella Stuart Gardner Museum, Boston.

73. Stephen Gardiner, Bishop of Winchester, tried to implicate Cranmer and Katherine Parr with Anne Askew, but Askew's martyrdom kindled a Protestant reaction.

74. Clippingdale, Medical Court Roll, 1: 23, LRCS; Munk, *Roll* 1: 22.

75. Vivian Nutton, "Medicine, Diplomacy, and Finance: The Prefaces to a Hippocratic Commentary of 1541," in *New Perspectives on Renaissance Thought*, ed. John Henry and Sarah Hutton (London: Duckworth, 1990), 230–33.

76. His *De Morbo Gallico* was published in 1566. Arrizabalaga et al., *The Great Pox*, 267–68; Clippingdale, Medical Court Roll, 1: 23, LRCS. Brasavola wrote a tract on aphrodisiacs published in 1728. Member of a prominent Italian medical family, Brasavola also ministered to Charles V

and several popes. He indexed all the works of Galen and was an expert on syphilis. See Arrizabalaga et al., *The Great Pox*, 267–68.

77. Munk, *Roll* 1: 35.

78. Bullein's *Bulwarke of Defence against All Sicknes, Sorenes and Woundes* (London: John Kyngston, 1579). Bullein, a Protestant rector from Suffolk, travelled abroad after Henry's death and took a medical degree: see John Fines, *Biographical Register of Early English Protestants* (Oxford: Sutton Courtenay, 1981), A-C. William Hilton, brother of his patron, Sir Thomas Hilton, accused Bullein of murdering Sir Thomas, but Bullein was acquitted and married the dead man's widow, whom he had cured of a "tympany." See Clippingdale, Medical Court Roll, 1: 23, LRCS; Raven, *English Naturalists*, 149–51.

79. John Caius, quoted in Carolly Erickson, *Bloody Mary* (Garden City, N. Y.: Doubleday, 1978), 24.

80. From Boorde's *Dyetary*, cited in W.S.C. Copeman, *Doctors and Disease in Tudor Times* (London: Dawson's, 1960), 88.

81. Costum is an aromatic plant (*costus arabicus* or its powdered root), which is often used in costly unguents, in this case with olive oil as a salve.

82. Porter and Rousseau, *Gout*, 25–26.

83. See Boorde's *Introduction and Dyetary with Barnes in the Defense of the Berde*, ed. F. J. Furnivall (London: Trubner, 1870) for both works.

84. *The Treatise Answering the Book of Berdes* can be found in the Furnivall edition of Boorde's *Introduction and Dyetary*, 305–16.

85. Boorde accumulated stories while in Montpellier, stories that were credited to him and later published as *Scogin's Jests*, "a preservative against melancholy." This comedic book and another ascribed to him, *Merry Tales of the Mad Men of Gotham* (London: Thomas Colwell, 1565), led to his well-known nickname. See H. Edmund Poole, *The Wisdom of Andrew Boorde* (Leicester, England: E. Backus, 1936), and my entry on Boorde in the *New Dictionary of National Biography* (Oxford: Oxford University Press, forthcoming 2004).

86. Antonia Fraser, *The Wives of Henry VIII* (New York: Alfred A. Knopf, 1992), 335–36.

87. One historian has found extraordinary bills for rhubarb in *L. & P.* 21/2: 768; see Lacey Baldwin Smith, *Henry VIII: Mask of Royalty* (Boston: Houghton Mifflin, 1973), 2. Antonia Fraser suggests that the nineteen year-old queen may have then made the fatal decision to look elsewhere for romantic pleasure. Katherine Howard was executed for adultery in February 1542 on the same spot where her cousin Anne Boleyn had died almost six years before. Fraser, *Wives of Henry VIII*, 336, 353.

88. Scarisbrick, *Henry VIII*, 211; see also Ove Brinch, "The Medical Problems of Henry VIII," *Centaurus*, 5/3–4 (1958), 339–69.

89. See A. S. Currie, "Notes on the Obstetrical History of Catherine of Aragon and Anne Boleyn," *Edinburgh Medical Journal* 38 (1888): 1–34.

90. One Henrician biographer suggests that the king's maltreated varicose veins became thrombosed. See Scarisbrick, *Henry VIII*, 485. Sir Hector MacLennan also rejects the syphilis diagnosis: see MacLennan, "Gynecologist," 68.

91. See MacNalty, *Henry VIII*, 159n.

92. See Susan Maclean Kybett, "Henry VIII—A Malnourished King?," *History Today* 39 (September 1989): 19–25.

93. His book is *A Meet Diet for the New Ague*: see Raven, *English Naturalists*, 69n.

94. Weir, *Six Wives*, 521.

95. Munk, *Roll* 1: 50.

96. Munk, *Roll* 1: 32. Munk cites Sir William Petre's criticism of Huicke's treatment of his wife.

97. Quoted in Raven, *English Naturalists*, 70n. The full title of Turner's work is *The New Booke of Spirituall Physick for Dyuerse Diseases of the Nobilite and Gentlemen of Englande*, printed in Rome by Marcus Antonius Constantius.

98. *L. & P.* 1: 20, 414.

99. *L. & P.* 5: 36, 365; 7: 1122; 13/2: 734; 14/2: 264.

100. *L. & P.* 1: 1224, 4390; Talbot and Hammond, 207; Jessie Dobson and R. Milnes Walker, *Barbers and Barber Surgeons of London* (London: Blackwell, 1979), 137.

101. *L. & P.* 2: 889, 890, 2066.

102. *L. & P.* 2: 1586.

103. The red and white barber pole alludes to the bloodier services—like tooth pulling—performed by barbers.

104. Vicary was paid £20 per year for the assignment. Young, *Annals*, 522; Beck, *Cutting Edge*, 183.

105. Cecil Wall, *History of the Surgeons' Company* (London: Oxford University Press, 1937), 18–21. Clark notes that the Act concerning surgeons is separated from that concerning physicians on the Statute Roll by one that "decides which innholders may bake horse-bread within their houses." Clark, *Royal College of Physicians* 1: 82.

106. In 1745 two separate corporations were established.

107. Quoted in Beck, *Cutting Edge*, 177. Stubbs has the wrong year for the communication: Stubbs, "Royal Recipes," 794.

108. Clark, *Royal College of Physicians* 1: 85. The union of the Barber-Surgeons lasted until 1745 when the surgeons separated to form their own organization.

109. For an updated edition containing a life of Vicary, see F. J. Furnivall and Percy Furnivall, eds., *Anatomie of the Bodie of Man* (London: Trubner, 1888).

110. A seventh edition of *The English-Man's Treasure* appeared in 1626 containing almost "a thousand approved waters and medicines, meete and necessarie for physicke and chyrurgerie." It could be purchased at B. Alsop's bookstore in Grub Street "neere the Lower Pumpe."

111. Henry VIII also left Ayliffe one hundred marks in his will: Beck, *Cutting Edge*, 183.

112. John Stow, *Survey of London* (New York: Dutton, 1912), 256–57.

113. Young, *Annals*, 90.

114. *L. & P.*, 3/2: 1562.

115. Munk, *Roll* 1: 57.

116. Quoted in Porter, *Medicine*, 32.

117. Dobson and Walker, *Barbers and Barber Surgeons*, 32.

118. D'Arcy Power, "Some Notes on Edmund Harman, King's Barber," *Proceedings of the Royal Society of Medicine* 9 (1916): 67–88. An inventory by Harman of the king's wardrobe and barber's stock can be found in the Royal Rolls: Ro 1413 (47), British Library.

119. Matthews, *Royal Apothecaries*, 64.

120. Matthews, *Royal Apothecaries*, 63.

121. In 1519, for instance, he received 22s. 10d. per quarter. Matthews, *Royal Apothecaries*, 65.

122. Matthews, *Royal Apothecaries*, 66.

123. Benjamin is the popular term for benzoin.

124. Fraser, *Wives of Henry VIII*, 373.

125. Matthews, *Royal Apothecaries*, 63–68.

126. Royal Rolls 7c, folios 98–99, British Library.

127. For a balanced assessment of Henry VIII's reign, see Scarisbrick, *Henry VIII*, 498–526.

Chapter 2

Doctors to the "Little Tudors": Medicine in Perilous Times (1547–58)

Edward VI, the son for whom Henry VIII had moved heaven and earth, became king of England at the age of nine.[1] "God's imp" was intelligent with scholarly tastes and a Protestant zeal that benefited the council of regency that governed in his name, but he had been overprotected and coddled as Prince of Wales. The walls and floors of his apartment were washed down three times a day to protect him from disease and his food was carefully prepared by servants appointed to tend to his every need. Great care, however, had to be taken with royal children, given the frightening rate of mortality for youngsters in Tudor England.[2] Edward was slight of build, pale-complected with auburn hair, and although he manifested a slightly deformed shoulder he was not a sickly child. Though never rambunctious, Prince Edward completely recovered from a bout of fever in 1541 and was an active boy. His first love was intellectual pursuit, but he participated in fencing, horsemanship, and hunting despite increasing short-sightedness.[3]

Edward's tutor from 1544 was John Cheke, classical scholar and humanist of the first rank. An early devotee of Protestant doctrine at Cambridge, in 1540 Cheke became Henry VIII's first Regius Professor of Greek at that university and under his influence Cambridge became the center of the "New Learning" in England. He lived on a pension in lieu of a canonry and devoted himself to educating the prince. A strong bond of affection existed between them and at Edward's accession Cheke was granted a number of royal favors including a knighthood and the post of Provost of King's College, Cambridge. Cheke, one of the most erudite men of his generation, would also play an important role in effecting religious changes in the new reign.[4]

During the final months of Henry VIII's life, a clique of lords with Protestant sympathies emerged as the dominant faction at court. When Henry made his will in December 1546, he left the government in the hands of a Council of Regency composed of sixteen men equal in status and commanded them to rule jointly in Edward's name until he came of age. He also instructed his son to esteem these "entirely beloved" executors and assist them in their charge.[5] Among the more prominent members of the Council, renowned for their military prowess, were Edward's uncle, Edward Seymour, Earl of Hertford, and John Dudley, Viscount Lisle. When Henry VIII died, however, Hertford had no intentions of sharing the government of the kingdom with the others and as the boy's uncle argued effectively that he should be Lord Protector. Enough of the other councillors agreed with him that the regents needed a leader and, disregarding Henry's will, proclaimed Hertford Governor of the King's Person. On the day following the funeral of Henry VIII, Edward Seymour was created Duke of Somerset and John Dudley became Earl of Warwick. Their rivalry became the dominant motif of Edward's short reign.

Somerset initiated the Edwardian reformation with an Act of Uniformity which enforced the use of Archbishop Cranmer's *Book of Common Prayer* (1549).[6] Containing the liturgy of the Church of England, it replaced the Latin services with ones in English and designed a compromise doctrine aimed somewhere between conservatives and radicals, pleasing neither. Comparatively mild penalties were imposed for violating the Act, but an uprising of Roman Catholics in the west of England marred Somerset's settlement. Even more upsetting to Somerset's regime was a 1549 peasants' revolt in Norfolk over enclosures. Led by Robert Kett, the rebellion was directed at landowners who fenced common pasture lands to raise their own sheep. Somerset felt sympathy for the plight of the peasants, but in expressing compassion he incurred the wrath of the powerful landowners, who turned to his rival, Warwick. The rebels, numbering sixteen thousand, wanted the abolition of private ownership of land; they achieved some success before being subdued by Warwick, Lord Lieutenant of the Army.[7] Imprisoned in 1549, Somerset was released the following year, but Warwick finally overthrew him, engineering a second treason charge against him in 1551; Somerset was sentenced to death. Warwick took control, now virtually ruler of England. Just before Somerset's execution, John Dudley raised himself to Duke of Northumberland.[8]

Northumberland's government advanced the Protestant Reformation with a revised *Book of Common Prayer* (1552) and a new church creed (1553). Like the first prayer book, the second, more radical version was the work of Archbishop Cranmer, another key adviser held over from the reign of Henry VIII. *The Book of Common Prayer* removed all references to the Mass and to the altar, revised the Holy Communion office, and required that simple surplices rather than traditional vestments be worn during services. A new Act of Uniformity laid down more severe penalties for noncompliance with the liturgical changes as well as fines for nonattendance at church. The forty-two articles of religion followed a Calvinist pattern, rejecting the Catholic doctrine of transubstantiation and recognizing only two sacraments—Baptism and the Eucharist. Young Edward fully supported both plans to transform the Church of England into a Protestant church and Northumberland's more extreme religious amendment.

Besides the "beloved" councillors and church officers whom Edward VI inherited through his father's testament, he also acquired physicians from his father's household—Drs. Owen, Wendy, Huicke, Bille, and Boorde. In addition to these, the adolescent king was tended by John Caius, one of the most eminent physicians of the sixteenth century.[9] Born in Norwich in 1510, Caius took his arts degrees at Gonville College, Cambridge and then, like Linacre, to whom his contemporaries compared him, Caius studied medicine from 1539 to 1543 at Padua, where he attended the classes of the physician Johannes Baptista Montanus and of the great Flemish anatomist, Andreas Vesalius.[10] As part of Renaissance humanist medical training, which venerated classical authors like Galen, the study of anatomy was deemed essential for all doctors; Caius began to collect surgical treatises and perform dissections himself. Caius received his M.D. in 1541 and, after teaching Greek for a while at Padua, returned to England. Even after Vesalius discredited Galenic anatomy, however, Caius never abandoned his faith in tradition and because of that has been deemed an anachronism in his own lifetime.[11] Caius became a Fellow of the College of Physicians in 1547, rising to the office of President, which he held in 1555–60, 1562–64, and 1571. He spearheaded the adoption of new statutes that consolidated the best of the Linacre tradition with newer continental models; he championed new College examinations based on Galenic texts. Caius was a vigorous advocate of the College of Physicians' rights against surgeons. In March 1572 he argued that physicians ought to be treating serious conditions like sciatica, the "French pox," and ulcers; the ecclesiastical high commission sitting at the Guildhall unanimously agreed with him.[12] Caius revived the study of anatomy among the Fellows and taught it for twenty years, not at the College's premises, but at the Barber-Surgeons' Hall. Under his leadership, the College obtained permission in 1564 to dissect four corpses a year.[13]

A classical scholar of the first rank, Caius also wrote a treatise on English dogs and a book on the rare animals that he had seen in various aristocratic menageries.[14] *De Canibus Britannicis Libellus* provided a wealth of information on different dog breeds, demonstrating that dogs performed a vast array of roles and were well integrated into English society and culture. Caius based his canine categories on function, as opposed to lineage and appearance; hence, he carried on the ancient organizational classifications of hunting, pet, and working dogs.[15] In *De Rariorum Animalium atque Stirpium Historia*, he described and drew a cheetah and a lynx kept at the Tower, as well as North African specimens that he owned, including a Gentulan hound, a civet cat, and Barbary sheep. A beast brought from Norway, which Caius called a "hippelaphus", probably an elk, reportedly drank English ale without getting drunk or manifesting any ill effects.[16] In 1552 Caius penned in the vernacular an influential book on sweating sickness, based upon his own observations, which dealt with the external and internal causes of the disease as well as how to avoid it when well and how to cure it when infected. He recommended keeping warm during the "sweat" but avoiding sleep; a victim should be kept awake by hitting him with a rosemary branch. He suggested letting those infected smell apples. Unlike the Norwegian elk, Caius cautioned his patients against relying on English beer, seemingly a popular remedy.[17]

Though Caius functioned as a royal doctor to Edward, as well as his successors, Mary I and Elizabeth I, his adherence to Roman Catholic tenets had a bearing on his success with the Tudor siblings. In 1557 during the reign of Roman Catholic Mary, Caius received Letters Patent from the crown to re-found failing Gonville College at Cambridge as Gonville and Caius. He endowed the College with manors and advowsons, the right to name recipients of church benefices—a right considered property that could be sold; he gave the College plate and books, and became its Master the following year. Although imbued with the New Learning, Caius retained a love of tradition and preserved Gonville's old buildings. When a new court was built at the College in 1565, Caius ordained that it be three-sided to admit sunlight and fresh air; he also dictated standards of cleanliness and behavior. He was removed as Elizabeth's royal physician in 1568 because of his religion, and his spiritual preferences caused him grief even at the College named for him. Caius's rooms were raided in 1572 during a feud with the Fellows and other college Masters; destroyed in the disturbance were Catholic vestments and vessels, which he had safeguarded. John Caius died a few months later.[18]

In addition to his father's surgeons Sir John Ayliff, knighted by Henry VIII, and Thomas Vicary, architect of the Barber-Surgeons union, the Edwardian medical staff included veteran surgeon Nicholas Alcocke, Richard Ferris, and Henry Forest. Alcocke was admitted to the livery in 1523, a designation ackowledging his earned right to war the Company's regalia. Thus empowered by his colleagues, he took apprentices who served later monarchs in the same capacity as Alcocke served Edward. Beneficiary of a liberal education and a man of musical culture, in 1546 Alcocke obtained the right to publish the translation of a German herbal, *Magnus Herbarius*, which buttressed classical medical theory. He married into the Turner family, making noted botanist William Turner his in-law. Included in the famous Holbein drawing of the Barber-Surgeons, Alcocke made a substantial fortune during his career, and at his death in 1550, left one-third of his goods to his wife, one-third to his executors, and one-third to the Princess Elizabeth. He specified several precise bequests for the poor, for his maids' marriages, and for highways. One historian catalogs Richard Ferris as another Henrician-Edwardian surgeon who appears in the Holbein drawing, with a 1552 salary of £60 per annum, but later identifies him as Elizabeth's serjeant-surgeon. Less is known about Henry Forest, paid £40 per annum in 1552 for his surgical services. A respected London practitioner, Forest probably served in the household of Sir William Petre, a meritorious, veteran servant of the crown and eventually Elizabeth's Secretary of State, who brought Forest to the attention of the Tudors.[19]

Medical antiquarian Samuel Clippingdale affixed the name of Thomas Geminus, a friend of Vicary's and printer of an anatomy text by Vesalius, to his roll of Edwardian surgeons. Geminus, referred to as Italian or Flemish by differing sources, was a Stationer by trade and savvy entrepreneur at heart.[20] Without the approval of the author, Geminus borrowed most of the illustrations from Vesalius' *De Fabrica* (1543) and published the work in London under his own name. Vesalius bitterly protested that his book had been plagiarized in England "where the figures . . . have been copied very poorly and without skill in drawing." The first edition in Latin of *Compendiosa totius anatomiae delineatio* (1545), replete with pacesetting copperplate engravings, was dedicated to Henry VIII and signed by Geminus; a second was addressed to Edward VI and a third in 1559 to Queen Elizabeth I, these latter two in English. Geminus chose Nicholas Udall, a playwright and classical humanist, to translate the piece and turn it into a working manual. Despite the plagiarism, one scholar calls Geminus "typically Renaissance in his versatility" and adds that the compendium became an important tool for teaching anatomical knowledge.[21] Another publication associated with Geminus is *Tectonicon* (1556), a work on mensuration. The register books of the Stationers' Company refer to Geminus as "a stranger" when he transgressed the rules.[22] Geminus was an artist of some merit; however, there is no evidence at all that he was a legitimate surgeon or a licensed doctor. The successful publication of his anatomy manual probably tempted him to try out his skills as an empiric. In fact, in 1556 he was prosecuted by the College of Physicians for practicing without its authorization and fined.[23]

Patrick Reynolds and Thomas Alsop continued their household service as Edwardian royal apothecaries, and Alsop also retained the title of serjeant of the King's Confectionary. When Reynolds passed away in 1551, John Hemingway filled his slot and received a grant for life with wages of forty marks yearly. Apparently, Alsop and Hemingway used their influence to procure the appointment of relatives to the Confectionary, including Hemingway's son Edward. Alsop's position at court improved his standing in the Grocers' Company and in 1552 he became warden of the guild. A third appointment to the household from Christmas 1546 to 1553, George Carlton, likewise received forty marks, guaranteeing that one apothecary would always be available to provide medicines and indicating that there was an unusual need for medication in Edward's court.[24]

While there was every hope that the young king would live to beget a whole line of Tudor sovereigns, pandemics continued to endanger the lives of royals and their subjects alike. John Stow registered the effects of a pestilence that swept London in 1548 and caused "great mortality": people were forbidden to bury the dead before six o'clock in the morning or after six at night.[25] Throughout the summer of 1551 England was again in the grip of a sweating sickness epidemic, this one even worse than the outbreak in the 1520s. Fifty thousand people throughout England succumbed to the illness, including a few servants in the Princess Mary's principal residence, Newhall in Essex. According to Stow, the contagion began in Shrewsbury in April and struck London in July, killing its victims, mostly middle-aged men, within a day of infection.[26] The young king escaped contamination and, working temporarily without his tutor, decided to devote himself exclusively to the learning of statecraft.[27] Clearly, he thought he would soon be king in his own right. He assumed complete responsibility for the primary business of full Council meetings in February and

March of 1552. His interests ranged over the broad spectrum of government and he planned to reorganize and reform the Privy Council itself.[28]

Edward's health, however, while never hardy, began to fail in April 1552. He contracted almost simultaneously diseases reported as measles and smallpox, although observers were optimistic that recovery from those scourges indicated a salutary cleansing of unhealthful humors. Weakness lingered, however, and made him more susceptible to other diseases. The king went on a punishing schedule of progresses the following summer, and by August he was exhausted. Thereafter, he complained of "continual infirmity of body . . . rather as an indisposition in health then any set sicknesse."[29] The Duke of Northumberland, who had remained in London, was shocked by Edward's appearance when he saw him and summoned the Milanese doctor and astrologer, Giralamo Cardano.

Dr. Cardano was a magus—a fashionable physician, a popularizer of science, a dabbler in spiritualism, and an alchemist. The variety of his learned undertakings reveal the complexity of Renaissance thought and the interrelationship of magic, science, and religion.[30] Regarded by many as second only to Vesalius among European physicians, he was sought after by papal and imperial households, but rejected the life of a court physician as fraught with dangerous intrigue. He did accept a lucrative mission to minister to John Hamilton, Archbishop of St. Andrews and brother of the Scottish regent, James Hamilton. The Archbishop suffered from severe attacks of asthma and turned to Cardano for help; Cardano traveled to Edinburgh early in 1552. A friend of Edward's tutor, John Cheke, Cardano was staying in Cheke's London house on his return trip later that year when he was called to court.[31] He met with the young king and found him to be well informed on intellectual matters; Edward was familiar with Cardano's work, *De Varietate Rerum*, and they conversed in Latin about comets. Prior to his visit, Dr. Cardano, famed for his astrological horoscope of Christ, cast Edward's horoscope and discovered omens of a great calamity.[32] Since it was treason to predict the death of a king, he publicly predicted a long life, describing ailments that would afflict Edward at age fifty-five. For the king's current infirmities, Cardano recommended rest from his burdens.[33]

But respite from responsibility did not revive the young king, and he began to show obvious signs of consumption or phthisis, the wasting disease for which there was no cure. Throughout the autumn and winter Edward suffered from fevers, racking coughs, and loss of appetite; his body became bloated and he spat blood, symptoms of a classic case of acute pulmonary tuberculosis. He grew worse in January 1553, but his physicians thought it merely another of the colds or catarrhal maladies he often endured. Princess Mary was summoned to visit him for the Candlemas festivities, February 2, but after three days of waiting found him flushed and unable to breathe. She heard rumors that Edward was being slowly poisoned, and the Spanish ambassador, who had accompanied her, reported that the king's right shoulder was now much higher than his left.[34] Preparations used to treat phthisis in the sixteenth century and likely prescribed for the king included powders of precious gems, oil of ants, vegetable syrups, bile, the excreta of various animals, the sloughed skin from a snake, and moss from the skull of a person who had died violently.[35]

In the spring Edward caught a chill that worsened his condition, and he could not ride to Westminster in March to open Parliament; its members came to him in Whitehall for the official opening. Despite the frantic ministrations of the king's physicians, it was evident that he would not live much longer. Other secret horoscopes predicted the king's demise and portentous signs troubled Englishmen, who whispered of "prodigies" like monstrous births and the ominous capture of twelve huge dolphins in the Thames.[36] Edward's physicians gave up hope and to protect themselves from later recriminations warned the Council that Edward was in peril and that if any other severe illness supervened he would not survive. In April his state was grave; the Imperial ambassador, Jehan Scheyfve, reported that an anonymous royal physician confided to him that the king would be dead within weeks. The physician was probably John Banister, a twenty-year-old student doctor and the son of a minor official in the royal household, whose undated and unsigned Latin letters to Scheyfve have been identified by Tudor historian S. T. Bindoff.[37] During the first two weeks in May, Edward felt somewhat better and the government proclaimed that he was merely run down; the cruel, sporadic expectations for recovery that distinguish tuberculosis had produced mistaken hope in the royal patient.[38]

But on May 28, in his longest missive to the Imperial ambassador, Banister wrote that the king was ceaselessly deteriorating:

> He does not sleep except when he be stuffed with drugs . . . but the doctors do not exceed twelve grains at a time . . . and then only if the patient be in great pain or racked by violent coughing . . . the sputum which he brings up is livid, black, fetid and full of carbon; it smells beyond measure . . . his feet are swollen all over . . . to the doctors, all these things portend death, and that within three months, except God of his great mercy spare him.
>
> Today the Duke called the doctors together and asked them what the king's chances were. They answered that . . . when autumn comes it will end his life. The Duke told them not to slacken their efforts . . . ; meanwhile, he said, you will all be paid your fees every month, at a rate of 100 crowns.[39]

Concerned about the Catholicism of Mary and the dubious legitimacy of Elizabeth, and encouraged by Northumberland, the young king had already decided to ignore his father's plans for the Tudors, as well as a parliamentary Act of Succession, and exclude his half-sisters from the throne in favor of the offspring of Lady Jane Grey. Granddaughter of Henry VIII's younger sister though not next-in-line even within that dynastic branch, Jane was a devout Protestant and gifted scholar. Edward himself insisted that his councillors should agree to a new "device" for the succession and Northumberland applauded the plan, having compelled Lady Jane in May 1553 to marry his son, Guilford Dudley. Now, armed with the unanimous verdict of Edward's doctors that the king would not survive the year, Northumberland needed time to persuade the

Lord Chief Justice and other key judges that the young king's device was constitutional; he also altered the document to include Jane Grey herself.[40]

Accordingly, he dismissed Edward's vanquished physicians and installed a mysterious female quack who claimed that she could cure the king with a special potion that almost certainly contained arsenic. These weird elixirs and concoctions might prolong life, but would cause additional pain and suffering in the patient. Even Barrett Beer, a historian friendly to Northumberland, acknowledges the appointment of three new physicians early in May, one of whom was a woman characterized as a conjuror and a quack. He identifies another as Northumberland's doctor, but the man in question might have been Thomas Smith, the duke's personal apothecary.[41] By July 2, the king's body had swollen like a balloon, despite his not having eaten since June 11, his pulse was weak and irregular, and his hair and nails were falling out. It was reported that the laundress who washed his shirts lost her nails and the skin of her fingers.[42] Racked by agonizing pains, Edward's extremities were being eaten away by gangrene and, as a result of prolonged immobility, his body was covered in ulcerous bedsores. He lay in feverish delirium as Northumberland effected compliance at home and abroad with the new succession. Recalled by Northumberland, the royal doctors prescribed new medicines including one that contained spearmint syrup, fennel, liverwort, turnip, dates, raisins, celery, mace, and pork from a nine-day-old sow.[43] Accomplishing the imposition of a new heiress presumptive, however, did little to revive the afflicted king. With Dr. Owen and friends Sir Thomas Wroth and Henry Sidney in attendance, Edward VI expired at Greenwich Palace on July 6, 1553.

Desperate to retain power after Edward's death, yet still uncertain what Princesses Mary and Elizabeth would do, Northumberland convinced the Council to conceal the king's death for two days. By then Mary had eluded Northumberland's forces and taken flight through Norfolk to the coast. Despite an intemperate sermon given on July 9 by Bishop Ridley in London, which bitterly denounced her fervent Catholicism, spontaneous support for Mary among the ruling classes erupted and Northumberland's hope for the peaceful succession of Lady Jane Grey evaporated. Northumberland informed Jane of Edward's device and had her proclaimed queen on July 10, 1553; she reigned for only nine days before troops loyal to Mary routed Northumberland's men and installed their candidate on the throne.[44] When Edward's death was finally commemorated on August 8 by the authority of Queen Mary, a complete list of the household staff was made, to determine the amount of black cloth needed for court mourning. Senior officials were allotted seven yards or more; lesser assistants received four yards each. Gross yardage was copious and the somber black-clothed household must have created a melancholy atmosphere. Mary commanded that Edward's sealed coffin be ferried upriver and buried according to the rites of the old faith, but, fearful of public displeasure, she settled for a private Mass sung for him in the Tower chapel. Archbishop Cranmer preached the funeral sermon at Westminster Abbey, and Edward VI, the last Tudor king, was buried there under the high altar in Henry VII's chapel.

History has been unkind to England's first queen, branding her with the sobriquet "Bloody Mary" and ridiculing the passions that ruled her life. Yet, until the elder daughter of Henry VIII came to the throne, no woman had governed the kingdom in her own right. True to her faith, she restored the Roman Catholic religion throughout the realm and reinstituted doctrine, ceremony, and the old heresy laws. True to her mother's Aragonese heart, she married Philip II of Spain in 1554, binding England to an alliance that led to war with France and the loss of its last continental possession, Calais. True to her duty as a dynast, Mary tried desperately but futilely to produce an heir, prompting critics to sneer that her reign was as barren as her womb.[45]

Petite and thin, Mary I had a fragile demeanor, and, according to one biographer "the tragedies that marred Mary's life were reflected in her face."[46] Poor eyesight made her stare, thin lips stretched to cover a mouth largely devoid of teeth, and she suffered from chronic ill-health. In the midst of the most dangerous time of her youth, when Henry VIII divorced her mother and rejected her, she was surrounded by courtiers whom she could not trust. One upon whom she did rely was her longtime tutor and physician's assistant, Richard Featherstone, a transmitter in 1534 of messages from her in Latin to the Imperial ambassador.[47] No doubt she chose to count on Featherstone because he knew her frailties and vulnerabilities well. Although Henry VIII humiliated Mary on multiple occasions, even he was concerned about her periodic sicknesses and sent his own surgeon to bleed her, prescribe for her, and draw her teeth. Henry also dispatched Dr. William Butts to monitor her condition. She complained to him of toothaches, neuralgia, heart palpitations, and headaches. Butts, whose wife had earlier been in the Princess's entourage as a gentlewoman, suggested that Mary should be allowed to stay with her mother, who might nurse her back to vitality, but the king refused. She was seriously ill during the Christmas season of 1537 and again in the spring of 1542, then debilitated by a curious fever and heart palpitations. Because the onset of puberty coincided with her parents' separation, Mary endured several sporadic sicknesses that were probably psychological in origin, including premenstrual tension and erratic periods.[48]

Nonetheless, as early as 1536 and despite her own fragile constitution, Mary Tudor participated in the regal miracle of healing known as touching for the "King's Evil." The King's Evil was the English name given to scrofula, a disease of early life often characterized by slowly suppurating abscesses and fistulous passages, which could be cured, it was thought, by the sacred touch of a divinely chosen potentate. In so doing, Mary continued the practice of her father, her grandfather, and prior kings of England dating back to Edward the Confessor in the eleventh century, thus bolstering her own legitimacy and popularity.[49] After she came to the throne, Queen Mary continued the protocol as a magical "doctor" who healed people afflicted with scrofula, which was actually primary tuberculosis of the cervical lymph nodes and the most common form of tuberculosis in preindustrial Europe. Scrofula was probably caused by infected milk, and a significant number of deaths from the Evil was recorded throughout England in the sixteenth and seventeenth centuries. During Mary's reign, the royal thaumaturgy took place on Good Friday, but observances could also be held on Easter Sunday, Pentecost, and the Feast of Michaelmas. In the touching ritual, elaborate liturgical elements included a reading of two passages from the Gospels: the verse from St. Mark referred to miracles performed by the Apostles, and the words from St. John were often used in blessings or exorcisms. A church official brought the scrofulous person directly to the seated sovereign, who laid hands on the sick and made the Sign of the Cross over the "patient's" sores. Making the hallowed gesture, Queen Mary actually caressed the raw wounds several times.[50] After completing the first touching, she then brushed the person's sores with a gold coin or amulet (usually prepierced and threaded onto a ribbon), which was then placed around the sufferer's neck. Around the edge of the Marian coin ran the words: "This was the Lord's doing, and it is marvellous in our eyes." In the minds of the English, these coins, called "angels" because they depicted the figure of St. Michael, became instruments of the monarch's sacerdotal power. A Venetian witness recorded that Mary made each patient promise never to part with the gold piece "except in case of extreme need."[51]

Mary's healing force could prevent illness, too. At the same Good Friday service, to the right of the high altar, the queen blessed containers of rings, some expressly obtained by her for this purpose and others provided by their owners, marked with their names for later retrieval. Mary prayed and passed her hands over the receptacles, separating and fingering the gold and silver bands, which were then distributed. Her subjects cherished these cramp-rings, as they were known, regarding them as talismans containing the power intrinsic to the touch of an anointed monarch. Mary's sanctified rings were uncommonly coveted, not only in England but in foreign courts as well, especially in Scotland.

But this monarch often needed healing herself, and for that she employed the established court doctors: Caius, Wendy, and Owen. Queen Mary's life was lived out in court, dominated by public ceremonies, dignified audiences, and entertainments. Her sex, however, altered the structure of the Privy Chamber and had ramifications for the entire household, as men could hardly fraternize as freely with a female sovereign as they could with a male. All of the most coveted Privy Chamber offices fell to women, and access for men to the Person was reserved to a small group of household officers. Moreover, men did not speak to the queen "but in adoration and kneeling, all persons of the realm [were] bareheaded before [her]."[52] These formal requirements coupled with concern about sexual propriety must have complicated the usual doctor-patient interactions. So, too, did the conspicuously public lives led by kings and queens. Even the most private moments in life, such as weddings, births, and deaths, took place before a throng of onlookers. There were few secluded spaces in Tudor palaces, few withdrawing rooms into which the monarch could retreat from the crowd. When Mary did escape to her private apartments, all of her body servants were women. The intimate information needed from the sick person by doctors for proper medical care could hardly be forthcoming in this oddly public, yet also female, environment. Thus, the peculiar difficulties facing the doctors of the new Tudor monarch were exacerbated by her gender.

Mary I's "personal physician" throughout most of the reign was Thomas Hughes (or Huys), the man who hurried to her house in July 1553 and informed her of Edward's death.[53] Hughes received an M.D. in 1548 from Merton College, Oxford, became a Fellow of the College of Physicians in 1550 and consiliarius the following year. Caesar Dalmaris, however, attended the queen most frequently.[54] A native of Italy, Caesar Dalmaris got his M.D. from Padua and settled in England at about the time Mary ascended the throne. A Roman Catholic naturalized by the queen, he joined the College of Physicians in 1554 after an initially rough reception. In April 1553 the College fined him for illegal practice, but he provided testimonials about his Padua degree which mollified the Fellows.[55] Caesar Dalmaris was well-accepted by his new colleagues and countrymen: the Fellows elected him College censor in 1555 and his London neighbors made him an alderman for Bishopsgate. The queen valued his expert medical opinion, appreciatively giving him a tax immunity in 1558. Caesar Dalmaris's 240–page recipe book, dated 1563 and written in Latin, discusses his adherence to Galen and Hippocrates; he attributed lumbago to humors that needed purging.[56] Elizabeth I also consulted him.

George Holland was Mary I's serjeant-surgeon, appointed around 1557, and her apothecary was John de Soda II.[57] Mentioned in Henry VIII's will, Holland had an illustrious career as a member of the Barber-Surgeons' Company, rising to become its Master on three occasions; one guild historian refers to him as "king's surgeon," indicating that Holland's assignment might have been to Philip.[58] John de Soda I, the French-born apothecary who had served Catherine of Aragon, had tended to Princess Mary's household after 1536 with an annuity of forty marks. When asked in 1542 by the French ambassador if Mary's health might prevent her from being a suitable wife for Francis I's son, de Soda replied that he only gave her light medicines and those usually at the instructions of Henry VIII.[59] But the truth is that Mary was frequently sick, and she often summoned de Soda from his house in East London. Since the Tudors had been generous to him, granting him licenses to export wheat and malt, he came when called. Besides, the aging apothecary had real affection for Princess Mary, and in his will he left her "my little coffer with cordial powder and confections."[60] De Soda made the sweet waters that Mary favored to perfume her rooms and to fortify herself against malodors. One Tudor-era aromatic formula called for a boiled blend of rosewater, sugar, musk, ambergris, and civet to make the household smell like cloves.[61] John de Soda II, the old apothecary's elder son, gifted Mary with coronation presents upon her accession to the throne. Grateful, perhaps, for his appointment as her royal apothecary in 1554 and the chance to follow in his father's footsteps, the younger de Soda gave her six boxes of marmalade and cordials, a gift he repeated on New Year's Day in 1557. The queen in turn sent him a gilt saltshaker weighing nine and one-half ounces.[62]

Mary I of England and Prince Philip of Spain (who became King Philip II in 1556) married at Winchester in July 1554. He was a reluctant bridegroom, a young widower urged by his father to marry the queen of England, eleven years his senior. It was an unpopular union, for although the new joint sovereign had no formal authority under the marriage treaty or from Parliament, Mary as his wife was expected to defer to his judgment in all matters.[63] Moreover, xenophobic courtiers and malicious Londoners resented the Spanish retinue that accompanied Philip to England for the nuptials and caused ugly demonstrations that embarrassed Mary. Nonetheless, marriage pleased the queen and in September her doctors confirmed that she was pregnant. She displayed all the normal symptoms: her periods had stopped, her breasts and abdomen had swollen, and she experienced nausea in the mornings. She told her attendants that she felt the baby leap in her womb.[64] In November she announced the two triumphs that she believed fulfilled her destiny: an expected heir to the throne and reconciliation with Rome.

Mary's health had clearly never been robust and pregnancy only aggravated her debilities while multiplying her concerns. The queen's own doctor felt she ate too little to keep a child alive, but physicians bickered over the proper diet for a mother-to-be. Aiming for humoral balance required the ingestion of appropriate foods such as orange juice, egg yolks, and wine mixed with running water. Forbidden foods included salads, lentils and beans, baked pies and meats, milk, cheese, and fish, the latter perceived as being too phlegmatic to be wholesome. The only nourishment commonly thought fortifying was toast. Taken dipped in wine (or even applied externally), a pregnant woman was advised to eat toasted bread every day "so that nothing would grow to the child."[65] Mary's anxieties were fed better than she was, especially with additional worries that horrid frights and sights could cause peculiarities and marks in unborn children. Since the mother's imagination was also believed to act upon the fetus, pregnant women often took potions to ward off fears; one such concoction combined two drams each of mastic and frankincense, plus half a scruple each of dragon's blood (resin from the dracaena), myrtles, bolearmoniak, and Hermes berries, ground together in chicken broth.[66] To make matters worse for the already agitated queen, whatever passion existed in the royal marriage was all hers. Philip grew restless in England, but because of her age and medical history, Mary feared a difficult birth and wanted him near. He felt an obligation to support his father's war against France and was anxious to leave for the Low Countries; Mary begged him to stay, and his vacillation hurt her immeasurably. Her own misery mirrored the nation's, its distress caused by the queen's policies.

As a corollary to the papal absolution restoring England to Holy Mother Church, the government of England began to punish religious apostasy, empowering bishops in December 1554 to investigate cases of suspected heresy and enforcing their decisions with sentences of burning at the stake. Philip had been a champion of the Spanish Inquisition and had himself presided over mass executions called Acts of Faith, but the responsibility for persecutions under the Marian heresy law is Mary's. Believing it was her Christian duty to punish those who had sinned against God's church with a foretaste of hell on earth, Mary ordered the fires lit.

Suffering discomfort from her condition and the perceived neglect of her husband, eyewitnesses called Mary "melancholy" in February 1555, but her own unhappiness did not cause her to reflect on the anguish of others and to forgo the burnings. She never once extended clemency to a heretic and never wavered in her support of the Counter-Reformation. The first victim of the Marian persecution, John Rogers, a married priest, perished at the stake on February 4 at Smithfield in London. When Rogers was not allowed to say goodbye to his wife and children, the London crowd protested angrily and, following subsequent immolations, a number of which were particularly gruesome, a public outcry ensued. Unprecedented numbers of men and women spoke out against the persecutions that spring, and many of these people were pilloried for uttering perfidious words against the queen and her Council. Mary was oblivious to the remonstrances against her, having retired from public life and into the privy apartments at Hampton Court for a delivery expected on May 9. Swaddling cloths were laid out in readiness; midwives, nurses, and "rockers" were retained and lodged. In the birth suite, physicians gathered the accoutrements that they required: tables, benches, and bowls, as well as sweet perfumes to scent the air during delivery. The baby never came.

Though Mary showed all the signs of pregnancy in the earlier months of her confinement, these signs disappeared in May and observers believed she had deluded herself into thinking she was with child. Other diagnoses have been put forward. Unsympathetic sources insinuated that deceit lay in the heart of the expectant mother, who schemed to smuggle in a suppositious child at the opportune moment and claim that an heir had been born. French ambassador Antoine de Noailles opined that the swelling of the queen's belly was caused by a tumor or dropsy and some modern historians have concurred.[67] A French envoy recounted gossip to Henri II that Mary had given birth in April to a hideous lump of flesh, perhaps a hydatidiform mole.[68] In such a condition, caused by chromosomal irregularity, the placenta develops into a benign tumor and deprives the growing embryo of nourishment; the embryo dies but the mole continues to grow. Mary, however, did not experience the heavy bleeding associated with expulsion of such a mole, which in any event occurs much earlier than six or seven months after conception. Nor does it seem possible that the queen suffered an inter-uterine death and the subsequent bloody discharge of the fetus without her knowledge. She endured simulated contractions in late May, had another false alarm in June, and in July still insisted that she was with child. Based upon the information available to us today, it seems likely that her contemporaries were right and that the queen experienced a phantom pregnancy.[69]

Why might Queen Mary have thought she was with child? The obvious answer is that she missed several periods, presumably due to the onset of perimenopause. Mary was only thirty-eight in 1554, but menopause came earlier for women in the sixteenth century, usually between the ages of forty-two and forty-five.[70] Moreover, she was too thin, described by observers as emaciated, maybe even anorectic, a factor that could also temporarily inhibit menstruation. The missed periods doubtless led her to hope she was pregnant, producing psychosomatic symptoms like a distended abdomen and swollen, lactescent breasts. Believing herself to be with child was surely preferable to contemplating disease as the cause of her amenorrhea, and she would not have thought of herself as too old for parenthood; her grandmother, Isabella of Spain, had given birth at fifty-two to Catherine of Aragon. Additionally, Tudor physicians viewed abnormal stoppage of menstruation as very serious, leading to "swellings, imposthumes, ulcers; [and] . . . feavers, obstructions, evil habits, loathing, dropsie, heart-ache, cough, short breathing, fainting, sore eyes, madness, melancholly, joynt-gout, and the like" could also be a consequence of cessation.[71] Authorities today believe that a woman with a history of menstrual inconsistency, like Mary Tudor, is more prone to produce unusual gynecological symptoms under pressure than a woman with a normal cycle.[72] The queen was certainly under unimaginable pressure to produce a Catholic prince for her younger husband before the royal biological clock ran down. Hence, her pathetic self-delusion is easily understandable.

What was the diagnosis of Mary's medical staff?[73] Did her doctors really think she was pregnant or were they just telling her what she wanted to hear? It is certainly true that as late as July the queen's doctors still affirmed that she was carrying a child, but that she must have miscalculated the date of conception by two or three months and the birth might not take place until September. Perhaps they thought that the baby would be a princess; it was commonly asserted in the sixteenth century that gestative times for males and females were different, with longer formative time essential for girls. Prominent English physicians argued that ten, eleven, even twelve months were needed for the completion of a daughter, on the ancient grounds that females were weaker, even in the womb.[74] Moreover, the cessation of the menses was not considered particularly important by Tudor-era physicians as a sign of pregnancy, and although uroscopy had fallen into discredit, it was still used by many practitioners for pregnancy diagnosis. According to some texts, in pregnant women the urine ought to appear white with a cloud floating on top that, if shaken, looked like wool. Others described an experiment in which a needle turned red when left overnight in a basin of urine from a pregnant woman, black when the woman had not conceived.[75] Regardless of these signs, enough uncertainty existed to make precise predictions of gestation risky, especially for a queenly mother-to-be. If Mary's doctors doubted the reality of her pregnancy, therefore, they held their tongues and reassured her. A paid informant told the French ambassador that the queen's midwife, discerning that Mary was not pregnant at all, nonetheless comforted her with encouraging words.[76] But however complicitous in the queen's delusions her doctors might have been, Mary's stubborn insistence that she would have a child was their best excuse.

In the sixteenth century, physicians regarded pregnancy as somewhere between sickness and health, a condition best left to nature and not to men.[77] Tudor gynecology was an amalgamation of ignorance about internal medicine, bias against women, and almost complete belief in classical medical texts. Physicians believed that menstruation was essential because women led such sedentary lives and that the womb caused all female diseases from headaches to consumption; in Galenic nomenclature, the stream of blood rid the body of ill humors. Doctors considered sexual intercourse a proper cure for obstructed flow and apothecaries devised a solution of ground steel to be taken orally as an emmenagogue, but medical professionals resorted to other measures when necessary. Remedies for non-menstruation included hot baths, fumigations for virgins and pessaries for married women, or blood letting from the foot during the waxing of the moon. More drastic correctives entailed bleeding, cupping, and scarification of the breasts or venesection of the woman's thighs.[78]

No wonder that the majority of women patronized neither physicians nor apothecaries for their female problems; indeed, convention actually prohibited such consultation and most physicians merely theorized about women's conditions.[79] Actually gazing upon the female body produced an occasion of sin and anatomical drawings of women were omitted from medical texts. Male doctors were resolutely barred from childbirth throughout Europe. Authorities executed a Hamburg physician in 1522 for posing as a woman in a lying-in chamber, and as late as 1657 Percivall Willughby, who wrote a book for English midwives, was obliged to crawl on his hands and knees into a darkened room when called to a patient.[80] Complete examination of one's female sovereign was even more problematical than for an ordinary woman. Even the most common word used for menstruation in Tudor times, "flowers," shows an attempt at polite circumlocution.[81] Midwives were the caregivers of choice, and they relied primarily on magic and herbs to treat female complaints. After 1540 they had a good handbook in English, a translation of Eucharius Rosslin's *The Birth of Mankind*, published in 1540 and reissued under the same title by Thomas Raynald in 1545.[82] Because of her low social class and the stigma of her profession, most doctors avoided interference in the midwife's practice. Besides, since physicians were forbidden to examine female genitalia, midwives had knowledge that physicians lacked. However, professionals paid little attention at all to menopause and most women viewed their body cycles as private.

When her menstruation resumed in August, Mary had to admit to herself that she had been terribly mistaken, but she never alluded to her catastrophic "pregnancy" in public. Mortified by his wife's error, Philip announced that he was leaving England without further delay, compounding her desolation and hardening her heart. The queen would not see her husband again for over eighteen months. Meanwhile, the unprecedented burnings of religious dissenters continued, killing three hundred in four years and producing a permanent backlash against Catholicism and the queen. Compared to her grandfather, who burned ten heretics in twenty-four years, and her father, who incinerated eighty-one in thirty-eight years, Mary was now seen by her subjects as a heartless persecutor of martyrs.[83] Most of those exterminated during the Marian persecutions were preachers, artisans, or peasants, hardly major targets for the state; more important schismatics like the Protestant bishops John Ponet and John Bale had already fled abroad.[84] In October 1555, however, the Protestant bishops Latimer and Ridley went to the stake in the ditch outside the walls of Oxford, and in February 1556, Mary signed the death warrant for Thomas Cranmer, by then formally dismissed from his primacy at Canterbury. Though Cranmer tried to recant, the queen refused to relent, recalling not only his policies and prayer books but the role he had played in nullifying the marriage of her parents and bastardizing her. Cranmer went to his death courageously, rallying those who were repulsed by the fires.

Heretics were not the only souls blazing in England during the Marian reaction. Between December 1555 and October 1556, London endured an epidemic of "burning fevers" that killed seven of the City's twenty-six aldermen and persisted for the better part of a year, principally attacking older people.[85] During this same period there were nearly simultaneous outbreaks of influenza and typhus, presenting the kingdom with a mortality crisis of major proportions. No sooner had the populace recovered from these epidemics than a quartan ague (with paroxysms recurring every seventy-two hours) struck the community, also particularly devastating to the elderly and persisting for well over a year. Malaria is one of the oldest diseases known to humanity; certain environmental conditions produce recurrent bouts of malaria and the east coast of England had long been a trouble spot. Because of the long incubation period that the disease displays, quartan fever peaked in the English winter, while summer and autumn infections caused additional outbreaks every spring.[86] According to historian Dale C. Smith, ague manifests three classes of fevers: continued, periodic, and eruptive; he has further subdivided periodic fevers into intermittent, remittent, and malignant types. Intermittent fevers rarely killed in any of their forms—quotidian (every twenty-four hours), tertian (every forty-eight), or quartan, but remittent fevers were much more severe, with higher levels of fatality than simple ague. Sufferers exhibited fever from the outset, as well as vomiting, diarrhea, and thirst; their miseries could end in delirium, cramps, and convulsions. Moreover, no complete respite from the symptoms gave relief to victims of remittent fevers. Malignant fevers, however, were fiercest, registering many deaths following delirium and coma. Tudor doctors tried to determine the sort of ague from which their patients suffered by timing febrile recurrence, by gauging the color of the patient's skin, and by administering special remedies.[87] One preferred ague cure in Tudor England, taken twice a day, was a decoction of snails, boiled in milk sweetened with sugar and candied eryngo, to which cut-up earthworms were added; many ague prescriptions called for spiders' webs or pellets of opium poppy juice.[88]

Protestants said that God had sent these various plagues to punish the queen for her sins, and one of the most notable victims of ague in 1558 was Cardinal Reginald Pole, the Archbishop of Canterbury, a zealous proponent of the suppression of heresy. As for Mary herself, some historians have suggested that the queen's already delicate constitution might have been weakened by the same malarial fever.[89] At the peak of the contagion, she received a present of Dr. Stevens' Imperial Water, a tonic made of spices in Gascoigne wine, guaranteed to lengthen life. Its inventor, who himself lived to a ripe old age, had pledged that the brew would also restore good health. Nevertheless, all that the queen wanted was for her husband to return to her.

Philip finally arrived in England in March 1557 to persuade Mary and her Council to declare war on France. He must have noticed how his wife had aged in his absence. One courtier reported that she was wrinkled, melancholy, and often needed "to be blooded, either from the foot or elsewhere, which keeps her always pale and emaciated."[90] The queen slept badly, had incessant problems with what teeth remained to her, and wept copiously. Although she was able to convince her councillors to declare war on France in June, she could not have been buoyed by Philip's departure for the continent the following month.

Six months after his departure, Queen Mary announced that she was expecting a child, having explained to her husband that she was absolutely certain this time and had delayed the announcement so there would be no mistakes. This time, however, she did not even appear pregnant, even though she was supposedly at the end of her second trimester; likewise, her courtiers made no elaborate preparation for a royal lying-in as they had in 1555. Mary had probably entered menopause and her periods had ceased altogether. No sooner had the queen broadcast the happy tidings than word reached England that the French had taken Calais, the last remaining piece of English territory in France. Philip's war had cost Mary dearly, and she regarded the loss of Calais as the worst failure of her reign. Her "pregnancy" went no better, and in February 1558 observers remarked that although her belly was distended, the queen looked ill rather than gravid.[91] She was the object of derision and scorn, including John Knox's famous vituperative attack, *First Blast of the Trumpet against the Monstrous Regiment of Women*, and everyone pressured her to name Princess Elizabeth as her heir. She did so in late March 1558, still believing herself pregnant.

By late May, suffering from erratic fevers and intense melancholia, Mary lay in her rooms at Richmond as if in a stupor. The fires still consumed heretics, as seven were burned in one fire at Smithfield in June; in August the queen personally rebuked those sheriffs who suspended the executions of recanting heretics. She then moved to London and, to appease the Council, her doctors argued that her usual autumnal indispositions might actually eliminate her malaise; the queen cooperated with their advice, but despondency made her disorder intensify. In October, Dr. Caesar Dalmaris, using all his skills, managed to bring her out of despair temporarily and she ordered that he be paid £100 as a reward. Mary then wrote a codicil to her will acknowledging that she would have no offspring to whom to leave her crown.

During her last illness, courtiers and councillors ebbed away from Queen Mary to accumulate around Princess Elizabeth at Hatfield House; Elizabeth would note for future reference the speed with which allegiances could shift once a successor had been designated. Mary sent a poignant message to Elizabeth at the end, beseeching her to sustain the Roman Catholic faith. The queen died on November 17 at St. James' Palace, three months short of her forty-third birthday. She presumably succumbed to the disorder that had produced two phantom pregnancies, but she was evidently free from pain in the final days, leading to speculation that she might may have been felled by the same strain of influenza that kept her subjects, even members of Parliament, in their sickbeds.[92] The delivery to Elizabeth of Mary's treasured betrothal ring along with official word from the Council signaled the transfer of power from one daughter of Henry VIII to another.

Notes

1. For more on the juvenile king, see John Hayward, *The Life and Raigne of King Edward the Sixth*, ed. Barrett L. Beer (Kent OH: Kent State University Press, 1993). Sir John Hayward was a late Elizabethan-era lawyer and a major historian in the early seventeenth century. For the first years of Edward's reign, W. K. Jordan, *Edward VI: The Young King* (London: George Allen and Unwin, 1968).

2. Of all sixteenth-century deaths, 34.4 percent were recorded as those of children under ten years of age. Life expectancy varied between thirty-five and forty years, relatively high for Europe. Schofield and Wrigley, "Infant and Child Mortality," 61–96.

3. Alison Weir, *The Children of Henry VIII* (New York: Ballantine Books, 1996), 123. There is considerable disagreement among historians about the health of Edward VI. Leslie Matthews argues that a third apothecary was appointed to the Henrician household in 1546 because the boy was frail, but Barrett Beer notes that Tudor chronicler John Stow "never suggested that the king was sickly or suffered from ill health before January 1553." Matthews, *Royal Apothecaries*, 69; Barrett L. Beer, *Tudor England Observed* (Stroud, England: Sutton, 1998), 110.

4. For Cheke, see C. H. Garrett, *The Marian Exiles* (Cambridge: Cambridge University Press, 1938).

5. Quoted in Weir, *Children of Henry VIII*, 26.

6. See M. L. Bush, *The Government Policy of Protector Somerset* (Montreal: McGill-Queen's University Press, 1975).

7. Kett was hanged. For more on Edwardian protest, see Barrett L. Beer, *Rebellion and Riot: Popular Disorder during the Reign of Edward VI* (Kent, Ohio: Kent State University Press, 1985).

8. See Barrett L. Beer, *Northumberland* (Kent, Ohio: Kent State University Press, 1973).

9. Munk, *Roll* 1: 37.

10. Henrician physician William Bullein, in an imagined dialogue between two men, Sorenes and Chirugi, praised Caius for revealing Galen's emphasis on surgery, like a "seconde Linacar." The dialogue follows Bullein's chapters of simples, also in dialogue form. See Bullein's *Bulwarke of Defence*.

11. For a more critical view of Caius, see O'Malley, *English Medical Humanists*. By Caius's time, Galen was also under attack from Paracelsus, who burned Galen's works in a notorious 1528 bon-

fire, thereby also igniting the lengthy conflict between Galenic and chemical doctors. Clark, *Royal College of Physicians* 1: 111.

12. Clark, *Royal College of Physicians* 1: 121.

13. For a revisionist appreciation of Caius, see Nutton, "John Caius and the Linacre Tradition."

14. The pieces were published together in 1576. Caius knew the great Swiss scientist Conrad Gesner well and collaborated with him on Gesner's five-volume *Historia Animalium*, considered to be the foundation of zoology. Charles Webster, *The Great Instauration: Science, Medicine and Reform in England 1626–1660* (New York: Holmes and Meier Publishers, 1976), 122; Nutton, "Conrad Gesner and the English Naturalists," 96–97. Incidentally, Gesner been credited with publishing the first work on chemical therapy in England, *The Treasure of Euonymus*, in 1559 when the College of Physicians was still conservative and a Galenic stronghold. See Allen G. Debus, *The English Paracelsians* (London: Oldbourne, 1965), 52.

15. Caius referred to all large dogs as mastiffs, though they were not necessarily precursors of today's English Mastiff breed. I am grateful to Jennifer Vermillion for this canine information.

16. Raven, *English Naturalists*, 141–42.

17. For the various writings of Caius, see E. S. Roberts, ed., *The Works of John Caius, M. D.* (Cambridge: Cambridge University Press, 1912).

18. Shakespeare ridiculed Caius in "The Merry Wives of Windsor" and one medical antiquarian wrote that Caius died after "sucking milk from a wet nurse as an infant would." See Macmichael, *Lives of British Physicians*.

19. Young, *Annals*, 527; Beck, *Cutting Edge*, 183, 197. For more on the Devon-born Petre, who listed twenty physicians and surgeons in his accounts, see F. G. Emmison, *Tudor Secretary: Sir William Petre at Court and Home* (Cambridge: Cambridge University Press, 1961). "Forest, the king's surgeon," cured the "flux" in Petre's leg in 1548, initially charging him 33s. 4d. for looking at the ulcer, with a final bill of 53s. 4d. for healing it: Emmison, *Tudor Secretary*, 250. Susan Kybett says that scurvy caused Petre's ulcerous legs and springtime attacks: Kybett, "Henry VIII," 24.

20. One authority argues that Geminus was also known as Lambrit and hailed from Flanders: Leonard Payne, "A Plagiarist Plagiarized," *Journal of the Royal College of Physicians of London* 19 (1985): 44. Another pinpoints Geminus's birthplace as Liche in the diocese of Liège: Beck, *Cutting Edge*, 179. See also Sanford V. Larkey, *Vesalian Compendium of Geminus and Nicholas Udall's Translation* (London: n. p., 1933).

21. Caius may have aided Geminus in publishing a "pirated" work: Larkey, *Vesalian Compendium*, 369.

22. Clippingdale, Medical Court Roll, 1: 29; *Dictionary of National Biography*. Young has no record of a Thomas Geminus in the Barber-Surgeons' *Annals*.

23. Payne, "A Plagiarist Plagiarized," 47. At about the same time, the College rebuked Oxford University for granting medical degrees to Simon Ludford, an apothecary, and David Lawghton, a coppersmith, both illiterate men. Annals of the Royal College of Physicians, vol. 1, f. 8b, LRCP.

24. Matthews, *Royal Apothecaries*, 69. Sir William Petre referred to Carlton as "the prince's apothecary" in his account books of 1544: Emmison, *Tudor Secretary*, 249.

25. Stow quoted in Beer, *Tudor England Observed*, 49–50. Beer calculates a mortality rate for London parishes of 8 percent.

26. One historian proffers the notion that this epidemic may have been attributable to an arbovirus transmitted by mosquitoes. Paul Slack, *The Impact of Plague in Tudor and Stuart England* (London: Routledge and Kegan Paul, 1985), 70. The Princess Mary, suffering from a variety of maladies, was so ill "that she could hardly reply to letters from [Edward's] Council": H.F.M. Prescott, *A Spanish Tudor* (New York: AMS Press, 1970), 178.

27. Edward's tutor, John Cheke, was caught up in the net that brought in Somerset, and he retired for a season to Cambridge; he returned to London after a few months. Edward's formal education ended in June 1552 when Cheke fell seriously ill. For the last part of Edward's reign, see W. K. Jordan, *Edward VI: The Threshold of Power* (Cambridge, Mass.: Harvard University Press, 1970).

28. Jordan, *Edward VI: Threshold of Power*, 440–53.

29. Hayward, *Life and Raigne*, 168.

30. For more on the Hermetic tradition, an attempt to work with the forces of nature through magic, see Keith Thomas, *Religion and the Decline of Magic* (London: Weidenfeld and Nicolson, 1971); Frances Yates, *Giordano Bruno and the Hermetic Tradition* (Chicago: University of Chicago Press, 1964); and Ingrid Merkel and Allen G. Debus, eds., *Hermeticism and the Renaissance* (Washington, D.C.: Folger Library, 1988).

31. Among Cardano's London acquaintances was John Dee, a magus in his own right. Peter French, *John Dee* (London: Ark, 1987), 51.

32. Cardano recorded twelve "nativities" or horoscopes of Edward in a 1555 book published in London, *Geniturarum exempla*. He also made a careful, critical observation of the young king's appearance. Jordan, *Edward VI: Threshold of Power*, 409–10. For more on Christ's horoscope as read by Cardano, see Wayne Shumaker, *Renaissance Curiosa* (Binghamton: State University of New York Press, 1982).

33. Dr. Cardano was sufficiently embarrassed by the erroneous casting that he felt obligated to pen an explanation: "What I Thought of the Matter Afterward." He said he could not gauge things accurately because he was unable to view the sun and moon while in audience with the king. Oystein Ore, *Cardano* (New York: Dover, 1953), 39; Jordan, *Edward VI: Threshold of Power*, 410n.

34. Erickson, *Bloody Mary*, 284; Hester Chapman, *The Last Tudor King* (London: Jonathan Cape, 1958), 267–68.

35. J. Arthur Myers, *Captain of All These Men of Death* (St. Louis, Mo.: Warren Green, 1977), 26. Barrett Beer asserts that, given these foul medications, "few can still believe that Northumberland . . . poisoned Edward VI." Barrett L. Beer, "Northumberland: The Myth of the Wicked Duke and the Historical John Dudley," *Albion* 11 (1979): 9.

36. Hayward, *Life and Raigne*, 168–69. Hayward opined that having "assured his own deuices, nothing remained by that the King should not longer suruiue, lest haply his sickly judgement might be over-ruled by sounder aduice." Ibid., 176.

37. S. T. Bindoff, "A Kingdom at Stake, 1553," *History Today* 3 (1953): 647.

38. Myers, *Captain of All These Men*, 26.

39. Quoted in Bindoff, "Kingdom at Stake," 647.

40. Bindoff, "Kingdom at Stake," 648. John Cheke was appointed a Secretary to the Council in May 1553, partly because several of the government's chief ministers were absent due to "illness" and partly because Cheke agreed with the direction that the Church of England had taken under Northumberland: Jordan, *Edward VI: Threshold of Power*, 502–3.

41. Weir, *Children of Henry VIII*, 146–50; Beer, *Northumberland* (Kent, Ohio: Kent State University Press, 1973), 150; David Loades, *John Dudley, Duke of Northumberland* (Oxford: Clarendon Press, 1996), 306. Weir says that the crone was probably murdered, as she disappears from the records after Edward's death; Chapman and Erickson concur. Chapman, *Last Tudor King*, 280; Erickson, *Bloody Mary*, 285. Of course, the "improvement" noted in Edward's condition might have been yet another manifestation of tubercular deception.

42. Chapman, *Last Tudor King*, 285. Sir Arthur MacNalty posits that Edward's pulmonary tuberculosis was accompanied by Raynaud's disease: MacNalty, *Elizabeth Tudor*, 223.

43. Reported in Weir, *Children of Henry VIII*, 152, but described by Jordan as a remedy given by Lord John Audley to William Cecil in the State Papers. See Jordan, *Edward VI: Threshold of Power*, 502.

44. Jane Grey lodged in the Tower during her reign, resolutely denying the Dudley family demands that her husband be declared king. After Queen Mary's accession, Jane was sentenced to die but Mary suspended the punishment; the following year Jane was beheaded for a connection to Wyatt's rebellion. For more on Jane Grey, see Hester Chapman, *Lady Jane Grey* (London: J. Cape, 1962.

45. G. R. Elton, *England under the Tudors* (London: Methuen, 1956), 214. Forceful criticism of Mary began in 1563 with Protestant hagiographer John Foxe's English-language indictment of her rule and policies, *Acts and Monuments of These Latter and Perilous Days*, usually called *The Book of Martyrs*, for the next century the most widely read book after the Bible. Foxe's severe judgment of

the queen continued through the centuries in histories by John Strype, J.A. Froude, A.F. Pollard, and Elton. See Foxe, *Acts and Monuments*, 8th ed., 3 vols. (London: Company of Stationers, 1641); Strype's *Ecclesiastical Memorials*, 3 vols. (London: B. Aylmer, 1721); Froude's *The Reign of Mary Tudor* (London: J.M. Dent, 1924); and Pollard's *History of England from the Accession of Edward VI to the Death of Elizabeth* (London: Longmans, Green, and Co., 1929). More recent scholars, however, have been sympathetic to Mary and have found her Parliaments effective. See, for instance, David Loades, *Mary Tudor* (Oxford: Basil Blackwell, 1989); and Jennifer Loach, *Parliament and Crown in the Reign of Mary Tudor* (Oxford: Oxford University Press, 1986).

46. Weir, *Children of Henry VIII*, 4. She had a low-pitched, resonant voice, however, that carried well in a large room: Erickson, *Bloody Mary*, 176.

47. Prescott, *Spanish Tudor*, 49. Prescott quotes Imperial ambassador Eustace Chapuys describing Featherstone as "a physician who formerly was her tutor and usual doctor." Erickson calls Featherstone Butts's "assistant and apothecary": Erickson, *Bloody Mary*, 62.

48. Prescott, *Spanish Tudor*, 52–53. Weir says that Mary's recurrent autumnal symptoms appear to have been seasonal affective disorder: Weir, *Children of Henry VIII*, 5.

49. Because of the coins given to the sick, records about the healing rituals of Henry VII and Henry VIII would have been kept in the Almonery books, now lost. Henry VII started the practice of giving a gold coin to those whom he touched. Edward VI touched occasionally, despite his disdain for superstitious images and idolatrous practices. Ironically, he contracted the virulent pulmonary form of tuberculosis. Marc Bloch, *The Royal Touch* (London: Routledge, 1973), 181, 189; Thomas M. Daniel, *Captain of Death: The Story of Tuberculosis* (Rochester, N.Y.: University of Rochester Press, 1997), 24. See also Thomas, *Religion and the Decline of Magic*, 227–35.

50. Erickson, *Bloody Mary*, 443.

51. Quoted in Bloch, *Royal Touch*, 182. Bloch noted that the coin's inscription had been "O Christ, Redeemer, save us by Thy cross" until Mary Tudor's reign.

52. Thomas Smith, quoted in John Cannon and Ralph Griffiths, *Oxford Illustrated History of the British Monarchy* (Oxford: Oxford University Press, 1988), 306. For court adaptations in Mary's reign, see John Murphy, "The Illusion of Decline: the Privy Chamber," in *The English Court from the Wars of the Roses to the Civil War*, ed. David Starkey et al. (London: Longman, 1987), 140–41.

53. A. G. Dickens, *The English Reformation*, 2nd ed. (University Park: University of Pennsylvania Press, 1991), 312; Dale Hoak, "Two Revolutions in Tudor Government," in *Revolution Reassessed*, eds. Christopher Coleman and David Starkey (Oxford: Oxford University Press, 1986), 95. Mary's New Year Gift List of 1557 shows that she presented Owen, Wendy, and Hughes with two pots of conserve each and received from each of them a fourteen-ounce gilt jug. Loades, *Mary Tudor*, 365.

54. Variations on the spelling of his surname include Adelmare, a Dalmaris, and Dalmariis; he signed a letter to Lord Burghley "Casar Adelmarius." Munk, *Roll*, 1: 53; Clippingdale, Medical Court Roll, 1: 30, LRCS; Additional Manuscripts (Add. MSS) 12497, British Library.

55. Annals of the Royal College of Physicians, vol. 1, p. 12, LRCP.

56. Add. MSS 12497. Adelmaris' son, Sir Julius Caesar, became a doctor of canon law, Chancellor of the Exchequer, and Privy Councillor to James I and Charles I.

57. David Loades mentions a Miguel de la Soa, a physician to Princess Mary in 1536 and formerly to her mother, Catherine of Aragon. See Loades, *Mary Tudor*, 352.

58. Beck, *Cutting Edge*, 183; Young, *Annals*, 5.

59. Erickson, *Bloody Mary*, 214. Meanwhile, Mary's own attendants feared that her ailments would surely kill her: Prescott, *Spanish Tudor*, 110.

60. Quoted in Matthews, *Royal Apothecaries*, 70.

61. Frederic Madden, ed., *Privy Purse Expenses of the Princess Mary* (London: W. Pickering, 1831), 68, 208, 269.

62. Matthews, *Royal Apothecaries*, 70.

63. Parliament resisted all of the queen's attempts to have Philip made king of England. John Guy, "Tudor Monarchy and Political Culture," in *Tudor and Stuart Britain*, ed. John Morrill (Oxford: Oxford University Press, 1996), 232.

64. Weir, *Children of Henry VIII*, 285–86; Prescott, *Spanish Tudor*, 368. A delegate from the Duke of Savoy related that he had personally seen the queen sick to her stomach and had received positive assurance that she was with child; Erickson, *Bloody Mary*, 386.

65. Audrey Eccles, *Obstetrics and Gynaecology in Tudor and Stuart England* (London: Croom Helm, 1982), 63–64.

66. This is famed midwife Jane Sharp's potion, quoted in Eccles, *Obstetrics and Gynaecology*, 65. A scruple equaled twenty grains; three scruples made one dram. Mastic resin came from an evergreen tree of the cashew family; myrtle leaves are still used by herbalists as a vaginal douche to protect against prolapse of the uterus.

67. An ovarian cyst or tumor might account for another delusional pregnancy in 1557: Loades, *Mary Tudor*, 251. Carolly Erickson refers to Mary as "entering the terminal stage of ovarian cancer" and identifies Frederick Chamberlin (in *The Private Character of Henry the Eighth*, [New York: Washburne, 1931], 27) as the first to posit ovarian dropsy as her problem. See also Erickson, *The First Elizabeth* (New York: Summit Books, 1983), 159; *Bloody Mary*, 505, n.9.

68. Monstrous births were of intense interest to sixteenth-century commentators, who felt they were caused by illicit acts and signaled widespread calamity. If a monarch delivered a fleshy mass that resembled a bunch of grapes, the portent was even more ominous. For more on birth deformities and their interpretation, see Retha M. Warnicke, *The Rise and Fall of Anne Boleyn* (Cambridge: Cambridge University Press, 1989).

69. Pseudocyesis is the verdict of most mainstream historians and Mary's biographers. See James A. Williamson, *The Tudor Age* (London: Longman, 1979), 240; Prescott, *Spanish Tudor*, 397–98; Weir, *Children of Henry VIII*, 314; Cannon and Griffiths, *Oxford Illustrated Monarchs*, 332. Loades, who supports the idea of a cyst or tumor, also considers the idea of delusional pregnancy, as does Erickson. See Loades, *Mary Tudor*, 232; Erickson, *Bloody Mary*, 205.

70. Patricia Crawford, "Attitudes to Menstruation in Seventeenth-Century England," *Past and Present* 91 (1981), 67. Menarche came earlier than today, usually between fourteen and sixteen.

71. Quoted in Eccles, *Obstetrics and Gynaecology*, 74.

72. Sir Hector MacLennan wrote that pseudocyesis is "common in elderly sterile women," and would now be diagnosed early. He also posits that Mary's ailment could have been a fibroid or ovarian cyst. MacLennan, "Gynecologist," 70. See also Irving Fischer, "Hypothalamic Amenorrhea: Pseudocyesis," in *Psychosomatic Obstetrics, Gynecology and Endochrinology*, ed. William S. Kroger (Springfield, Ill.: Thomas, 1962), 291–97.

73. Other doctors mentioned in various places as Mary's physicians include Drs. Roper and Vagham in 1555, cited in the College's records: Annals of the Royal College of Physicians, vol. 1, f. 12. A Dr. Calagila is referred to without further identification in Weir, *Children of Henry VIII*, 307; and Erickson, *Bloody Mary*, 415.

74. The foremost English physician who cited examples of such alarmingly lengthy pregnancies was William Harvey. Eccles, *Obstetrics and Gynaecology*, 44–45.

75. Eccles, *Obstetrics and Gynaecology*, 60. When surgeons began using uroscopy, the College of Physicians officially cast doubt on this method of diagnosis long-established among doctors, requiring in 1601 that it not be the only procedure for determining a patient's condition. Roberts, "Personnel and Practice: London," 225.

76. Prescott, *Spanish Tudor*, 397.

77. Michael K. Eshleman, "Diet during Pregnancy in the Sixteenth and Seventeenth Centuries," *Journal of the History of Medicine* 30 (1975): 29.

78. See Hilda Smith, "Gynecology and Ideology in Seventeenth Century England," in *Liberating Women's History*, ed. Berenice A. Carroll (Urbana: University of Illinois Press, 1976), 97–114.

79. Thomas G. Benedek, "The Changing Relationship between Midwives and Physicians during the Renaissance," *Bulletin of the History of Medicine* 51 (1977): 551.

80. R. L. Petrelli, "The Regulation of French Midwifery during the Ancien Régime," *Journal of the History of Medicine* 25 (1971): 276–92; Arthure, "The Midwife," 1–9.

81. Other euphemisms for menstrual periods included "terms," "courses," and "wonted grief." Crawford, "Attitudes to Menstruation," 49.

82. Rosslin, whose book was for the instruction of official town midwives, was state physician of Worms and Frankfurt-am-Main. Eccles, *Obstetrics and Gynaecology*, 11–12. Jacoba Felicie, a Parisian physician, argued that women doctors were better able to deal with female problems in the existing moral climate. Another Frenchwoman, Louise Bourgeois, was the first woman to write a book about midwifery, published in the early seventeenth century. See Benedek, "Changing Relationship," 551–58; and Robert E. Roush, "The Development of Midwifery," *Journal of the Nurse Midwife* 24/3 (May-June 1979): 27–37.

83. Also counted in the Marian carnage should be the ninety who were executed for their part in Wyatt's rebellion, including poor Jane Grey and her husband, and thirty more who died after two other conspiracies. Mary's successor, Elizabeth, would burn only five souls in forty-five years. Weir, *Children of Henry VIII*, 355.

84. Some eight hundred English Protestants had been allowed to emigrate to Frankfurt, Zurich, and Geneva. They waged a relentless crusade of anti-Catholic propaganda against Mary's government, which tried to refute the subversion as best it could. Edward's tutor, John Cheke, recanted and retired to the countryside, where he died in 1557.

85. Richard Grafton, *A Chronicle at Large*, 2 vols. (London: H. Denham, 1569), 2: 1351. Stow noted that five of the seven had been mayor of London: Beer, *Tudor England Observed*, 50.

86. Hackett, *Malaria in Europe*, 31, 205, 213. Hackett argues against economic conditions affecting malarial regression; wealth is no preventive.

87. Dale C. Smith, "Quinine and Fever," *Journal of the History of Medicine* 31 (1976): 344–45. The search for an antifebrile led to many ingenious approaches: one indirect remedy called for the urine of the patient to be mixed with dough, formed into seventy-seven small cakes, and put on an anthill before sunrise. When the cakes were all gone, the fever should vanish. Three drops of blood from a cat's ear in peppered brandy drunk by the sufferer was another, more direct, method. For more on the search for a cure, see M. L. Duran-Reynals, *The Fever-Bark Tree* (Garden City, N.Y.: Doubleday, 1946).

88. For some antimalarial recipes, see W.S.C. Copeman, *Doctors and Disease in Tudor Times* (London: Dawson's, 1960), 132.

89. Beer, *Tudor England Observed*, 50; Prescott, *Spanish Tudor*, 495. Beer notes that the population of England declined by at least 6 percent between 1556 and 1560.

90. Giovanni Michieli, quoted in Weir, *Children of Henry VIII*, 342–43.

91. Nonetheless, Princess Elizabeth brought Mary a layette of handmade baby clothes at the end of February, after which the queen took to her chamber to await the birth of her child. Weir, *Children of Henry VIII*, 351.

92. Loades, *Mary Tudor*, 310–11.

Chapter 3

The Medical Personnel of Elizabeth I (1558–1603)

Born in 1533 to Henry VIII and Anne Boleyn, Elizabeth Tudor was a lively, active child and, apart from teething problems as an infant, experienced robust health until adolescence. Despite the traumatic loss of her mother to the executioner's sword while still a toddler, Princess Elizabeth showed no evidence of illness until puberty. Then, a series of disturbing events triggered a cycle of chronic ailments that overshadowed her teenage years. The death of her father in January 1547 precipitated a change in her abode and before long the princess found herself living with Henry's widow, her stepmother Katherine Parr, and Katherine's new husband, Thomas Seymour, at their house in Chelsea. Attractive to women, Thomas Seymour was the brother of Protector Somerset; he was also Edward VI's younger maternal uncle, and Lord High Admiral after February 1547. Rumors joined his name to Elizabeth's, but just five months after the king's death, Seymour married the Queen Dowager, previously an object of his affections, in a secret ceremony.[1] Seymour was jealous of his brother and conspired against him with John Dudley and others. Somerset initially opposed the hasty marriage of the Lord Admiral to Katherine, but was later reconciled to it by the young king, with whom Thomas had ingratiated himself.

According to depositions from members of the household at Seymour's later trial, strange behavior characterized the interactions of the Seymours and their innocent, inexperienced guest, conduct that sometimes took the form of physical, semi-sexual frolics in the princess' bedroom in the early morning hours. On one bizarre occasion in the garden of their residence at Hanworth, Seymour ripped Elizabeth's dress while Katherine held her fast. After Katherine absented herself due to advancing pregnancy, the rough-housing between the Lord Admiral and Elizabeth sometimes got out of hand.[2] Servants told Katherine that her husband made overtly lecherous advances towards Elizabeth, and Katherine herself may have caught them in an inappropriate embrace. The princess soon left the Seymours to stay with Sir Anthony Denny at Cheshunt in Hertfordshire, under the shadow of embarrassment and in the face of multiple complaints.

Elizabeth's symptoms included migraine headaches, irregular menstrual periods, digestive problems, jaundice, and episodic anxiety attacks; she was ill throughout the summer of 1548 and into the fall. Although she avoided alcohol and followed a frugal, sensible diet, the princess remained debilitated and often bedridden. Katherine died in September 1548 after having given birth to a daughter the week before, doubtless inducing further afflictions in the princess. The Lord Admiral continued to pursue her, however, as part of his schemes against his brother. Accused of treason, by January 1549 the Lord Admiral was in the Tower and prosecutors interrogated Elizabeth for evidence against him; she acknowledged no wrongdoing on his part. Denied an open trial, Thomas Seymour died two months later on the scaffold. Though we cannot assess Elizabeth's feelings for Seymour, at the very least she learned how dangerous a position she was in and it made her sick again. Elizabeth's shift from wellness to infirmity paralleled crises in her personal life and produced a lifelong pattern of tension-induced infirmity. She was always susceptible to illness at the height of emotional stress.[3]

When the uproar over Elizabeth's relationship with Thomas Seymour had diminished by the following year, Protector Somerset sent Edward's physician Thomas Bille to Cheshunt to tend to her. After her recovery under Dr. Bille's supervision, Elizabeth thanked him for his services.[4] Though much improved, the princess still complained from time to time of headaches so ferocious that she could not read or write. Given the arduous regimen of reading demanded of Elizabeth by her tutor, Roger Ascham, her headaches might have been due to eyestrain, although there is no evidence that she ever wore spectacles. After 1580, when she was forty-six, her headaches appear to have ceased. She had an attack of what was probably scarlet fever in 1553 when she was twenty years old.

Elizabeth fell ill in early 1554 while at Ashridge with what may have been nephritis. Suffering from painful swelling in her extremities and head reminiscent of Edward's fatal illness, she probably wondered if her bloating might be due to poison. When Queen Mary summoned Elizabeth to court out of concern over anti-Spanish plotting, the princess replied that she was too sick to come. Mary sent her own doctors to check on Elizabeth's infirmity, and they determined that with care along the route and warm, dry quarters awaiting her at the end of the journey, Elizabeth might travel.[5] Those who saw her when she arrived at Westminster were shocked, remarking that she was distended, exhausted, and wraithlike. Sending the princess to the damp and infamous Tower of London during Wyatt's rebellion hardly improved her condition, especially since it was there that her own mother had been imprisoned. Elizabeth survived the crisis and was released on May 19, exactly eighteen years after Anne Boleyn's execution. Elizabeth left for Woodstock, a dilapidated medieval house near Oxford. At the time of her liberation, Dr. Owen wrote a letter to Vice-Chamberlain Bedingfield relating to Elizabeth's medical circumstances, commenting on her chronically sore eyes.[6]

In June, her face still swollen and her back sore, a disconsolate Elizabeth asked to be bled by Mary's physicians whom she trusted—Owen, Wendy or Huicke. When the queen's Council told her to find someone in Oxford to do the task, Elizabeth averred that only the royal doctors would do. Her stubbornness wore down the Council and she got the physicians and the treatment of her choice. Under their supervision, she was bled from the arm and foot by a barber-surgeon; the bleeding was to be repeated in autumn to prevent recurrence of the illness.[7] Another illness was recorded in the summer of 1556, an attack of jaundice with intermittent breathlessness which the French ambassador attributed not to the unusual heat but to anxiety over the queen's mistreatment of Elizabeth. The Venetian ambassador specifically remarked on to her olive skin, perhaps a sign of infectious hepatitis or some other disease.[8]

And then, in November 1558 she became queen at the age of twenty-five. Elizabeth assumed the mantle of an English monarch and the supernatural powers that went with it. Despite ridicule from some free-thinking foreign religious reformers who thought kingly "healing" superstitious and silly, she perpetuated the royal touch for curing scrofula. Elizabeth "carefully preserved the traditional ceremonial, merely cutting out from the liturgy a prayer that mentioned the Virgin and the saints, and probably translating into English the Latin ritual of the previous ages."[9] She even made the Sign of the Cross over the affected parts of the sick. Catholics rejected Elizabeth's powers on the grounds that she was an excommunicated heretic, but her healings were cited as proof that the Papal Bull of Excommunication had failed to take effect. Puritans thought the practice irrational and absurd. In response to their challenge, official preachers defended the ancient privilege of the English monarchy against unbelievers. Elizabeth's chaplain, William Tooker, penned the first book in praise of the royal miracle, and at the end of her reign, one of the queen's surgeons, William Clowes, provided an apologia for the wonder-working virtue of English rulers. Though she maintained the touching ceremonials, at the beginning of her reign Elizabeth quietly ceased to distribute cramp-rings on Good Friday, essentially halting that ancient rite. Despite her own health concerns and mindful of royal prestige, the queen retained the ceremony that brought her into direct contact with her suffering subjects and jettisoned the one that did not.[10]

Whatever were the concerns about Elizabeth's health that prevailed before her coronation, they centered afterward on her reproductive abilities. Her contemporaries remarked that she was always too thin and bony, insufficiently robust to withstand the rigors of governance, let alone childbirth. In June 1559 her physicians bled her from the foot and arm, a familiar treatment for menstrual irregularity; the Spanish envoy Count de Feria reported that his spies told him the queen could not bear children.[11] In August she developed a burning fever that lasted for several weeks. Contradictory gossip circulated constantly, that the unmarried queen was pregnant or that she knew she was incapable of bearing children and would remain unwed. In October 1562 a crisis brought the quandary of the succession into focus: Elizabeth contracted smallpox.

Smallpox is explosively contagious as it ranges through the air. Virus-laden specks of moisture in the mouth are propelled outward when their host speaks, and a single inhalation can lead an individual to come down with the disease. Although smallpox is less easily transmittable than measles, it is more so than mumps. Several women at court had gotten smallpox in the weeks before the queen's illness, and a few had died. Smallpox disfigured those whom it did not kill, leaving the skin of once handsome men and beautiful women hideous with pits and sores. Sufferers who survived bore the angry red scars that refused to heal and resisted medicinal and cosmetic treatment, though some found relief from groundup, roasted maggot-drippings.[12] But the facial spots that were the bane of smallpox were also the sign of improvement in the patient; the raging fever that accompanied the contagion abated only when the characteristic red spots appeared, usually on the fourth day of the course of the disease. Ordinarily, during the first three days of smallpox slight eruptions can be discerned on the victim's trunk. Then a papular eruption envelops the face, hands, and feet, vesiculates, and becomes opalescentally pustular, signaling the disease's progression. It is an excruciating progression, however, as the skin actually tears horizontally, splitting away from its underlayers. Normally in smallpox, the pustules eventually crust, scab, and drop off, leaving depressed and depigmented scars. But in Elizabeth's case, there was no sign of the usual transition to the second stage of the disease, and her court physicians feared the onset of pneumonia or other deadly complications.[13]

Her doctors did what they could and followed the practice of installing red cloth over the windows to filter out harsh light and prevent scarring, insisting on the maintenance of a warm fire, and swaddling the royal victim in red cloth. Her fever continued to rage for seven days, she lost the power of speech, and she slipped into unconsciousness; the court prepared to go into mourning. Because the queen had not made a will or acknowledged a successor, her ministers were frantic with fear for themselves and the nation. Then Elizabeth's fever broke and the spots appeared. Afterward, Elizabeth sequestered herself for more than a week until the scabs fell off, and dealt with the ravages done to her complexion, but the crisis had passed. Although she and her councillors had encountered a terrible threat to the country's security when smallpox felled her, Elizabeth had withstood yet another ordeal.

The next year in England was hardly more felicitous. The College of Physicians' Annals noted that colds and catarrh spread throughout England, followed by fever and pleurisy. For the first twelve days of December 1563, the air was "smoky and dank" and a "dense and fetid gloom" hung over London; "everywhere was full of woodlice." The Fellows determined that all cats and dogs should be killed.[14] Imagine the pressures endured by ordinary physicians during such a time and the exponentially more ominous urgencies visited on the royal doctors.

Two factors influenced the therapies authorized by doctors at the court of Elizabeth I—the growing influence of Paracelsian medicine in England and the length of the queen's reign. It is hard to overestimate the impact of Paracelsus, the sixteenth-century physician and teacher, on medicine and science, not just the laboratory aspect of his studies, but, as we shall see, on their political and institutional aspects as well. Paracelsus subscribed to the Neoplatonic cosmology taught by Marsilio Ficino in Florence, with its doctrine of macrocosm and microcosm: the body and soul of man replicate in miniature the body and soul of the world, a correlation that the philosopher or magus can comprehend and master. Since Paracelsus believed that the universe was chemically controlled, it followed for him that the human body could be altered and cured by the chemical treatment of a medical magus, rather than by trivial herbal remedies. Paracelsus constructed a bridgehead between magic and science; there are elements of both in his endeavors.[15] Because of his peculiar amalgam of the occult and the experimental approaches to nature, Paracelsus is neither ancient nor modern. Physician to Erasmus, he defined the bases of medicine as philosophy, astronomy, alchemy, and ethics. As an anti-Aristotelian, Paracelsus contemptuously discarded the four humors of Galen, impugning the lack of patient examination and symptom observation characteristic of Galenic theory (classically-trained doctors did, however, examine patient's urine, in a process termed "water-casting"). Paracelsus argued instead that disease emanated from external causes and became localized in particular organs. He termed his urine analysis "chemical dissection" and carried his patient's weighed urine in a gauged cylinder shaped like the human body.[16] Although famous for his use of chemical remedies such as mercury, lead, arsenic, and antimony, he did not neglect vegetable simples or preparations made from them.

Despite his affinity for laboratory experimentation, Paracelsus still endorsed certain mystical treatments such as an ointment made of usnea (moss from skulls), bear grease and boar fat, dried boar brains, red sandalwood, calcined worms, and bone or tissue matter from a mummy. The ointment, called weapon-salve, was a treatment for injuries; it was, however, to be applied not to the wound but to the instrument that had caused it. Healing would occur by the power of sympathy.[17] According to Paracelsus, disease was a material entity that could be made apparent and detectable, in contrast to the classical notion of humoral imbalance. Disease, in chemical terms, was the product of coagulation caused by some exogenous substance introduced with food or drink and specific or fixed as a process, influenced by some local environmental factors. Among other things, his convictions provided Paracelsus with a new explanation for gout, which he advanced in 1531. Water supply, he argued, could cause chemical deposits like bodily tartar to cluster around a joint.[18] Paracelsus also touted the natural healing processes of the human body, recommending milder doses of medication and opiates like laudanum, a word he invented, to relieve pain. Whether his theories were correct or not, his patients and those of his followers recovered and handled their recoveries better.

Though he fits no more easily into a sectarian category than he does into an ideological one, Paracelsus directly challenged institutional authority with his seditious ideas. He disliked Luther for embracing secular authority as much as he disliked the Roman Catholic ecclesiastical establishment; Paracelsus made no secret of his blessing on the German Peasants' Revolt in 1525. As city physician of Basel, he lectured in German rather than Latin, suggesting a popular audience for his views. Paracelsus disdained traditional medicine and tossed the works of Hippocrates and Galen, as well as the canon of Avicenna, into the St. John's Day bonfire at Basel in 1527. After the death of its founder in 1541, Paracelsianism became as much a social threat as an intellectual heresy, especially to privileged practitioners with vested interests to protect. It "encouraged the subject classes of the medical profession, the surgeons and apothecaries, to claim rights above their station."[19] By the first decade in the reign of Gloriana, the confrontation on the continent between Galenists and followers of Paracelsus became fierce, in part due to the dissemination of Paracelsian works supported by the Elector of Cologne. As the medical conflict migrated to the British Isles, the patronage of princes would be necessary to overcome opposition to the subversive nature of Paracelsus' teachings. The London College of Physicians, however, after flirting with Paracelsianism in the 1580s, remained a stronghold of conventional Galenic doctrine until the end of the Elizabethan era. Though some of her courtiers championed the new medicine, the queen herself "clung to established ways."[20]

While few English physicians manifested public admiration for mystical or occult works in medicine and alchemy during the mid-Tudor era, interest in chemical medicine ran high. However, no real chemical therapy evolved in Great Britain until the 1559 publication of Conrad Gesner's *Treasure of Euonymus*. Just the next year John Geynes spoke out against Galen's teachings and was summoned to discuss his contentions with the College Fellows or face imprisonment. Geynes asserted that he found twenty-two errors in Galen, but after three days of debate the Fellows remained firmly on the side of the ancients. The College Annals note that Geynes then repented.[21] Despite the outcome of that disputation, physicians trained in the experimental aspects of Paracelsian-influenced curricula began to make their way to England. The Oxbridge majority in the College of Physicians responded by tripling its fees for Fellows with foreign degrees.[22]

Historian Allen Debus labels Richard Bostocke, practicing around 1585, the first English Paracelsian. Bostocke wrote *Difference betwene the Auncient Phisicke . . . and the Latter Phisicke*, which noted the historical antecedents of chemical medicine, from Adam to Hippocrates, and pointed out that herbs and plants comprised a valuable part of a doctor's repertoire when treated chemically before being administered. Bostocke warned, however, that doctors should not experiment on men.[23] Hugh Trevor-Roper bestows the historical honor of introducing "the sophisticated form of Paracelsianism into England" on Thomas Muffet (Moffet), an Anglicized Scotsman who transferred in 1578 from Galenist Cambridge to the University of Basel where he absorbed the new medicine.[24] Upon his return to England, Muffet, a former pupil of Caius, cultivated noble patrons and illustrious patients including Sir Francis Drake, Sir

Philip Sidney, and Sir Francis Walsingham, Elizabeth's Secretary of State. He sat in Parliament and joined the College of Physicians. Spurred by a new spate of Paracelsian publications after 1570 and the lobbying of Dr. Muffet, the College contemplated a section on chemical medicine for its proposed pharmacopoeia. Though the College did not complete its plans for the pharmacopoeia and a period of conservativism ended the century, by 1589 one-third of the Fellows had graduated from universities with chemical therapy among their requirements and the numbers of such Fellows would surely increase in the next generation.[25] Toward the end of the Elizabethan era, an implicit doctrinal truce existed within the English medical profession; in the reign of the Stuarts would come new impetus for change.

Despite occasional fevers that bedeviled her for days, a troublesome leg that caused her to limp on occasion, and persistent rumors of female disorders, Queen Elizabeth lived into her seventieth year. Her longevity and numerous discomforts necessitated the employment of an unusually large medical staff, one that had to cope with the changing needs of an aging monarch. The older she got, the thinner she became: so thin that one physician in 1566, after examining her gaunt and skeletal body, feared that she was becoming consumptive and developing kidney stones.[26] Quite understandably, the doctors who attended her tried to elude serious accountability for keeping such a frail creature alive, hinting that her constitution was too weak even for their medical mastery. She outlived them all.

At least fifteen physicians and seven surgeons have been listed as attached to the Elizabethan household.[27] Some, like John Caius, Caesar Dalmaris, and Thomas Vicary, were holdovers from the Marian era; Dr. Robert Huicke had attended Princess Elizabeth for many years at Hatfield and stayed at his post after her accession to the throne, the first doctor designated physician-in-ordinary. Others were new to the job and to the queen, and more than one was controversial in his own time. Elizabeth appears to have favored the medical counsel of Oxbridge graduates, but Roderigo Lopez was an exception. Chief physician at St. Bartholomew's Hospital and a Portuguese Jew, Lopez corresponded with the Spanish court and was accused of conspiracy against Elizabeth. Robert Jacob had the perilous task representing England at the court of Ivan the Terrible. Politics mattered more to these appointees than to their predecessors in the medical household, and the queen even found it necessary to dismiss John Caius in 1556 for his religious preferences.

Elizabeth's doctors received £100 board and other perquisites.[28] Described as the "queen's physician" by all his contemporaries, Robert Huicke continued as a physician to the Protestant Tudors after the Marian interruption. As a participant in the instruction of future doctors mandated by the Physic Act, Huick debated medical theory in 1564 at Cambridge and in 1566 at Oxford with the queen in attendance. Elizabeth rewarded Huicke with a mansion, White Webbs House in Middlesex.[29] From about 1568 until his death in 1574, Chester native Thomas Francis attended the queen as physician-in-ordinary.

He began his studies at Christ Church, Oxford, in theology, but switched to medicine, receiving his M.D. there in 1554. Regius Professor at Christ Church, then in 1561 Provost of Queen's College, Francis was not a popular choice as Provost and resigned after two years. In 1560 he became a Fellow of the College of Physicians and its President in 1568. While serving in that office, Francis ran into trouble with Eliseus Bomelius, a quack the College prosecuted for practicing without a license. Bomelius did not go quietly, however, and drew Elizabeth's chief minister, William Cecil, later Lord Burghley, into the confrontation, offering to expose Francis' ignorance of Latin and astronomy.[30] The queen stood by her doctor despite these professional problems.

Walter Bayley enjoyed the comfortable if busy life of a successful physician, priest, and professor. Born in Dorsetshire, son of an attorney, and educated at Winchester, Bayley was a member of the growing circle of Oxford medical alumni, receiving his degree from New College. Like Francis, he also had a religious vocation. He became prebendary of Dulcote in Wells, proctor of Oxford university in 1558, and three years later the queen's professor of medicine there. Bayley belongs on the cusp of medical change in England; indeed, he embodies the professional compromise that took place within that citadel of the medical establishment, the Royal College of Physicians.[31] By the time that Bayley became a Fellow of the College in 1581, many of the Fellows had earned their degrees from more progressive continental universities and were influenced by a Paracelsian curriculum. Bayley had already carved out a successful career and had established associations with scientists who advocated radical methods of medical analysis. Though himself a product of a medical curriculum so traditional that attendance at Galenic-centered lectures was required by law for graduation, Bayley practiced a more experimental type of medicine. His interest in the study and analysis of mineral waters was typical of the followers of Paracelsus, but also characteristic of the Paracelsians was publishing medcial informationin the vernacular, which Bayley did, though he hedged his bets by writing his own prescriptions in arcane Latin.

In 1587 Bayley published an account in English of the medicinal waters at Warwickshire's Newnham Regis in which he identified the waters' composition by distillation and encouraged their use in summer. He filtered and analyzed the spa's minerals by taste, color, and reaction to fire, concluding that limestone, alum, nitre, and iron were present.[32] He wrote a brief treatise on eyecare in the vernacular, emphasizing the importance of air and nourishment. Included in his aphorisms is "southern winds do hurt the sight." Among his cures for the 113 diseases of the eyes and "eye liddes," Bayley sanctioned washing the eyes with the urine of a child and the liquor from the liver of a goat. He also wrote a piece on peppers; diatrion pepper warms the tummy while diacalaminthe penetrates further than diaspoliticon, "which keepeth the belly loose." His books were printed privately and without his name attached to them, to be given away as New Year's greetings. Bayley's advice for camomile ointment rub, "given to one who had an inveterate consumption of the lungs, shortly after a dropsy," described the malady in English but gave the prescription for it in Latin, usually a sign that the doctor in question wished to preserve some of the secrets of the profession.[33]

John Dee, England's first Hermetic magus or alchemist, was a close friend and colleague of Bayley. At the center of the English Renaissance, Dee traveled extensively on the continent, meeting and conversing with other philosophers and scientists, and gathered at his house at Mortlake the greatest collection of books and manuscripts in the nation.[34] Dee's influence on Bayley was significant, and it transported the physician beyond the limits of his conventional medical education. Both Bayley and Dee were linked with Elizabeth's personal favorite and councillor, Robert Dudley, Earl of Leicester. Leicester, son of the Duke of Northumberland, patronized certain physicians and other men of letters who had a progressive, pragmatic attitude toward learning. As a proponent of more widely available medical knowledge, Bayley displayed the eclectic spirit that Leicester supported.[35] Bayley was in Leicester's service throughout the 1570s, accompanying him to the Peak District for three consecutive summers to take the waters at Buxton. Leicester smarted from pain and swelling in his leg, and Bayley, whose enthusiasm for mineral waters was well-known, persuaded him that the warm, constant temperature of the spring would be beneficial. Leicester wrote to Sir Christopher Hatton in early May 1578, assuring the future Lord Chancellor that Dr. Bayley was still keeping him in hand "because the late hot weather had returned again."[36]

Bayley's first opportunity to serve Queen Elizabeth came in late 1578. Elizabeth suffered from painful toothaches so disabling that she twice canceled audiences with the French ambassador in September of that year.[37] After a consultation with Bayley at Elizabeth's command about the excruciating pain in the queen's teeth, Dee was sent by Leicester and Secretary of State Walsingham, to whom he also ministered, to Germany to confer with learned physicians.[38] Bayley probably accompanied Dee to Frankfurt-on-the-Oder. Though their mission was to discuss toothache and the rheumatism thought to cause it, some of Dee's biographers have speculated that there may have been a secret political purpose to this trip as well.[39] The queen rewarded Bayley upon his return with a twenty-one-year lease on Stanlake in Oxfordshire. With a career that required almost constant travel among university, cathedral, and court, Bayley became Elizabeth's physician-in-ordinary in 1581.

Bayley was certainly connected in the public mind to Leicester after the appearance in 1584 in Antwerp of a book attacking the earl and accusing him of multiple murders. Titled *The Copy of a Letter Written by a Master of Arts of Cambridge to his friend in London . . .* , the appellation by which the volume has come to be known is *Leicester's Commonwealth*.[40] Probably emanating from lay Catholic exiles based in Paris who were partisans of Mary Stuart, the queen of Scotland long imprisoned in England, the book claimed that conspirators like Dee, Bayley, and Martin Culpeper, Vice-Chancellor of Oxford University, had aided Leicester in eliminating anyone who stood in the way of his passage to greater wealth and power. Bayley and Culpeper were described as "once papists, now galenists," poisoners so subtle "they can make a man die of any sickness they will and as long afterwards as they like."[41] Since Leicester's first wife, Amy Robsart Dudley, had perished in a mysterious fall in 1560, the book recalled the suspicions many had expressed at the time of her death.

The anonymous author, thought at the time to be the Jesuit Robert Parsons, wrote that Leicester was made cunning

> by the counsel of his Dr. Bayley, a man not a little studied (as he seemeth) for his art. For I heard him once myself in a public act in Oxford (and that in the presence of Leicester, if I be not deceived) maintain that poison might be so tempered and given as it should not appear presently, and yet should kill the party afterward at what time should be appointed.[42]

Bayley and Culpeper were also named as Leicester's agents in Oxford, letting him know when properties near the university became available and, when he praised their diligence on his behalf, becoming "so much the fitter for my lord's humor".[43]

The effect of the book was enormous in its time, and it survived to be translated, reissued, and treated as if it were documentary material. Leicester's nephew, Sir Philip Sidney, produced a passionate but unprinted rebuttal against the conspiracy theory based on common sense. Sidney ridiculed the attacker for accusing living persons who could presumably repudiate the charges made, and hinted that Bayley would be more than willing to testify for Leicester. Sidney, however, did not answer the exact accusations.[44] A twentieth-century work repeated the aspersion that Amy Dudley might have been murdered by "Leicester's hirelings," but exculpates Bayley as the source of a deadly potion.[45] Walter Bayley continued to enjoy a large practice in spite of the gossip engendered by *Leicester's Commonwealth*, published his medical theses, and died in 1593. He was buried in the inner chapel at New College. His son-in-law, Anthony Aylworth, succeeded him as Regius Professor of Physic and physician-in-ordinary to Queen Elizabeth.[46]

A contemporary of Bayley, Richard Master similarly held clerical office and a position of high regard in the minds of his peers. Born in Kent around 1525, he attended All Souls, Oxford, and after joining the Church of England thought he might become a clergyman. Instead, he returned to Oxford to study medicine and obtained a license to practice around the university. Master's medical epiphany may have come about as a result of an eighteen-month bout with a quartan fever in 1549, following which he obtained an M.D. from Christ Church College (later incorporated at Cambridge) and a Fellowship in the College of Physicians; in the ensuing years he filled the offices of censor (1556–60) and President (1561).[47] In June 1559 Elizabeth made him her personal physician. Evidently the earnings and bouche compensating royal doctors left Master a little short and in 1562 he accepted the post of prebendary of York. Property came his way, too, with his purchase of the site of a monastery in Cirencester for £590. Married to a Lincolnshire woman, Master had seven sons. He passed away in 1588 in his house on Silver Street in London.

Roger Gifford or Giffard was another of Elizabeth's many physicians. Born in Buckinghamshire, Gifford attended Merton and All Souls Colleges, Oxford, receiving his medical degree in 1566. According to Munk, Gifford was "created doctor of All Souls by Walter Baylie" at the instigation of a directive from the college convocation, the assembly of its graduates.[48] He served as President of the College of Physicians from 1581 to 1584, during which time he received a permanent dispensation for his dissection work. He succumbed to hematemesis in 1597 and was buried in St. Bride's, Fleet Street. Clippingdale calls Gifford a politico, a label he also applied to multidimensional John James, Member of Parliament. A native of the Isle of Wight and educated at Trinity College, Cambridge, James became the first English medical graduate of Leiden in 1581, three years after getting an M.D. in England; the College of Physicians made him a Fellow in 1584. Dr. James is recalled as an avid collector of plants, particularly the wild pea, which he sought with fellow Cambridge naturalist and mentor Thomas Penny, on the slopes of Mont Mole in Savoy.[49] James represented St. Ives, Cornwall, in the House of Commons in 1585 and Newcastle-under-Lyme in 1592–93. James tended to Leicester and to the Sidney household; he doctored Sir Philip Sidney in the fall of 1586 after Sidney was injured in a minor skirmish at the siege of Zutphen and the wound turned fatally gangrenous. Elizabeth named John James physician to her household in 1595; he died in 1601.[50]

Robert Jacob, described as a midwife-physician or man-midwife in the parlance of Elizabethan times, lived a life no less exciting than some of the famous English seadogs. He became a physician at the court of Russia's Ivan the Terrible. A native of London, Jacob received his undergraduate and graduate degrees by 1573 from Trinity College, Cambridge. He completed the medical program at Basel and, as was the custom to facilitate licensing by the Royal College of Physicians, his degree was incorporated at Cambridge in 1579. A physician to Queen Elizabeth, Jacob was held in the highest esteem for his skill as an accoucheur and for dealing with gynecological problems. After corresponding in Latin with Tsar Ivan IV about Jacob's talents, in the summer of 1581 the queen sent the doctor, "our physician," to the Russian royal household to attend Tsarina Maria Nagaia, largely on the recommendation of Englishman Jerome Horsey, a clerk of the Muscovy Company who had become a Russian court favorite.[51]

Jacob, accompanied by his brother, traveled in a convoy of thirteen Muscovy Company vessels, which was bringing sulphur, saltpetre, gunpowder, lead, and copper to the Company's depot on Rose Island, near present-day Archangel. Jacob then traveled overland to Moscow where he was greeted warmly and allowed to minister to the tsarina, who was troubled by difficult childbearing. Jacob had been given a hundred rubles by the Company upon his arrival, which sustained him until Christmas when the tsar awarded him a salary.[52]

Ivan IV was interested in establishing a permanent nexus with England, and as early as 1567 may have proposed marriage to Elizabeth.[53] Even though the tsar was already married, Dr. Jacob was consulted on a marital alternative to the queen herself, and he extolled to the tsar the qualities of thirty-year-old Lady Mary Hastings, daughter of the Earl of Huntingdon and a kinswoman to the queen on the Boleyn side. In 1583 Ivan sent a representative, Theodore Andreievitch Pissemsky, to England to negotiate an alliance, to propose marriage to Lady Mary, and to get all the physical minutiae on his latest potential fiancée. The tsar made it clear that his wife would have to convert to Orthodox Christianity and would have to accept monetary appanages for any offspring of the union rather than the throne itself. If no such agreement could be arranged, then Pissemsky should return to Moscow.[54]

In the face of the tsar's enthusiasm for an English bride, the queen displayed her consummate gift for delaying matters, but when Lady Mary learned the disturbing marital history of her suitor, she balked at the proposal. Elizabeth sent an official envoy, Sir Jerome Bowes, back with Pissemsky to dissuade the tsar from his choice and to smooth negotiations for a treaty specifying privileges for the Muscovy Company.[55] Luckily for everyone, Ivan died not too long after Bowes's arrival in Moscow, and Dr. Jacob, whose brother had died in Russia the previous year, returned to England with Bowes in March 1584. Once home, Jacob found that he was in trouble with the Muscovy Company, which rebuked him for trading on his own account while in Russia. The physician had evidently sent a large quantity of wax to England for his own profit, angering the Company and endangering its monopoly.[56] The censure was not serious enough to prevent Jacob at that time from being licensed by and admitted into the Royal College of Physicians.[57]

The charges were not unusual, however. Even Jerome Horsey, the former clerk of the Company and now a knight, was accused upon arriving in England with illegal trading. But Horsey had the queen's ear, and drew her attention to the medical needs of the new royal family in Moscow. He had a letter from Prince "Boris Fethorwich" (Boris Godunov) asking expressly for the return of Dr. Jacob.[58] Once again the queen called upon Jacob to go to Russia, this time with an unnamed midwife, to attend the spouse of the new tsar, Feodor I. Elizabeth wrote to Tsarina Irenia on March 24, 1586, praising Irenia's excellent qualities, to which Jacob had attested:

> We have not only sent you (as you lovingly requested us) an experienced and skilful midwife to assuage the pains of childbirth by her science, but We also send you with her the aforesaid Doctor Jacob our physician who has been wont to take care of our health (a man previously known to you, full of faith in the medical art in which he excels), in order that he may superintend the operations of the midwife, and faithfully tend your health. [59]

Accordingly, Jacob traveled again to the court of the tsar, as part of a new deputation sent from the queen and headed by Horsey.[60] Jacob arrived safely in the north and journeyed south overland to the capital, but the midwife was detained at Vologda, and was not permitted to enter Moscow. She returned to England in 1587 never having seen the tsarina.[61]

Jacob stayed on at the court during a difficult time. Due to differences in customs and attitudes about absolute sovereignty, the Russian leaders often took umbrage at the manner of their treatment by English emissaries. In a letter to Horsey, Prince Boris expressed amazement at what he deemed boorish foreign behavior, explicitly ungrateful, he commented, given his graciousness and protectiveness towards the English. The Prince Protector, as he was styled during Feodor's reign, specifically remarked that he "shewed mercy upon Robart [Dr. Jacob], [and] pardoned his offences."[62] Whatever the fuss, no more is heard of Dr. Robert Jacob. He died in Russia in the first half of 1588; his will was probated in England in June of that year.

No less thrilling is the career of Roger Marbeck, considered the chief of Elizabeth's royal physicians.[63] Marbeck was son of John Marbeck, who from 1541 was the organist of St. George's Chapel at Windsor. John Marbeck, a Calvinist, opposed the conservatism of Henrician church doctrine. When the king's commissioners in 1543 found heretical books in his lodgings, they dispatched Marbeck to Marshalsea Prison. He was interrogated by the Bishop of Winchester, tried by a jury at Windsor, and sentenced to die at the stake for heresy. The crown pardoned him because of his musical talents. Roger Marbeck, born in 1536, was educated at Eton and Christ Church, Oxford, graduating B.A. in 1555 and M.A. in 1558. Though there is no record of his ordination, he was appointed prebendary of Withington in Hereford Cathedral in 1559, Provost of Oriel College in 1564, and canon of Christ Church in 1565.

He may have left Oxford because of an unhappy or "disgraceful" marriage, but he took up medicine after his wife died.[64] After getting both his undergraduate and graduate medical degrees at the same time in 1573, Marbeck joined the College of Physicians in 1578, became its first registrar, and was elected to that post for life. He received 40s. per year and a bonus of 3s. 4d. for each new member brought in during his tenure; moreover, he collected when fines were paid and held other College offices simultaneously. As Elizabeth's physician to the household, Marbeck collected £134 6s. 8d. plus bouche and five dishes at each meal. Despite his rather lucrative position, in 1587 Marbeck begged off holding the College's feast in his house and paid a fine of £5 for this. At the age of fifty-three he was admitted to Gray's Inn, an honorary distinction reflecting his standing in medicine and the frequency of litigation involving the College registrar as the institution pursued illicit practitioners.[65] Marbeck's rather humdrum life took an adventurous turn in 1595 when he went with Leicester, his patron, to the Netherlands and in the following year he accompanied Lord High Admiral Charles Howard to Cadiz, leaving an account of the latter expedition.

Over a hundred pages of his handwritten Latin recipes for purgatives, tablets, hydragogues, and vomitories can be found in the Sloane Manuscripts;

among his correctives was a beverage for melancholy made with grated lemon, sugar, and borage.[66] In 1602 Marbeck published *A Defense of Tobacco*, one of the first English endorsements of the New World medicaments, such as ipecacuanha and cinchona, which would revolutionize English pharmacy. In it he argued that tobacco fit into the Galenic vision of four balanced elements in nature, providing the hot and dry components needed for good health; Marbeck touted tobacco's virtues as a purgative if used moderately and in an orderly fashion. His work was just the opening salvo in a prolonged debate over tobacco that included a future king. Roger Marbeck died in 1605 and was buried in London at St. Giles', Cripplegate.

Perhaps the most notorious of Elizabeth's doctors was Roderigo Lopez, executed in 1594 for joining a plot against her. Dr. Lopez, educated in Portugal and fluent in five languages, settled in England in 1559 and rapidly rose to prominence. Neither his Iberian origin nor his Jewish descent hindered his professional success. Moreover, Lopez was baptized and became a professing member of the Church of England. First house physician to St. Bartholomew's Hospital in 1567 and its resident officer (for which he received 40s. per year, "billets and coals"), Lopez was scheduled to read the anatomy lecture at the College of Physicians in 1570, but declined the assignment. The Fellows fined him for his refusal and probably harbored ill feelings toward him as a result. That same year the College forced Lopez to return £7 he had been paid for ostensibly healing a man with a swollen tibia, when the Fellows determined that the doctor had done nothing.[67] Despite these problems, the doctor numbered among his patients Sir Francis Walsingham, a man never in very good health, and was appointed medical adviser to the large household of the Earl of Leicester. *Leicester's Commonwealth* (1584), the libel on the earl and his cohort, Dr. Lopez, described as "the Jew," was credited like Drs. Bayley and Dee with skill in envenoming. He also served as an intelligence agent first for Walsingham, then after Walsingham's death for Lord Burghley, and "like many Marranos, he was deeply involved in secret diplomatic intrigues."[68] Lopez had a good practice, a sizable home in Holborn, a son attending Winchester College, and a promising monopoly importing aniseed and sumac. His father-in-law was Purveyor and Merchant for the Queen's Majesty's Grocery; another of his wife's relatives was vizier to the Sultan in Constantinople and England's "point man in the Sublime Porte."[69] Elizabeth made Lopez her physician-in-chief in 1586.

At war with Spain, England offered asylum to Philip II's enemies including in 1585 the bastard pretender to the Portuguese throne, Don Antonio, who lodged at Eton College near Windsor Castle while trying to raise support for his cause. Dr. Lopez became his intermediary with the queen and the center of a circle of Portuguese émigrés. He also became a spy for Spain against Don Antonio.[70] Portuguese double agents regularly stayed at Lopez' London house, and before long, their communications with the Spanish ambassador in Paris were intercepted by the English government. Although there is no extant evidence that Lopez conspired against Elizabeth, his Spanish connection proved catastrophic for him.[71] In 1593 at a party one night at Windsor, his tongue loosened by wine, Dr. Lopez maligned the sexual tastes of Elizabeth's darling, Robert Devereux, Earl of Essex, Leicester's successor as head of the war party. Informed of the slander, Essex determined to avenge himself.

Essex accumulated cryptic evidence against Lopez as a pro-Spanish provocateur, but Burghley considered the accusations against the doctor preposterous and the queen herself rebuked Essex for his suspicions. Letters, probably forgeries, further incriminated Lopez, but he maintained his innocence and argued that Walsingham had known of his plans, which were really aimed at double-crossing Spain. Unwilling to accept defeat, Essex prevailed when Lopez was implicated in skulduggery by two Portuguese agents, who confessed under torture that they were involved in a conspiracy to poison the queen. Xenophobic Englishmen found it hard to believe a Jew from Portugal, even one who had lived among them for thirty-five years, especially after Essex had Lopez detained at Essex House for investigation and then transferred to the Tower for further examination. Threatened with torture, Lopez confessed, a confession he later retracted but one that guaranteed his indictment.

Lopez' trial was held in the Guildhall on February 28, 1594, before a special commission presided over by Essex; throughout, Lopez insisted on his innocence. His denials meant little to prosecutor Sir Edward Coke who labeled him "a perjured, murdering villain and a Jewish doctor worse than Judas himself . . . [not] a new Christian . . . [but] a very Jew."[72] Coke's rhetoric convinced the commission, which convicted Lopez of high treason. Queen Elizabeth delayed signing the death sentence for several months, but on June 7 Lopez was taken to Tyburn Hill, site of the London gallows. When Lopez announced that he loved the Queen as he loved Christ, the assembled crowd hooted in derision. According to chronicler John Stow, Lopez and two others were then "hanged, cut downe alive, holden down by strength of men, dismembered, boweled, headed and quartered, their quarters set on the gates of the city."[73] Despite the forfeiture of Lopez' property upon his attainder, the queen deliberately permitted Sarah, the doctor's widow, and his family to retain a beneficial lease and his assets; Elizabeth also supported Lopez' son at Winchester through the grant of a parsonage of £30 per year. Not incidentally, Christopher Marlowe's *The Jew of Malta* began rehearsals in London on the same day that Lopez was taken to Essex House and William Shakespeare modeled his Shylock in *The Merchant of Venice* after Lopez, the only royal doctor to be executed in England.[74]

Prudently, most of Elizabeth's doctors tried to stay away from hazardous court machinations and concentrate on their professional lives. William Gilbert and Edward Lister attended Elizabeth in the last years of her reign; at the same time Gilbert continued his practice among the aristocracy of London, where he had settled in 1573. The Essex-born Gilbert, a 1569 graduate of St. John's, Cambridge, is well-known for his work with magnets, initiating the modern science of electricity, a word he invented, while remaining true to the traditions of "natural magic." Galileo, whose own work was inspired by Gilbert, spoke of him as "great to a degree that might be envied"; a more recent writer has called Gilbert "a mathematical practitioner."[75] Influenced by Caius and Gifford, Gilbert became known at court, thanks to his friendship with Leicester and Walsingham; he attended Lady Cecil in her last illness and later ministered to her husband. A lifelong bachelor, he received armorial bearings in 1577. At the time of the war with Spain, the Privy Council consulted him along with Elizabethan physicians Marbeck and Lancelot Browne for enlightenment on various diseases identified with naval service. A decade later, geographer and propagandist of overseas expansion Richard Hakluyt inquired of Gilbert about tropical sicknesses that might adversely affect travelers.[76]

Assisted by a pension from the queen, Gilbert conducted many experiments, leading to the publication in 1600 of *De Magnete*, the most important work on magnetism before the nineteenth century. In this work, Gilbert describes the methods for strengthening natural magnets and for using them to magnetize steel rods by stroking. Gilbert concluded that the earth behaves like a giant magnet with its poles near the geographic poles. He spent freely on laboratory investigation including an experiment using seventy diamonds to determine if a lodestone loses its powers. Despite his own fascination with magnetite, Gilbert denounced the use of lodestones in *De Magnete* as "evil and deadly advice."[77] Paracelsians found his work compatible with their cosmology, especially the part played by sympathetic or magnetic influences in treating wounds with weapon-salve.[78] An active Fellow of the College of Physicians, Gilbert was allocated a section on pills for its planned pharmacopoeia and sat on the editorial board in 1589. Though the compilation failed to come to fruition, Gilbert recorded in a written opinion that he approved the use of iron to treat anemia.[79] Besides his work on the pharmacopoeia, Gilbert provided leadership to the College as censor, treasurer, consiliarius and President in 1600. He cared for Elizabeth in her last illness. William Gilbert died in 1603 at age fifty-nine, probably of plague, leaving his valuable library of books, globes, and instruments to the College; the College buildings containing Gilbert's bequest were destroyed by the great London fire in 1666.

Yorkshire-born Edward Lister hailed from a distinguished medical family, progressing up the professional ladder via Eton and King's College, Cambridge, where he received his arts degrees and his M.D. in 1590. Fellowship in the College of Physicians followed in 1594; he was treasurer from 1612 to 1618. Married to Ann Farmery, a doctor's daughter, Lister continued his service to the crown as physician-in-ordinary to James I. He died in 1620 and was buried in St. Mary the Virgin, Aldermanbury. Lancelot Browne, a Yorkshireman like Lister who bridged the Tudor-Stuart dynasties, became Elizabeth's first physician toward the end of her reign. Browne had matriculated at St. John's, Cambridge, earning his arts degrees by 1566; he became a Fellow of Pembroke College and its proctor in 1573. Munk says that he was created an M.D. in 1576 and membership in the College of Physicians followed in 1584.[80] Browne was involved in 1594 in the College's prolonged attempt to create a pharmacopoeia, helping to prepare it for publication, but the undertaking failed to materialize. Briefly continuing his service as household physician after the queen's demise, he died in 1604. Lancelot Browne's daughter married famed Jacobean doctor William Harvey.

One "irregular" whom Elizabeth consulted was the eminent magus, John Dee. Author of seventy-nine works, Dee was well acquainted with the philosophical currents of Renaissance magic and was inspired by rediscovered Hermetic texts to work with the forces of nature through magic.[81] Something of an anomaly among English humanists, Dee sought the complete community of all beings and objects. Though not a medical doctor, Dee was a founding Fellow of Trinity College and the recipient of a law degree from Louvain; more pertinent to Elizabethan times, Dee was tutor to the Dudley household, the boyhood teacher of Leicester. He had been imprisoned during the Marian reaction on false charges of treason, but was acquitted to enjoy happier times under Gloriana and was welcome at court as the queen's philosopher. That position included astrological and mystical responsibilities, such as choosing the most propitious day for the queen's coronation or counteracting harm intended against her. Moreover, explorers consulted Dee about their impending voyages, politicians sought his guidance about affairs of state, and in 1583 the queen asked him to reform the Julian Calendar for Britain, a project that failed.

As a "physician," Dee embraced Paracelsian medical innovations, many of which had their roots in the alchemical traditions of the Middle Ages. In particular, Dee applauded Paracelsus's search for a "universal dissolvent" or "liquor Alkahest" and his distillations and "projections."[82] Dee himself searched for the philosopher's stone. Internationally celebrated for his diverse studies but always in financial distress, Dee hoped to obtain permanent financial support from Elizabeth to sustain further scholarly work; in 1564 he received the grant of a deanery in Gloucester, but not until 1596 did he acquire wardenship of Christ's College, Manchester. As mentioned earlier, Dee accompanied Walter Bayley to Germany in 1578 to discuss the queen's bothersome dental problems with continental specialists. In appreciation, Elizabeth accorded Dee rectories at Upton and Long Leadenham, but, in the midst of work on calendar reform, the distracted magus neglected to procure attachment of the Great Seal to the legal documents awarding him the properties. He estimated that the oversight cost him £1,000 that he could ill afford.

On the continent from 1583 to 1589, John Dee befriended a disreputable occultist and conjurer, Edward Kelly; evidently, he and Kelly exchanged wives. While he was abroad, a mob, believing Dee to be a sorcerer, broke into his house at Mortlake and destroyed many of his books and instruments. Though discredited by his association with Kelly's frauds, Dee remained in demand as a magician and Elizabeth herself asked him to return to England. His magic mirror, made of polished cannel coal, fascinated believers and skeptics alike. Perhaps out of loyalty to the Earl of Essex, Leicester's stepson, Dee testified against Roderigo Lopez in 1594. Despite the sympathies of the queen, the public regarded Dee as a necromancer. After her demise there was no support for him at the court of a new king terrified of wizards. At the end of his own career, Dee was miserably poor and perished in poverty in 1608. J. O. Halliwell edited John Dee's diary in 1842.[83] His eldest son and fellow alchemist, Arthur Dee, would enjoy a happier career as recipient of James I's tribute and as physician-in-ordinary to Charles I.

The venerable *Dictionary of National Biography* (first published 1885–1901) refers to Elizabethan doctor Edward Atslowe as "one of her physicians" whom the queen sent (along with royal surgeon Robert Balthrop) to minister to John Dee when the magus fell ill. Atslowe was likely an ad hoc appointee for that assignment, but he was certainly well-known for his medical skill, devotion to Catholicism, and ardent support of Mary, Queen of Scots. Educated at Winchester and New College, Oxford, Atslowe received his M.D. in 1566. That same year he disputed before the queen when she visited the university. He joined the College of Physicians in 1569, accepted several of its offices, and became the household doctor of Thomas Radcliffe, Earl of Sussex. However, Atslowe's enthusiasm for the Scottish queen and his involvement in plots to liberate her doubtless ended whatever court blessing he might have held and may have put his patron in jeopardy, for after the physician visited Mary Stuart at Tutbury in 1570, Elizabeth suspected Sussex of disloyalty.[84] Atslowe was racked in the Tower, but released. His politics probably got him into trouble with the College of Physicians, although its records indicate only that he owed £60 to the institution, probably accumulated fines for refusing to attend meetings in 1582. The following year Atslowe attended Sussex throughout a long illness that ended in death and in 1587 he ministered to Henry Percy, Earl of Northumberland, during Northumberland's own fatal sickness. Atslowe died in 1594.[85]

An even more irregular medical consultant to the queen than Dee was Margaret Kennix, described in the College of Physicians' records as "an outlandish, ignorant, sorry woman."[86] In 1581 Francis Walsingham requested of the Fellows on behalf of Queen Elizabeth that Kennix be allowed to administer "her small talent and craft" in medicine. He entreated them:

> Whereas heretofore by her Majesties commandment upon the pityful complaint of Margaret Kennix, I wrote . . . signifying how that it was her Highness pleasure that the poore wooman shoold be permitted by you quietly to practise and mynister to the curing of diseases and wounds, by the means of certain Simples, in the applieing whereof it seemeth God hath given her an especiall knowledge, to the benefit of the poorer sort, and chiefly for the better maintenance of her impotent husband, and charge of Family, who wholy depend on the exercise of her skill.

Evidently, the Fellows had been moving against Kennix as an "empirick and unlicensed practiser," contrary to Elizabeth's preference. Such cases usually involved fines and imprisonment. Walsingham insinuated to the Fellows that, unless they let her be, Kennix would renew her complaint to the queen and "further inconvenience" might befall the College. Though the Fellows politely refused Walsingham's entreaty, there appears to have been no royal repercussion against them.[87] Nonetheless, Elizabeth's exceptional intervention in the business of the College, however restrained, reveals the queen's close tie to Margaret Kennix, possibly as a recipient of the wise woman's care.

Besides her physicians, after 1560 two serjeant surgeons cared for the monarch's health, and from time to time supplementary appointments were made with the title of serjeant- surgeon extraordinary, a post that usually carried with it a reversion to the principal serjeant-surgeoncy on the next vacancy. Elizabethan surgeons included Thomas Vicary, a holdover from her father's reign who still dominated the Barber-Surgeons' Company, Richard Ferris, Thomas Gale, and Robert Balthrop (Balthorp), Nicholas Alcocke's apprentice. Bequeathed one hundred marks by Henry VIII, Ferris attended Elizabeth I briefly as serjeant-surgeon in 1562 when he was probably felled by illness; he expired four years later, remembered for an illustrious career in the Barber-Surgeons' Company. Ferris' name is on the frontispiece of an illuminated manuscript called "The Lanterne of Hygiene," a Galenic text of 234 folios with marginal notes that might be Ferris's. It contains recipes and instructions for setting broken bones.[88]

Born in 1507, Thomas Gale, a contemporary of Vicary's and apprentice to Ferris, served in Henry VIII's army in France in 1544 and described the horrifying conditions he himself witnessed in the campaign for Boulogne. Sowgelders, tinkers, and cobblers took on the duties of surgeons, dressing and treating wounds with dreadful concoctions made from grease used for treating horses' hooves and shoemakers' wax. With these "medicines," even minor wounds turned fatal. Gale returned to London to a successful career as a writer and teacher. Master of the Barber-Surgeons in 1561, he wrote a volume in 1563 about battlefield surgery for bullet wounds, *An Excellent Treatise on Wounds made with Gunneshot*, dedicated to Leicester. That same year he produced his *Enchiridion of Surgery* and in 1566 he translated Galen into English because so few surgeons understood Latin. One historian of the surgeons believes that the paucity of surgical and anatomical books during Vicary's lifetime and the publication of several works immediately following his death point to control by Gale.[89] After a 1562 visitation of St. Bartholomew's and St. Thomas' Hospitals, Gale depicted in trenchant detail the woeful condition of over three hundred patients, many the victims of quack surgery and mischief by charlatans. Gale reported that at least 120 of them "could never be recovered without loss of a leg or an arm, a foot or a hand, fingers or toes, or else their limbs crooked so that they were either maimed or else undone for ever." Elizabeth recognized his leadership in the field and selected him her serjeant-surgeon.[90] Thomas Gale died in 1586.

Robert Balthrop was the queen's serjeant surgeon from 1562 to 1591 and Master of the Barber-Surgeons on a number of occasions. He accumulated a considerable estate and left a lengthy will disposing of his valuable surgical instruments and books. He died 1591 and is buried in the church of St. Bartholomew-the-Less within St. Bartholomew's Hospital, to which he was surgeon. His monument on the south wall of the church reads:

> Here Robert Balthrop lyes intombed, to
> Elizabeth our Queene,
> Who Serjeant of the Surgeons swore neere
> thirtye yeeres hath beene
> He died at sixty-nine of yeers December's
> ninth the daye
> The yeere of Grace eight hundred twice
> deducting nine a waye
> Let here his rotten bones repose, till angells
> trompet sounds,
> To warne the world of present chaunge, and
> raise the dead from grounde.[91]

Balthrop bequeathed a gold enameled lancet to William Gooderus (Guddridge), his immediate successor as Elizabeth's serjeant surgeon and Master of his guild in 1594; he willed his syringe and three silver pipes to George Baker, who became serjeant-surgeon in 1597.[92] Besides the queen, Gooderus doctored Leicester's ally Henry Herbert, Earl of Pembroke, and personally sought out whatever ingredients were needed for his cures. According to his friend and fellow naturalist Thomas Muffet, the surgeon killed a hoopoe, a sharp-billed, crested bird, in Clandon Park for Pembroke's health.[93] Gooderus, who attended the wounded in the expedition to the Low Countries in 1585 under the Earl of Leicester, in turn was followed by George Baker in 1597, although records indicate that Gooderus remained in aulic service until 1603 and into the reign of James I, perhaps because of Baker's death in 1600.[94]

Born in Kent in 1540, George Baker came on the medical scene in the 1560s, just as the war between Galenists and Paracelsians heated up. Baker walked an Elizabethan middle path by encouraging experimentation while denigrating Paracelsus as a physician compared to Galen. At the outset of his career, Baker clearly lambasted empirics and "Paracellistes" who had done great harm to their patients.[95] However, Baker himself experimented with distillations in 1574 while attached as surgeon to the household of Edward de Vere, Earl of Oxford, and concluded that dehydrated medicines exceeded all others in power and value. He wrote *The New Jewell of Health* in 1576, dedicating the work to the Countess of Oxford; in it, he claimed one could find "the most excellent secrets of physick and philosophy." He defended publishing his remedies in English, to which physicians objected, and lauded the Paracelsian alchemy that produced recipes for balms and oils, and instructions for the furnaces in which they were cooked. Baker provided the conduit through which Paracelsian remedies and chemical medicine received a favorable introduction to "the most enterprising and enlightened group of surgeons" in England.[96]

Inclined to endorse other popular manuals, an anti-establishment posture if ever there was one, Baker composed a preface to John Gerard's famous English herbal in which Baker is identified as "chief chirugion in ordinary."[97] In his own short treatise on "quicksilver," which he touted as a cure for smallpox, scabs, and worms in children, Baker denied that Galen had ever called mercury a poison. Moreover, Baker translated into English a pamphlet on a healing oil by a Morisco empiric, Aparicio de Zubia. Besides his support for alternative medicine, Baker's loyalty to the surgeons and determination to defend their prerogatives manifested itself on enough occasions to rile the College of Physicians. Master of the Barber-Surgeons, Baker refused a summons by the College beadle to appear before the Fellows, saying he was too busy and they should not bother him. The beadle related that he found Baker "saucie."[98]

Samuel Clippingdale reported that Baker and William Clowes, then surgeon at two London-area hospitals, quarreled at a Barbers' Company meeting in 1577 and carried their disagreement over to an adjoining tavern; later they so "misused each other that they fought in the fields together."[99] Their colleagues pardoned them so that they might become friends once again and, as evidence of their renewed accord, the two each edited a work by the other in 1579. The records do not make clear what the surgeons tussled over, but it may have been about the extent of Clowes's published criticism of other surgeons. Baker urged keeping the secrets of the surgeon's trade, if not the physician's, within the livery and supporting one's fellows, while Clowes advocated the exposure of incompetent surgeons, especially those in the military who, he opined in a manual, "A Proud Practice for All Young Surgeons," slew more than the enemy. This handwritten album contains Latin recipes for pills, clysters, suppositories, and an ointment made of puppy-dog fat.[100]

Clowes had the last laugh, emerging from the altercation with Baker to become according to some historians "the greatest surgeon during the reign of Elizabeth I," one who could distinguish "between proud, prattling Paracelsians" and the "good works of the right Paracelsians."[101] Born between 1540 and 1544, Clowes became another key member of the Leicester medical circle, having studied surgery under George Keble, Master of the Barber-Surgeons' Company, when John Caius taught anatomy to the members at their hall.[102] He then served for a period in the army and navy. Clowes's career as a surgeon owed much to his solid civilian training, but was shaped even more by his extensive wartime experience outside of England. In 1563 he began his affiliation with the Dudley family.

That year Clowes contracted to be surgeon to the ill-fated three-thousand-man army of Ambrose Dudley, Earl of Warwick, sent to Normandy to aid the Huguenot leader, the Prince de Condé, in his struggle against the French king. However, when the French factions reconciled temporarily, they turned collectively on the foreign interlopers and attacked the English garrison in Normandy. The training Clowes received during the siege was brutal but invaluable. However, because the English forces were trapped at Le Havre for months, plague and scurvy took their deadly toll. After surrender of the English forces, Clowes chose to remain on active duty, and based in Portsmouth, he worked on the queen's ships until 1569. During that time he became a specialist in treating syphilis; by 1570 he was back in London, and he developed a large clientele in the city.

Clowes's years of military service, coupled with wide reading and a willingness to accommodate continental techniques in his practice, made him successful in the capital. He wrote:

> if I find anything that may be to the good of the patients, and better increase my knowledge and skill in the art of surgery, be it either in Galen or Paracelsus; yea Turk, Jew or any other infidel: I will not refuse it, but be thankful to God for the same.[103]

He was appointed surgeon at St. Bartholomew's Hospital in 1575 and surgeon to children and the poor at Christ's Hospital the following year. He also began to publish, first a small book on syphilis in 1576, but his magnum opus was *De Morbo Gallico,* issued in Latin in 1579 and translated into English in 1585, which discussed the use of unctions in treating syphilis; a third edition appeared in 1585. Medical historian Norman Moore has called Clowes's work "the very best surgical writings of the Elizabethan age."[104] Clowes's prefatory address to the general reader of *De Morbo Gallico* demonstrates his recognition of a nascent medical marketplace no longer controlled by physicians with venerable secrets. In fact, the very act of publishing a medical treatise at all fuses Clowes with those surgeons and apothecaries wishing to make "Everyman" his own doctor. Powerful physicians denounced this affront to their prerogatives; most of the books published by members of the College of Physicians during Clowes's time were written by Fellows of marginal status.[105]

William Clowes epitomized the excellence of the medical men in the Leicester circle. However, despite his apprenticeship to Keble and his established reputation, Clowes was only a licensee of the Barber-Surgeons as late as 1580. The queen intervened and insisted on his full membership in the Company after an examination.[106] Clowes resigned his surgeoncy at St. Bartholomew's in 1585 to accompany Leicester to the Low Countries, a mission closely chronicled in Clowes's book, *A Prooved Practice,* first published in 1588.[107] Again Clowes was faced with the horrors of warfare made worse by plague and malaria. Again he gained enormous practical experience on a foreign field, which he described for future doctors. He learned of Jean Tagault's method for extracting an untracked bullet and put the new method to good use. He described for others who would be battlefield doctors the minimal contents of a military medical chest. In addition, he had to deal with incompetent "false surgeons" whom he expelled from Leicester's camp.[108]

Clowes received appointment in 1587 as Surgeon to the Fleet. Though there is no record to confirm it, Clowes was probably aboard Admiral Howard's flagship, *Ark Royal,* when the Armada was sighted the following year. He would later describe with great care treating sailors' fractured ribs, burns from gunpowder, *mal de mer,* and scurvy at sea. In recognition of his naval service and his preeminence within the medical profession, Clowes was chosen at age forty-four as one of the queen's "chirurgeons" in September 1588. His appointment was continued by James I.[109]

Clowes's *Book of Observations* was published in 1591 as was a second printing of *A Prooved Practice*. His son, William Clowes, Junior, was apprenticed to him at about that time and eventually became a royal surgeon himself.[110] In 1597 the veteran surgeon moved to the Essex countryside. The Barber-Surgeons' records indicate that many complaints against Clowes had been filed with the guild over the years, but with the monarch's approbation, criticism did not topple him from the apex of the surgical world. Clowes's *Treatise on the King's Evil,* published in 1602, did much to cement the monarch's favor. In this work, the surgeon argued for the monarch's touch for strumas when physic and surgery did not prove efficacious. William Clowes succumbed to plague in the epidemic of 1604.

Just as Elizabeth kept many physicians and surgeons busy during her long reign, she also relied on several apothecaries for her own and her household's pharmaceutical needs. John Hemingway, apothecary to Elizabeth's father and to her half-brother, attended the queen for many years, beginning when she succeeded Mary. He kept fastidious records, of which the register for a six-month period in 1664 survives, listing various medicines and fragrances supplied to the royal household. Hemingway perfumed certain rooms including closets, chambers, and chapels with rosewater and cloves; he scented the queen's elaborate, jeweled dresses with benjamin and storax. When Elizabeth began to lose her hair steadily after the age of twenty-five, Hemingway made pomades and salves. His unguents did not stop her hair loss, so she changed her hairstyle in 1664 and wore curls to cover the bald crown of her head.[111]

The court apothecary supplied urinals for the queen's councillors at a cost of 3d. each; his powders and rosewater kept public rooms free of disagreeable odors. Hemingway's records also make reference to orris powders and ten-ounce glasses of rosewater "for the perfume pan in the private chamber."[112] As Elizabeth moved from palace to palace, it was Hemingway's task to prepare royal residences in anticipation of the queen's arrival, supervising the airing and cleaning of rooms. He did not merely mask unpleasant smells for an overly fussy monarch, her nobles, and foreign dignitaries. Physicians regarded stench as unwholesome; corrupt air could cause illnesses like plague. Thus, Hemingway made certain that even the royal litter shielded Elizabeth from deleterious smells.

John Hemingway's account book indicates how demanding the Elizabethan household must have been, with so many members of the queen's retinue needing his services. With his son, Edward, as yeoman apothecary, he made their pills, plasters, powders, clysters, suppositories, and candy lozenges; he brewed spiced wine, mixed cosmetics and cold creams, and prepared aromatic, therapeutic baths in what seems to have resembled an enclosed wooden sauna. Two of the queen's doctors, Richard Masters and Robert Huicke, examined Hemingway's ledgers and verified the charges. Besides paying for his services, Elizabeth rewarded Hemingway in 1562 with a valuable thirty-year lease on former monastic property in Yorkshire, his native county.[113]

John Ryche became royal apothecary in 1576, probably at the time of John Hemingway's death, and maintained service to the queen until 1592 when he fell seriously ill. A member of the Grocers' Company, Ryche gained significant renown as a botanist, garnering the attention of no less a personage than botanist William Turner, Dean of Wells and a physician. Turner cited Ryche many times in his three-volume *Herball*, and he was evidently in correspondence with Ryche while botanizing along the Rhine. According to Turner, Ryche's physic garden yielded "good and strange herbs" not seen anywhere else in England.[114] Like other aulic servants, Ryche acquired considerable wealth and property—land, mills, and tenements—including a house in Deptford through which a water conduit ran. In his will, Ryche requested that the flow continue for the benefit of the community. At his death in 1593, he bequeathed money to the Grocers' Company to host a lavish dinner for its liverymen to be held on the day of his funeral.

Essex-born Hugh Morgan was an exceptional Tudor apothecary, perhaps the most illustrious of all.[115] Apprenticed to Londoner William Chikke for nine years, Morgan rose up through the ranks of his craft in the usual way, becoming a freeman of the Grocers' Company in 1543 and member of the livery in 1563. He set up a house and shop near Coleman Street and later, as prosperity permitted, increased his holdings with a house and garden in Battersea. Morgan was an evident leader among the Grocers; he attracted the attention of the College of Physicians in 1556 and again in 1559 when he was chastised by the Fellows for selling pills without a doctor's permission.[116] Their rebuke does not seem to have hurt his reputation. He served Queen Elizabeth from 1559 as a yeoman apothecary, and the date of her "discovery" of his talents may not be coincidental. That same year Morgan took a party of soldiers impressed by the Grocers' Company to Greenwich where they constituted one of the City-trained bands reviewed by the queen. In 1583 she made Morgan principal apothecary for the household, a position he held until her death.

Morgan's professional standards were impeccable and helped to raise public confidence that the apothecary-members of the Grocers' Company could police themselves. Morgan was often called upon to audit the accounts of the Company, and in 1564 at the behest of his comrades, he inspected for purity drugs sold by other apothecaries, especially rhubarb, wormseed, scammony, and manna.[117] Since he grew many specimens of herbs gathered by those who voyaged to Virginia, some of them very rare like the Judas Tree, Morgan was uniquely equipped to judge the utility of vegetable material. Moreover, he extended the scope of the physic garden by contacting many of the great continental pharmacists, exchanging seeds and samples with others interested in the medicinal aspects of herbs.[118] During his investigation of London drug stocks, Morgan found so many leaves, berries, and resins contaminated and unusable that the Company court ordered them burned in the fireplace of Grocers' Hall. The guild generally appreciated Morgan's efforts; he was elected a warden in 1574 and was to be Master in 1583 when the queen elevated him to the post of principal apothecary on her medical staff.

Despite Morgan's endeavors to assure the authenticity of various medicines, he squabbled with the Grocers' Company over treacle or theriacle. Paracelsus posited that poisons ranked among the most valuable medicines available if chemists removed the toxic qualities so that they might be administered internally. Morgan invented a mixture that depended to some extent on that principle. He claimed that his multi-ingredient formula, sanctioned by the College of Physicians, rivalled that of Venetian molasses, and that several members of the Company sold unacceptable treacle to the detriment of the health of Elizabeth's subjects. Morgan asserted that genuine theriacle, sometimes containing up to seventy substances mixed with honey, could protect victims from the bites of poisonous animals. He denounced the barrels of a "false and naughty kind of mithridatium and threacle" that entered England daily. After arbitration by the Lord Mayor, the Company accepted the truth of Morgan's charges and fined some apothecaries for selling inferior concoctions.[119]

Hugh Morgan passed away in 1613, possibly over one hundred years of age, after serving for a time as a sort of honorary apothecary extraordinary in the household of Elizabeth's Scottish successor, James I.[120] Morgan left money to the poor of several parishes, trinkets for his relatives, and a special ring for his former apprentice and successor in royal service, George Shiers. Another assistant apothecary destined for service in the next reign, William Weston, joined Elizabeth's staff in 1587 and by 1594 had secured a pension for life of £20 per year. One New Year's gift list includes Weston's present to the queen of three boxes of peaches.

During her dotage, the queen endured many physical afflictions typical of the elderly. She may have inherited her father's tendency to varicose veins and she suffered for many years from an ulcerated leg. Recurrent fevers bothered her and she endured a bout of chickenpox in 1572 and whooping cough in 1580. Tight-laced corsets made breathing and eating difficult, causing occasional attacks of faintness and digestive disturbances; her teeth and gums pained her constantly. Nonetheless, Elizabeth's constitution enabled her to live a long life; her decision to forgo purging and bleeding after about 1572 probably maintained her relatively good health. Given the startling mortality associated with childbirth, the Virgin Queen avoided a common cause of early death. Considering the era she lived in, when plague and other contagious diseases were rife, the ailments she endured and survived attest to her strength. The queen's last illness involved some disease of the throat, perhaps tubercular laryngitis, for she had trouble speaking and experienced marked swelling and excessive sputum. Sir Arthur MacNalty, however, argues for streptococcal infection of the tonsils and abscess, followed by a fatal attack of influenza.[121] In spite of a brave attempt to carry on with her accustomed activities, Elizabeth felt and looked haggard. She refused to go to bed and her mind was somewhat disordered; on March 24, 1603, the last Tudor monarch died.

Notes

1. The source for Seymour's purported February 1547 proposal to Elizabeth is the unreliable Gregorio Leti, *La vie d'Elisabeth reine d'Angleterre* (Amsterdam: Chez Henri Desbordes, 1714), 160–63.

2. Wallace MacCaffrey, *Elizabeth I* (London: Edward Arnold, 1993), 9.

3. Biographies of the Virgin Queen abound. Among the most recent and readable are MacCaffrey, *Elizabeth I*; Christopher Haigh, *Elizabeth I* (London: Longman, 1988); Carole Levin, *The Heart and Stomach of a King* (Philadelphia: University of Pennsylvania Press, 1994); Jasper Ridley, *Elizabeth I* (New York: Viking, 1987); and Anne Somerset, *Elizabeth I* (New York: Knopf, 1991). Physician-historian Sir Arthur MacNalty includes a chapter in his life of Elizabeth called "The Queen's Medical Case-Sheet": MacNalty, *Elizabeth Tudor,* 220–46.

4. Elizabeth's gratitude extended to the doctor's brother, William Bille, Edward's itinerant chaplain and Master of Trinity College, Cambridge, until his expulsion under Mary I. A decade after her cure by Dr. Bille, Elizabeth restored Master Bille to his post. Munk, *Roll* 1: 35.

5. Carolly Erickson, *The First Elizabeth* (New York: Summit Books, 1983), 116.

6. Add. MSS 34563, f. 65, British Library. Elizabeth had another attack of nephritis in 1561, but "never showed symptoms of the chronic form of the disease": MacNalty, *Elizabeth Tudor,* 245.

7. Weir, *Children of Henry VIII*, 270–71.

8. Weir, *Children of Henry VIII*, 334; Erickson, *The First Elizabeth*, 147. Sir Hector MacLennan posited that Elizabeth may have suffered from chronic nephritic toxemia: MacLennan, "Gynecologist," 70.

9. Bloch, *Royal Touch*, 190.

10. Bloch points out that "not a single genuine cramp ring has come down to us" and that ensuing generations doubted their secret virtues: ibid.

11. Cited in Erickson, *The First Elizabeth*, 417, n.3. The Spanish ambassador confirmed that Elizabeth's physicians thought she was too unhealthy to have children.

12. J. R. Clemens, "Notes on English Medicine," *Annals of Medical History*, New Series, 3 (January 1931): 308.

13. Elizabethan physicians knew that if the smallpox pustules converged, blanketing the body, the victim would die of shock; the virus had detached the whole skin.

14. Annals of the Royal College of Physicians, vol. 1, f. 22a, LRCP.

15. Charles Webster, *From Paracelsus to Newton* (Cambridge: Cambridge University Press, 1982). Webster says that French Paracelsianism was at its height between 1610 and 1650, English Paracelsianism after 1650. See also Eric Maple, *Magic, Medicine and Quackery* (S. Brunswick, N.J.: A. S. Barnes, 1968), 74; Hugh Trevor-Roper, *Renaissance Essays* (Chicago: University of Chicago Press, 1985), 156–57.

16. Debus, *English Paracelsians*, 30, 157.

17. Maple, *Magic, Medicine, and Quackery*, 72.

18. Porter and Rousseau, *Gout*, 25. Paracelsus offered no therapies, however, for tartarous diseases.

19. Trevor-Roper, *Renaissance Essays*, 159.

20. Trevor-Roper, "Court Physician and Paracelsianism," 91. Sir George Clark wrote that "until the statutes were revised in 1601 the corporate fidelity of the College to Galen was unimpaired": Clark, *Royal College of Physicians* 1: 165.

21. Annals of the College of Physicians, vol. 1, f. 22a, LRCP.

22. After 1585, those who finished their degrees at Oxford or Cambridge in less than normal time paid double fees; Annals of the College of Physicians, vol. 2, f. 46a, LRCP.

23. Debus, *English Paracelsians*, 24, 57, 62.

24. Trevor-Roper, "Court Physician and Paracelsianism," 90–91.

25. Debus, *English Paracelsians*, 24. Many renowned continental physicians converted quickly to Paracelsianism; these included Petrus Severinus, doctor to the king of Denmark, and Vesalius' teacher, Winter von Andernach. See also Trevor-Roper, *Renaissance Essays*, 160, 178.

26. Erickson, *The First Elizabeth*, 252.

27. A listing of Elizabeth's physicians can be found in MacNalty, *Elizabeth Tudor*, 261–64.

28. As recorded in John Nichols, ed., *Progresses and Public Processions of Queen Elizabeth*, 3 vols. (London: printed by the editor, 1788–1805), she gave gifts to her apothecary Hugh Morgan and to doctors Huicke, Master, Bayley, Browne, Lopez, Morecroft, and Browne. See 2: 73, 105, 209; 3: 140.

29. Munk, *Roll* 1: 32. Huicke's position made him the target of favor-seekers like a Mr. Ludford, who applied for admission to the College but who, in Huicke's view, lacked competency based on an examination: Add. MSS 5873, f. 97b, British Library.

30. Clippingdale, Medical Court Roll, 1: 36, LRCS.

31. According to Debus, "chemical therapy had won acceptance in England not by overturning the Galenic system, but by allying itself to it." Debus, *English Paracelsians*, 176. The Elizabethan compromise lasted until the mid-seventeenth century.

32. Allen G. Debus, "The Paracelsian Compromise in Elizabethan England," *Ambix* 8 (1960): 95. Bayley gave a copy of his *Brief Discourse* to Walsingham, who may have been his patient: Nati H. Krivatsy, "Walsingham's Copy of Bailey's *Brief Discourse*," *Library*, series 6, 1 (1979): 166–68.

33. SL MSS 1660, f. 29b, British Library. Bayley's three principal publications, all privately printed, are *Preservation of Eyesight* (1586), *Baths or Waters* (1587), and *Peppers* (1588). For more on Bayley, see L. G. Horton-Smith, *Dr. Walter Bailey* (St. Alban's, England: Campfield Press, 1952) and D'Arcy Power, *Dr. Walter Bayley and His Works, 1529–1592* (London: Royal Medical and Chirurgical Society of London, 1907). Power calls Bayley a Wykehamist, a follower of William of Wykeham, the vigorous clerical reformer who founded Winchester and New Colleges, the latter being Bayley's alma mater. Disputing Munk, Power also says that Bayley was not a Fellow of the College of Physicians. See Munk, *Roll* 1: 80; Power, *Bayley*, 438.

34. For an examination of Dee's life and work, see French, *John Dee*.

35. Eleanor Rosenberg, *Leicester: Patron of Letters* (New York: Columbia University Press, 1955), 35–36; Leslie G. Matthews asserts that both Leicester and Burghley were "favorable to empirics": "Italian Charlatans in England," 2–5.

36. Quoted in N.H. Nicolas, *Memoirs of the Life and Times of Sir Christopher Hatton* (London: Richard Bentley, 1847), 69. Buxton Spa, with its spring named for St. Ann, was on the Earl of Shrewsbury's property and was equipped with a row of houses used for bathers' lodgings. Elizabeth Jenkins, *Elizabeth and Leicester* (New York: Coward-McCann, 1962), 213.<notes>37. Jenkins, *Elizabeth and Leicester*, 237.

38. See the Bayley entry in the *DNB* by Norman Moore; Krivatsy, "Walsingham's Copy of Bailey's *Brief Discourse*," 167.

39. Clippingdale asserts that Dee was paid a regular salary by the Secretary of State for his espionage activities. Clippingdale, Medical Court Roll, 1: 436, LRCS.

40. For a recent, readable edition see D. C. Peck, ed., *Leicester's Commonwealth* (Athens: Ohio University Press, 1985).

41. Quoted in Milton Waldman, *Elizabeth and Leicester* (Boston: Houghton-Mifflin, 1945), 170.

42. Peck, *Leicester's Commonwealth*, 82.

43. Ibid., 116.

44. Jenkins, *Elizabeth and Leicester*, 294–95.

45. Arthur MacNalty, *The Doctor in Politics and Diplomacy* (London: privately printed, 1937), 6. More recent scholars have suggested that advanced breast cancer is very likely to have contributed to Lady Dudley's fatal fall; see, for instance, Erickson, *The First Elizabeth*, 197.

46. I have not found mention of Aylworth elsewhere, but MacNalty notes a memorial brass to him in the antechapel at New College: MacNalty, *Elizabeth Tudor,* 263.

47. Master's medical degree was incorporated by Cambridge University in 1571. Munk, *Roll* 1: 52.

48. Munk, *Roll* 1: 68.

49. Raven, *English Naturalists*, 160, 172–73.

50. Munk, *Roll* 1: 87.

51. Annals of the College of Physicians, vol. 2, f. 50a, LRCP, contains a letter from the queen to the Russian emperor and empress. See also J. Hamel, *England and Russia,* trans. John S. Leigh (New York: DaCapo: 1968), 236.

52. Hamel, *England and Russia,* 236.

53. Edward A. Bond, the editor of Horsey's journal, notes that there is no documentary evidence of this proposal. See Bond's introduction to *Russia at the Close of the Sixteenth Century* (London: Hakluyt Society, 1856).

54. Ibid.

55. The tsar was not pleased with the English response to his proposal, and treated Bowes rather badly while permitting him to represent England at court. See Ridley, *Elizabeth I,* 315.

56. Hamel, *England and Russia,* 237.

57. Munk, *Roll* 1: 88.

58. Bond, *Russia at the Close,* appendix II, 292. Boris Godunov was Feodor's brother-in-law.

59. Hamel, *England and Russia,* 235. The Latin text is appendix Z, 421.

60. See Horsey's account of his second and third royal assignments in Russia, in Bond, *Russia at the Close,* appendix II.

61. Hamel, *England and Russia,* 235.

62. Bond, *Russia at the Close,* appendix II, 293. Bond does not specify what those offenses are, but Jacob's earlier trading against the rights of the Muscovy Company might have been the problem.

63. Munk, *Roll* 1: 75.

64. A.G.W. Whitfield, "Roger Marbeck—First Registrar," *Journal of the Royal College of Physicians of London* 15/1 (1981): 59. Marbeck had no children and did not remarry.

65. Whitfield, "Roger Marbeck," 60.

66. SL MSS 1349, British Library.

67. Annals of the College of Physicians (English typescript), vol. 1, p. 47, LRCP.

68. William Meyers, "Shakespeare, Shylock, and the Jews," *Commentary* 101 (April 1996): 34. See also Margaret Hotine, "The Politics of Anti-Semitism: 'The Jew of Malta' and 'The Merchant of Venice,' " *Notes and Queries* 38 (March 1991): 35.

69. Arthur Dimock, "The Conspiracy of Dr. Lopez," *English Historical Review* 9 (1894): 440–41; Meyers, "Shakespeare, Shylock," 34. Lopez' in-laws were from Antwerp, source of the Leicester libel.

70. Trevor-Roper, "Medicine in Politics," 38. See also David S. Katz, *The Jews in the History of England, 1485–1850* (Oxford: Clarendon Press, 1994); and Lucien Wolf, "Jews in Elizabethan England," *Transactions of the Jewish Historical Society of England* 11 (1928): 1–91.

71. The debate over Lopez' guilt continues unabated. Dimock, Katz, and Shapiro find him guilty, but Dimock's scholarship is marred by late-Victorian anti-Semitism; Meyers, who vigorously rebuts Katz and Shapiro, and Margaret Hotine pronounce Lopez innocent; Trevor-Roper equivocates.

72. Quoted in MacNalty, *Doctor in Politics and Diplomacy,* 6–7, and more fully in Meyers, "Shakespeare, Shylock," 36. Dimock cites a letter from Robert Cecil, Burghley's son, acknowledging the soundness of the case against Lopez and the honor of the jurors: Dimock, "Conspiracy," 466.

73. Quoted in Meyers, "Shakespeare, Shylock," 32. The Venetian ambassador heard that Elizabeth supported Lopez even after his conviction and summoned him out of prison to attend her when she fell ill in March 1594: Hotine, "Politics of Anti-Semitism," 38.

74. Hotine, "Politics of Anti-Semitism," 36–37; Munk, *Roll* 1: 69.

75. Galileo, quoted in Munk, *Roll* 1: 77; Rattansi, "Paracelsus and the Puritan Revolution," 32.

76. For more on the Hakluyt-Gilbert connection, see A.L. Rowse, *The English Renaissance*, 2 vols. (New York: Scribner, 1971–72) 2: 233–38; and G. B. Parks, *Richard Hakluyt and the English Voyages*, 2nd ed., ed. James A. Williamson (New York : F. Ungar, 1961).

77. Silvarus P. Thompson, *Gilbert, Physician* (London: C. Whittingham, 1903), 11.

78. Allen G. Debus, *The Chemical Philosophy: Paracelsian Science and Medicine in the Sixteenth and Seventeenth Centuries*, 2 vols. (New York: Science History Publications, 1977), 1: 104.

79. Thompson, "Serjeant Surgeons to Their Majesties," 11.

80. Munk, *Roll* 1: 86.

81. French, *John Dee*, 50–51, 89. Most of Dee's writings were not printed in his lifetime.

82. Trevor-Roper, *Renaissance Essays*, 157.

83. J. W. Halliwell, ed., *The Private Diary of Dr. John Dee*, (London: Camden Society, xix, 1842).

84. Though Sussex was a friend to some of her opponents, he remained a loyal servant who gave her sound advice on what strategy to pursue with rebellious nobles. Somerset, *Elizabeth I*, 231.

85. Clippingdale names John Hatcher, Regius Professor of Medicine at Cambridge, an Elizabethan physician, but I can find no corroborating evidence, nor any for celebrated botanist Edward Bulleyn or for Leonard Poe, physician-in-ordinary to James I: Clippingdale, Medical Court Roll, 1: 41, LRCS. Nichols refers to a Dr. Julio in 1574 as a "great court physician to Queen Elizabeth" but without corroboration: Nichols, *Progresses of Elizabeth I*, 1: 61. Clippingdale also includes John Anthony Fenatius in his list of irregular physicians to the king, while at least one Richard Smith (from Cambridge) appears in another antiquarian work. See Kate Naylor, *Richard Smith, M.D.* (Lincoln, England: Governors of the Foundation of Christ's Hospital, 1951).

86. The Kennix episode is recorded in its entirety in the Annals of the College of Physicians, vol. 2, f. 7b, LRCP. The Annals feature many actions taken against female practitioners: about 15 percent of the Fellows' proceedings against unlicensed medicos in the Tudor-Stuart era involved women, most of them younger women. See Margaret Pelling, "Thoroughly Resented? Older Women and the Medical Role in Early Modern London," in *Women, Science and Medicine 1500–1700*, ed. Lynette Hunter and Sarah Hutton (Stroud, England: Sutton, 1997), 70–71.

87. For the traditions of healing women in English Renaissance drama, see William Kerwin, "Where Have You Gone, Margaret Kennix?" in *Women Healers and Physicians*, ed. Lilian R. Furst (Lexington: University Press of Kentucky, 1997), 93–113.

88. Young, *Annals*, 524; SL MSS 2463, British Library.

89. Beck, *Cutting Edge*, 200. Another historian questions Vicary's scholarly legacy. Despite a 1556 ordinance that a surgeon's apprentice must learn Latin, few did, and the mandate was rescinded the following year. D'Arcy Power, *The Education of a Surgeon under Vicary* (Bristol, England: Wright, 1921), 244.

90. Gale's report is quoted in Beck, *Cutting Edge*, 183, and his career is mentioned in Young, *Annals*, passim.

91. Quoted in Power, "Serjeant Surgeons of England," 82.

92. Young, *Annals*, 528, 530–31; Gustav Ungerer, "George Baker: Translator of Aparicio de Zubia's Pamphlet on the Oleum Magistrale," *Medical History* 30 (1986): 203.

93. Raven, *English Naturalists*, 177. Muffet, protege of the Earl of Pembroke and an avid collector of insects, was the father of Patience, Little Miss Muffet! Trevor-Roper, *Renaissance Essays*, 163.

94. Nichols, *Progresses of Elizabeth I* 1: 598. Sir John Sainty has found evidence (in the James Marshall and Marie-Louise Osborn Collection, Osborn MSS b. 39, at the Beinecke Rare Book and Manuscript Library, Yale University) that "Guddridge" was serjeant-surgeon as late as 1609; I thank Sir John for this information.

95. Debus, "Paracelsian Compromise," 76; Ungerer, "George Baker," 204. In *The English Paracelsians*, Debus argues that Baker chose Galen over Paracelsus but upheld the wisdom of chemical therapy; Ungerer says that Baker "embraced alternative medicine without abandoning traditional science."

96. Paul H. Kocher, "Paracelsian Medicine in England: The First Thirty Years," *Journal of the History of Medicine* 2 (1947): 458. Baker's table of contents encompasses balme of Rome, whose invention is attributed to Paracelsus, oil of garden spike, and potable gold.

97. John Gerard, *The Herball or General History of Plants* (London: John Norton, 1597). Dedicated to Lord Burghley, the 1,392–page herbal has a format that is easy to follow: description, place, name, nature, and virtues of the plants in question. Among the medicinal uses of plants, Gerard recommends sea onion for "provoking urine," saltwoort for "casting forth the dead childe," and Indian plum for the "French disease."

98. Annals of the College of Physicians, vol. 2, f. 68b, LRCP.

99. Quoted in Power, "Serjeant Surgeons of England," 83; Young, *Annals*, 428.

100. Add. MSS 43408, British Library. The pocket-sized manual, dated 1609, may have been written by someone else, perhaps Clowes's son and successor. It measures 1 3/4 inches by 5 1/2 inches by 1 inch. See D'Arcy Power, *Epoch-Making Books in British Surgery* (Bristol, England: n.p., 1928), which lauds Clowes's surgical writings.

101. Fielding H. Garrison, *Introduction to the History of Medicine*, 4th ed. (Philadelphia: W. B. Saunders, 1929), 227. For more on Clowes's life, see the introduction by F.N.L. Poynter, ed., *The Selected Writings of William Clowes* (London: Harvey and Blythe, 1948).

102. Poynter puts Clowes's birthdate at 1544 (not 1540 as reported in the *DNB* and Young's *Annals*), presuming that Clowes was the conventional twelve years old when apprenticed in 1556: Poynter, *Clowes*, 18.

103. William Clowes, *Treatise for the Artificiall Cure of Struma* (Amsterdam: Da Capo Reprints, 1970), introduction. Paul Kocher applauds Clowes's intelligent approach to medical theory, a pragmatism that facilitated the transmission of new, albeit foreign, ideas: Kocher, "Paracelsian Medicine in England," 470–71.

104. Moore, quoted in Garrison, *Introduction to the History of Medicine*, 227. Also see Norman Moore, *The History of the Study of Medicine in the British Isles* (Oxford: Clarendon Press, 1908), for vignettes from the careers of many key sixteenth- and seventeenth-century practitioners including Clowes.

105. See Bruce Thomas Boehrer, "Early Modern Syphilis," *Journal of the History of Sexuality* 1 (1990): 197–214; Robert G. Frank, Jr., "The Physician as Virtuoso in Seventeenth-Century England," in *English Scientific Virtuosi in the Sixteenth and Seventeenth Centuries*, eds. Barbara Shapiro and Robert G. Frank, Jr. (Los Angeles: University of California Pres, 1979). Incidentally, *Every Man His Own Doctor* is the title of a work by John Archer, published in 1671.

106. Bloom and James, *Medical Practitioners*, 16. Clowes's overseas assignments doubtless delayed his access to the livery.

107. This publication is different from the handwritten album mentioned above.

108. Poynter, *Clowes*, 25, 35–38.

109. Young, *Annals*, 536.

110. Young lists Christopher Frederick as Elizabeth's serjeant surgeon, but his appointment to James I's household can be definitively dated from 1609: Young, *Annals*, 551.

111. Matthews calls her new look a "semi calorite temperade." Matthews, *Royal Apothecaries*, 81, n. 51.

112. Ibid., 71.

113. Matthews reports that Edward Hemingway "gave place" to George Shiers as yeoman apothecary, with reversion of the office granted by Elizabeth herself. Matthews, *Royal Apothecaries*, 78.

114. Quoted in Raven, *English Naturalists*, 117. See also Eleanour Sinclair Rohde, *The Old English Herbals* (New York: Dover, 1971), 77; Matthews, *Royal Apothecaries*, 78.

115. See C. A. Bradford, *Hugh Morgan, Queen Elizabeth's Apothecary* (London: E. T. Heron, 1939).

116. Raven, *English Naturalists*, 116.

117. Rhubarb, scammony (a gum resin from the morning-glory), and manna (a sweet resin from the bark of ash trees) were used as mild laxatives, wormseed (dried flower-heads or seeds from the goosefoot family) as a vermifuge and emmenagogue. For an illustrated guide to the medicinal

uses of plants in Tudor and Stuart times, see David Potterton, ed., *Culpeper's Color Herbal* (New York: Sterling Publishing, 1983).

118. Morgan was also a correspondent of Turner's and figures prominently in the writings of the Flemish botanist Mathias de l'Obel, a visitor to London in 1569; John Gerard, author of the most popular *Herball* of all, called Morgan "a curious conserver of rare simples." Raven, *English Naturalists*, 116–17.

119. Quoted in Matthews, *Royal Apothecaries*, 75–77. Mithridatium worked upon the principle that ingestion of certain toxins built up an immunity to them. Morgan also must have been adept at legal maneuverings and comfortable with lawyers; he was admitted as a special member of the Middle Temple in 1608.

120. His brass in Battersea church describes him as "chief pothecary to Elizabeth" and includes the following epitaph:

And in his Science as he did excell,
In her high Favour he did always dwell.
To God religious, to all men kind,
Frank to the poor, rich in content of mind.
These were his vertues, in these dyed he,
When he had lived an hundred year and three."

Quoted in John Strype, ed., *A Survey of London and Westminster brought down from 1633 to the present*, 2 vols. (London: A. Churchill, 1720) 2: 740–41.

121. MacNalty thinks a septic infection, maybe dental in origin, best explains the queen's distress: MacNalty, *Elizabeth Tudor*, 242.

Chapter 4

Doctors to the Early Stuarts (1603–49)

The death of Queen Elizabeth without issue marked the end of the Tudor line, but, in fact, the ruling family started by Henry VII provided for continuation of the dynasty under a different royal surname. Prophesying that one day "the less [would] become subservient to the greater," in 1503 Henry Tudor had married his elder daughter, Margaret, to the Stuart (or Stewart) king of Scotland, James IV.[1] Their son, James V, fathered Mary, Queen of Scots. Despite a century of trouble between England and Scotland, Elizabeth arranged for a smooth, if complex, succession by bequeathing all her titles to James VI, the only son of Mary Stuart.[2] One sovereign prince ruled the whole of the British Isles for the first time in history. The Scottish crown passed to James Stuart in 1567, when he was only thirteen months old, coming to him after the murder of his father, Lord Darnley, and the forced abdication of his mother, who later fled to England for safety. After his coronation, the sickly boy-king was consigned to the care of a series of regents who fell victim to the violent atmosphere of still-feudal Scotland. In the midst of the chaos, James was brought up Protestant in the Calvinist mold and received an excellent education. In 1578 at age twelve, James VI nominally took the government into his own hands. By then, he had overcome the bodily weaknesses that beset him as a youngster through a rehabilitative program of vigorous physical activity. The emotional scars of his tumultuous childhood were harder to obliterate.[3]

Plainly susceptible to domineering influences, in 1579 James fell under the sway of a distant cousin, Esmé Stuart, an agent of the French king and a Catholic.[4] When James made Esmé Duke of Lennox and signaled his preference for him above all others, a group of Presbyterians called the Ruthven Raiders after their leader William Ruthven, Earl of Gowrie, kidnapped the king. The Raiders kept James imprisoned for months, extorting from him a proclamation that brought down Lennox, but in 1583 the king managed to escape his captors and took firm control of power. He knew he needed to diminish the clout of the Scottish nobles and the dangers of the Presbyterian faction; he also wanted to assert his claim to the English throne.[5] Thus, for a variety of purposes, James Stuart opted for an alliance with England, opening a rift with his mother who was incarcerated there by Elizabeth's command. Despite the poverty of his domain and the penury of the royal treasury, James ruled shrewdly after Mary's execution in 1587, firmly taking the reins of the Scottish Kirk while writing about the divine right of kings. James dutifully provided for his own succession in Scotland and made himself more attractive to Englishmen tired of kingly uncertainty when in 1589 he married by proxy a Lutheran princess, fourteen-year-old Anne of Denmark, who gave birth to their first son, Henry Frederick, in 1594.[6] James christened his daughter Elizabeth in 1596 and in 1601 wisely opened correspondence with Sir Robert Cecil, Burghley's son and then Elizabeth's Secretary of State, on how to persuade the queen to name him her successor.

Hence, before his accession to the throne of England as James I, King James VI had already ruled Scotland for thirty-seven years and had employed royal doctors in his household there. James manifested some health problems that were puzzling to them, but were excused as the consequence of childhood neglect: he ate sloppily and walked clumsily.[7] Designated "mediciners" ministered to royal health care in the northern kingdom in the sixteenth century. Owing to the absence of medical education and professional medical organization in Scotland, James VI's physicians had studied abroad and had little say over the qualifications of their peers.[8] While king in Scotland, James called upon the services of two physicians from Aberdeen, Gilbert Skeyne (Skene) and John Craig; the former was the king's mediciner from 1581 until his retirement in 1592 and the latter migrated to England upon James' coronation to serve the king and his family at a far richer court. The fourth son of a notary, Skeyne authored the first Scottish medical treatise to be printed, a 1568 tract on the plague; he also wrote another on the medicinal qualities of a well outside Aberdeen before James tapped him as Scottish court physician.[9] At the time of his appointment, Skeyne was Professor of Medicine at King's College, Aberdeen; he died in 1599. John Craig succeeded Skeyne as James' chief court doctor in Edinburgh; he was the first to be designated "principal" physician, and he continued in that post for several years in England.[10]

When James Stuart arrived at the capital of his southern kingdom in April 1603, he instituted household appointments similar to those of the Tudor monarchs who preceded him: one principal physician and two or three physicians-in-ordinary.[11] The Lord Chamberlain, principal officer of the court, hired all those brought into the presence of the king, and a committee known as the Board of the Green Cloth scrutinized household expenditures and authorized supplies. To handle the Stuart medical business in England, King James paid for the services of six to eight surgeons in 1616 alone. The queen, who had already given birth five times in Scotland, needed a midwife for two more pregnancies in England, and a range of apothecaries, whose bills were certified by the royal doctors, provided the court with drugs. Moreover, as a married monarch, James had to provide for separate households for Anne and for Prince Henry, heir to the throne. He also retained a personal physician and other medical staffers at his court in Scotland as did subsequent Stuart monarchs. Hence, over the course of his twenty-two-year reign, James I employed dozens of medical personnel. Some of Queen Elizabeth's doctors, including Roger Marbeck and Edward Lister, continued their household service to her successor. Two of James's personal appointees, Theodore Mayerne and William Harvey, were celebrities for different reasons in the field of medicine.

Interested in practical matters of health and science, James manifested skepticism about some elements of English custom. He scoffed at the miraculous ritual of touching for the King's Evil, nearly "dealing it a mortal blow." Despite James' written support for the divine right of kings, his Calvinism made him reluctant to participate in superstitious liturgy and he asked to be excused from the rite.[12] His advisers convinced him of the practical need to touch and he complied, albeit with some changes in the traditional ceremony, such as deleting the Sign of the Cross performed by the king over the afflicted subjects, and restyling of the "angels," which no longer bore the picture of a crucifix on them or the word "miracle." James sporadically performed the ceremony on progresses throughout the realm, as in 1617 when he touched several hundred scrofulous subjects *en route* to Lincoln and another several dozen in the minster itself.[13]

James I decried the use of tobacco in a powerful pamphlet, *A Counterblast to Tobacco*, published in 1604, two years after Roger Marbeck's apologia. He argued that smoking sprang from barbarism; that it had been begun by godless American Indians as a corrective against syphilis. Employing Galenic allusions, James described the body as analogous to four worldly elements, though he rejected the contention of some physicians that the heat of tobacco smoke could balance the wet, cold brain. Rather, tobacco soiled and infected the body with its malignant soot. In the same year that the *Counterblast* appeared, James imposed a duty of six shillings and ten pence on each pound of tobacco imported into England, an increase of 4,000 percent.[14] He soon discovered, however, that the tax produced smuggling rather than abstinence and, needing all the revenue he could get, lowered the duties. Undeterred by these difficulties, in 1619 he ordered the demolition of a tobacco shop that he spied adjacent to St. Paul's Cathedral, and when the Virginia Company's right to import its products into England duty free lapsed that year, the king demanded as high a tariff as possible. In July 1620, having obtained an opinion from the College of Physicians that domestic tobacco was more poisonous than that grown in hotter climates, he issued a royal proclamation that prohibited the cultivation of the noxious "weed of no necessarie use" in the realm. In September 1624, after encouraging Virginia planters to produce other crops, a Jacobean declaration permitted the importation of tobacco from Virginia and the Summer Islands (Bermuda), but not from Spanish territories.[15]

King James hated the practice of dueling, a dangerously fashionable custom that had become even more common after his accession in 1603. Chiefly troublesome to him was the frequency of dueling between Englishmen and Scots. He regarded the duelist as a willful murderer, blinded by an idiotic and archaic code of honor; dueling was also an affront to the king's authority. When two of his favorites, Sir George Wharton and Sir James Stewart, killed each other in a duel, the king commanded them buried in a single grave. Though no parliamentary statute dealt with dueling and common law required only punishment after the fact, James wanted prevention. He issued a proclamation in 1613 banning small daggers and short pistols, weapons whose use often led to duels, and another later in the year forbidding published challenges aimed at provoking a fight. In February 1614, King James explicitly outlawed dueling, establishing commissions to adjudicate quarrels and prescribing penalties for those who violated the interdiction. Though his endeavors did not end the practice altogether, the king's crusade produced a reduction in dueling.[16]

Though in later years, when James was secure on the English throne, he blasted witchcraft as superstitious nonsense, he had been terrified of the power of one "wizard," Francis Hepburn, Earl of Bothwell, while still in Scotland. Bothwell, deranged nephew of the man who had been the Queen of Scots' lover and third husband, became an enemy of the king and an outlaw at the time of James's marriage. Bothwell inspired some witches with whom he consorted to raise a storm at sea while the royal couple was *en route* home, hoping to imperil the lives of the newlyweds. When that scheme did not work, Bothwell twice attacked the king in his royal residences, stalking James to the entry of the private apartments, setting fire to his very door. Though he escaped, James remained in constant fear of capture until Bothwell went into exile in 1595. James subsequently wrote a tract in 1597 called *Daemonologie*, which advised that witchcraft should be punished, along with murder, incest, and counterfeiting, as an unforgivable crime.[17] Eventually, after coming to England James gradually relaxed his posture on witchcraft. Following personal investigations of frauds and hoaxes during which he was accompanied by competent doctors, he advised judicial caution in individual cases. Despite his earlier gullible attitude on witchcraft, King James came to promote a more rational approach to medicine and science through his court appointments; they in turn buttressed the theoretical compromise in the College of Physicians and in the English medical world as a whole.

Although she usually evinced only casual interest in affairs of state, James's Danish queen did take an active part in court life and may have altered the jurisdictional balance in the medical world when she championed the apothecaries in February 1617. Her own apothecary, Gideon de Laune, encouraged the separation of the apothecaries from the mere "tradesmen" of the Grocers' Company. Aided by Attorney General Francis Bacon and with the agreement of the College of Physicians, Queen Anne persuaded the king to grant the Worshipful Society of Apothecaries an autonomous corporate charter.[18] By 1623 the Apothecaries' Society had established its own laboratory for compounding the vegetable medicines then in use and de Laune later helped the new association purchase a suitable hall in Blackfriars Lane. Squabbles between apothecaries and physicians, even Paracelsians, escalated into full-blown turf war by the end of the seventeenth-century, spurred by the College of Physicians' policy of deliberate physician scarcity, a growing popular audience for published self-help manuals, and the discovery of amazing new medicines from overseas that apothecaries were not afraid to use. Surgeons factored into the equation, armed with practical techniques learned on the battlefield in Elizabethan times; they, too, sought a place for themselves in the medical marketplace. All three groups clashed in Jacobean London when surgeon John Gerard, James' herbalist and author of the famous *Herball*, angered the apothecaries after the College of Physicians made him curator of its new physic garden.[19]

John Craig the elder, James's continentally trained principal mediciner in Scotland, accompanied the king to London as his First Physician.[20] Born in the northern kingdom, Craig studied medicine at Basel and was a friend to Tycho Brahe and John Napier; Craig's work toward logarithms led to Napier's great mathematical discovery. Craig taught logic and mathematics at Frankfort-on-the-Oder from 1579 to 1582 before being chosen as the Stuart royal doctor. Despite his impressive foreign credentials, acceptance in 1604 by the Fellows of College of Physicians in London was not gained without questions being raised about Craig's national origin. Even though James ruled over both Scotland and England, Scots born before his accession had not been automatically naturalized in England as were those born after. The king indicated his intention to naturalize Craig, but asserted that "things are not between the two nations in such terms, as no man of judgement can accompt them two, but one."[21] The College agreed, substituting in 1606 *natione Britannus* for *natione Anglicus* in its statutes. Craig applied for incorporation of his medical degree by Oxford, which the university granted in 1605. James's choice of John Craig signaled that the king, himself a scholar, preferred learned physicians to men of superstition. Craig received £160 per year, bouche, and a "diet" of five dishes at per meal for daily attendance on the monarch; his gift to the king at New Year in 1606 was a box of marchpane. Craig's son, also Dr. John Craig (d. 1655) and a Fellow of the College, tended James I and Charles I, the former in his last illness; the younger Craig circulated rumors that King James died of poison.[22]

In Celtic Scotland, medicine rested principally in the hands of hereditary physicians in aristocratic households. Every nobleman had a personal retinue, which included the post of doctor, handed down for generations within the same family. As late as the mid-eighteenth century, chieftains kept these medical retainers as custodians of ancient learning and libraries.[23] The Beatons of Balfour in Fifeshire could boast of such a pedigree. A scion of that famed lineage, David Beaton, born around 1575, held a degree from Padua, a preferred university for Scotsmen wishing to learn medicine. Returning to Scotland from his studies around 1600, he became a physician to the royal court and, like Craig, went south with James in 1603. For all his merit, Beaton is a shadowy figure identified by little more than his surname and even that was recorded erratically as Bedwin, Beton, or Bethune. For over twenty years, the doctor is only a historical silhouette, but he was at James's deathbed in 1625 and the following year became senior physician-in-ordinary to Charles I.

Despite Craig senior's history of service with the king and Beaton's medical genealogy, Sir Theodore Turquet de Mayerne was the most influential Jacobean physician at court, if not the one judged by history as the most important to medicine. Geneva-born, Mayerne studied medicine at Paris and Heidelberg, and then iatrochemistry at the sophisticated Huguenot university at Montpellier, where he received his M.D. in 1597. While insisting that Galen was still the master of physicians, Mayerne strongly defended chemical remedies and the more experimental curriculum of continental practice, endearing himself to two neo-Paracelsians who held sway at the French court, if not to Parisian Galenists. After the promulgation of the Edict of Nantes, Mayerne became a French district *docteur* in 1600, rising to royal service as physician to Henri IV despite the king's conversion to Roman Catholicism. Mayerne traveled to Italy and Britain for purposes of finding new cures and promoting a pro-Protestant foreign policy; while he was in Oxford in 1606, his degree was incorporated there. Upon the recommendation of a peer whom Mayerne had treated in Paris, James made him physician to Queen Anne, but Mayerne returned to France. After the assassination of Henri IV, James I brought Mayerne back to England in 1611. Assisted by his surgeon, Master Naismith (Nesmith), Mayerne developed a large practice that included Robert Cecil, Earl of Salisbury; Robert Carr, Viscount Rochester, who consulted him for dyspepsia in 1611; Sir Henry Montague's daughter; and a Member of Parliament for Ely, Oliver Cromwell. In 1611 by Letters Patent under the Great Seal, Mayerne became first physician to King James.

Mayerne, an outstanding clinician, kept detailed case notes on both his English and French patients; one medical historian has called those the "medical annals of the Court of England."[24] His notations included a 1612 account, a model of its kind, of Prince Henry's losing battle with acute fever, probably typhoid. Mayerne attended to Queen Anne, treating her for coughs, dropsy, swollen feet and ankles, and redness in the face; he was with her at the time of her death at age forty-five in 1619.[25] Mayerne also had his hands full with the often-ailing James and maintained a register on the monarch's health, including observations of his sleeping, exercise, ailments, and disposition. The king had an intense fear of death, no doubt aggravated by the Gunpowder Plot of 1605, a conspiracy by disgruntled Roman Catholics to blow up James and the Houses of Parliament. Since King James was equally disdained by Puritans after rejecting most of their demands for reforms in the Anglican church, he dreaded retribution from them, too. Besides the king's anxieties, Dr. Mayerne treated him for physical maladies: renal colic and hematuria in 1613, an abscess of the arm that developed after a fall, gout, arthritis, and jaundice. James rejected many of the conventional remedies in a physician's repertoire including phlebotomy; Mayerne disclosed in his register that the king never allowed himself to be bled. He also confirmed that the king still had difficulty walking and riding.[26] James's kidney problems were exacerbated by alcohol and by his refusal to listen to his doctor's advice. As he lost his teeth, the king devoured his food without chewing, developed raging indigestion, and then "demanded relief from pain without considering the causes of his illness."[27] Moreover, James detested water as a beverage or a bath. Because he never washed, he itched constantly; because he did not change clothes until they wore out, he reeked of body odor. His uncleanliness offended even the least fastidious at court and occasionally tormented them; one lady at court complained that she and her companions got "lousy by sitting in [a councillor's] chamber" that James frequented.[28]

Both king and queen may have suffered from scurvy; Mayerne diagnosed Anne's ulcerated leg as "scorbutic," though he did not know a cure for the condition. In fact, he banned from the palace the fruits, berries, and legumes craved by James, but thought ignoble by English patricians.[29] Mayerne kept James's confidence despite the king's scornful dismissal of medicine and disbelief in the abilities of most physicians. An apostle of the chemical school, Mayerne engaged in countless experiments and while a royal physician brought the purgative calomel (mercurous chloride) and a mercurial lotion called "black wash" into use. As part of his chemical repertoire, Mayerne advocated the taking of unpalatable "steel" in powdered form for "the spleen" or melancholy; his other, nonmetallic treatments could be just as fearsome. For stupor and numbness he invented a balsam made of twelve boiled bats, three snakes, two suckling puppies, one pound of earthworms, hog lard, and white wine applied to the backbone; he advocated drunkenness once a month, probably one therapy to which the king did not object.[30] He believed that "the bitterest medicines . . . work the best," prescribing for a patient with respiratory problems "a syrup made with the flesh of tortoises, snails, the lungs of animals, frogs and crawfish, all boiled in scabrous and coltsfoot water, adding at the last sugar candy."[31] At the same time, Mayerne sustained faith in the Galenic expulsion of undesirable humors through bleeding, opening veins and keeping them open by means of "issues" or incisions prevented from healing by the insertion of small gold pellets.

The College of Physicians welcomed Mayerne as a Fellow in 1616, recognizing that his Paracelsianism was eclectic, compatible with much traditional practice. The College felt his influence immediately, as Mayerne, writing the preface, honored King James with the long-awaited *London Pharmacopoeia* in 1618. The pharmacopoeia, containing chemical and mineral medicaments as well as Galenic standbys, evinced the quiet syncretistic compromise effected by the Fellows in Elizabeth's reign and preserved until the Civil War.[32] Mayerne was responsible for much of its contents including the description of Thomas Muffet's Paracelsian medicines, which Mayerne had acquired after Muffet's death. Mayerne determined to publish Muffet's work on insects, originally dedicated to Queen Elizabeth, and rededicate it to James.

Financially confident and socially ambitious, Mayerne purchased a Swiss estate and became a baron, installed his daughter Louise in the court of James's daughter, Elizabeth of Bohemia, and affianced another daughter to the Earl of Huntingdon. Mayerne enjoyed the high life, especially rich and copious eating; a posthumously published cookbook of his, *Archimagirus Anglo-Gallicus*, testified to his status as a gourmand, as did his remarkable girth. Clearly, he had thrived in England. Inspiring other Huguenot physicians to follow him there, Mayerne continued his service to the Stuarts under Charles I and later. Medical historian Norman Moore calls Mayerne "one of the three great clinical observers in England."[33] His case books carefully document treatments imposed on Charles and his queen; for the latter he prescribed cosmetics and a dentifrice made from pumice stone, cuttlefish bones, powdered coral, pearl, and deer horn.[34]

Mayerne published with Thomas Cadyman in 1639, *The Distiller of London*, a digest of recipes and regulations for licensed distillers. Cadyman or Cademan, physician to the queen and a Catholic recusant, was the first Master of the Company of Distillers, an association whose split from the Apothecaries Mayerne had fostered. The Mayerne-Cadyman handbook contains the names of various waters: anise seed, angelica, wormwood, balsamint, and lavender, with more recipes for "strong waters, rich spirits," and vinegars made from "cider, perry, and buck." Norfolk-born, Cadyman procured his arts degrees from Trinity College, Cambridge, before moving to Padua for his M.D. in 1620. The College of Physicians' Annals record the Fellows' admonition of Cadyman in 1623 for assuming that his Italian degree enabled him to practice without a license in the English capital; at the same time they accused him of malpractice for bleeding a patient with petechial fever. In 1625 the Fellows formally charged, convicted, and fined Cadyman for malpractice in a gonorrhea case.[35]

Cadyman's Roman Catholicism probably hurt his career in England, though not with the Huguenot Mayerne, himself familiar with religious discrimination, nor with Charles I's queen. Henrietta Maria made Cadyman her physician sometime before December 1630, when the College of Physicians acquiesced and bestowed supernumerary status on him.[36] However, it was Cadyman's condensing various vinegars and waters that angered the London apothecaries, who petitioned against him. Mayerne stepped in and admonished the druggists to pay Cadyman and him more respect and to give their patients more attention.

Another distinguished physician in James' service was William Paddy, a native of Middlesex educated at the Merchant Taylors' School and then at St. John's College, Oxford, which reserved a few places each year for Merchant Taylors' boys. Paddy took his medical degree at Leiden and was licensed by the College of Physicians in 1590. His continental education made him an advocate of accurate anatomical training and in 1598 he was fined £4 for performing a public dissection in the Barber-Surgeons' Hall without the permission of the College President.[37] Esteeming Paddy as a physician, James I knighted him in 1603. Sir William had an illustrious association with the College of Physicians as its censor and four times President between 1609 and 1618. As the College's spokesman before the Lord Mayor and the Court of Aldermen, Paddy pleaded for the Fellows' immunity from service in arms. He must have been effective as an advocate, because the City granted exemption to collegiate members.[38] Those forensic skills also proved useful to Paddy as a Member of Parliament from 1604 to 1611, representing Thetford, Norfolk.

Paddy participated in a lively disputation for the king on a number of health-related questions in 1605 at Oxford. James enjoyed unorthodox speculation, and among the issues debated at Oxford was whether the morals of wet nurses are imbibed by infants along with breast milk; another was a perennial Jacobean polemic, the ill effects of tobacco. Paddy personified the fluctuations in James' antismoking campaign, as the publicity lent to tobacco by royal and scholarly concern only increased its fascination. Albeit himself a "great drinker of tobacco," the doctor insisted that its use was most deleterious.[39] A pragmatic Paracelsian like Mayerne, though unpublished, Dr. Paddy was sent for in 1625 when the king fell fatally ill. He did not receive a comparable appointment under Charles I. Loyal to the Stuarts and their personnel even in troubled times, Paddy spoke out for the High Church policies of Archbishop of Canterbury William Laud, a former President of St. John's. Dr. Paddy outlived James by nine years, dying at age eighty, and was buried at St. John's, to which he bequeathed an organ, £1800 for the choir, £1000 towards the commons, and books for the St. John's College library which his portrait still graces.

The other titan of the early Stuart medical world was James' physician extraordinary, William Harvey.[40] Medical historian Fielding Garrison avers that "no one save Vesalius influenced modern medicine more than he," but that Harvey was "an indifferent practitioner."[41] Born in Kent in 1578 into a successful merchant family, Harvey obtained a B.A. from Cambridge in 1597 before matriculating in medicine at Padua. There, he became interested in the general problem of how the blood flows through the body. Harvey was awarded his M.D. in 1602 at the age of twenty-four, but returned for more study in England; he received a second M.D. within a few months. Married to the daughter of Dr. Lancelot Browne, first physician to Queen Elizabeth, he began a London practice, joined the College of Physicians, and petitioned to become physician to St. Bartholomew's hospital in 1609, a stepping stone to professional distinction. Harvey became something of an expert on obstetrics and gynecology, his interest piqued by recent anatomical publications on female generative organs and by the practices of midwives. He advocated patience during childbirth rather than constant intervention.[42]

Harvey discerned that the color of a baby's lungs determined if it had been born alive, invented a dilator, and calculated the time of gestation at ten lunar months. The College saluted him in 1615 as Lumleian lecturer for life, and he began a series of anatomical addresses in which he concluded that the blood flows from arteries to veins, "in a perpetual motion of the blood in a circle" by means of the muscular action of the heart. Without a microscope, he deduced the existence of capillaries and published the results of his studies in 1628.[43] The importance of Harvey's achievement is not so much the discovery of the circulation of the blood as its quantitative or mathematical demonstration. With this display, physiology became "a dynamic science."[44]

Such remarkable work could hardly escape the notice of the crown. King James made Harvey his physician extraordinary in 1618 and the doctor involved himself in court business; however, not all of the Stuart courtiers accepted Harvey's recommended regimen of exercise therapy. Harvey's biographer, Geoffrey Keynes, finds it difficult to envision the coolly serious doctor as comfortable among the raucous royal minions, but John Aubrey, a seventeenth-century contemporary who boasted that he knew Harvey well, described him as "hott-headed [and] cholerique," given to wearing a dagger at the ready on "every slight occasion." Aubrey remarked that Harvey disdained "chymistrey, and was wont to speak against [chemical physicians] with an undervalue."[45] However, Harvey was a member of the committee responsible for the 1618 *London Pharmacopoeia*, and so must have given some support to the new therapies, even if he did not apply them at his patients' bedsides.

George Eglisham, a Scotsman whose medical degree came from Leiden in 1610, became James's personal physician in Scotland in 1616 at the recommendation of the Marquis of Hamilton. Eglisham dabbled in poetry, a likely indicator of the passion he brought to medicine and politics. While in Leiden, he denounced Arminian theologian and professor of divinity Conrad Vorst for atheism and published a pamphlet against him in 1612. Vorst promoted the idea of free will and undercut the Calvinist doctrine of predestination. King James had objected to Vorst's writings, had his books publicly burned in England, and pressured the Dutch with demands that Vorst be dismissed from his university post.[46] Eglisham challenged Vorst to a public debate, but the face-off never occurred. Certainly, Eglisham's denunciation of Vorst solidified his candidacy as a Jacobean royal doctor.

Eglisham next tried to get the University of Paris to pronounce his Latin translations of the psalms superior to that of the sixteenth-century Scottish humanist George Buchanan, hailed as one of the greatest poets and most erudite teachers of his generation. However, Eglisham only succeeded in generating satirical critiques of his own poems. In 1626 he wrote a tract accusing George Villiers, Duke of Buckingham, of killing the king.[47] *The Forerunner of Revenge* consists of two petitions about Buckingham: one to King Charles and one to Parliament. Describing himself as "physician to King James for ten years," Eglisham charged that the duke gave James, who was "misled by [his] favorite" and already sick with an ague, a poisonous white powder while the royal doctors were at dinner. Even Buckingham's mother was complicitous, wrote Eglisham, applying a mysterious heart plaster to the king, again while the king's physicians dined. Eglisham reported that James' body ballooned after death and that his nails loosened, proof of the foul deed.[48] However, the doctors who embalmed the king's corpse found no signs of poison, and William Harvey, who had been in attendance, dissociated himself from the charges. Proceedings were instituted against Eglisham for besmirching Buckingham's name, but the physician moved to Brussels to escape punishment and remained there until his death.

Dr. Henry Atkins, a long-lived practitioner, was a fellow and officer of the College of Physicians from 1588 until his death in 1635, serving as President on three separate occasions. Born in Hertfordshire, Atkins pursued his arts degrees at Oxford, then studied medicine on the continent, receiving his M.D. from the University of Nantes. He was already an officer in the College of Physicians when he went with the Earl of Essex in July 1597 on a naval expedition against Spain sailing to El Ferrol, the Galician port where informants indicated Philip II was preparing another armada. Unfortunately, the good doctor experienced incapacitating *mal de mer* and had to be put ashore; Dr. Thomas Moundforde took his place aboard ship.[49] Held in high regard by James I, Atkins served with Theodore Mayerne as a principal physician, often performing nonmedical services for the king, such as bringing young Charles to London from Scotland in 1604. Charles had been a sickly infant, suffering from rickets after weaning at age one, and left behind by his parents in the care of guardians until he was strong enough to travel. Atkins wrote to James that "the joints of his knees, hips, and ankles being great and loose are not yet closed, and knot together."[50] James appreciated Atkins' reports and his journeying southward with the boy; in his official remarks at the time of the establishment of the Apothecaries' Society, a grateful James referred to Atkins and Mayerne as "our discreet and faithful physicians."[51] Queen Anne was also Atkins' patient. During his presidency of the College of Physicians, the first *London Pharmacopoeia* was finally published and the apothecaries were established in a separate professional company. Atkins continued his service to the Stuarts under Charles I, acting as a regular conduit between the court and the College.

Leonard Poe's career demonstrates the professional mobility possible for a popular doctor with court connections. As early as 1590, Poe, whose family was from the Palatinate, was attempting to obtain approval from the College of Physicians to practice in London, specializing in the treatment of syphilis, fevers, and rheumatism. He was examined and found to be completely ignorant of basic medical information.[52] The College refused him a license despite the intervention of the Earl of Essex on Poe's behalf.[53] The Fellows did overlook, however, the earlier illegal practice of Poe in London, and so the man continued to treat patients without a College mandate. In 1596 Essex again put pressure on the Fellows, and this time a restricted license was granted, giving Poe permission to treat venereal, cutaneous, and calculous diseases.[54] But Poe ministered beyond those boundaries and got into trouble with the College for it. A certain Juliana Soulls accused Poe of giving her husband a purgative when the sick man was feverish, thereby causing his death. Poe rebutted the accusation, denying that he had administered diascordium or any other purgative. Apparently the Fellows believed the widow, for they censured Poe in January 1599.[55]

Despite his initial troubles with the College, Poe became a fashionable London doctor, and in 1606, at the suggestion of noblemen Southampton, Northampton, and Salisbury, all restrictions on his London license were removed. In 1609 Poe was appointed physician-in-ordinary to the royal household and admitted to the College, and in 1615 James I ordered Cambridge University to award Poe a medical degree. Poe attended Salisbury in his final illness, and was present at Orlando Gibbons' death in 1625.[56] Poe continued to take care of the royal household until his own demise in 1631.

The son of an Essex apothecary, Simon Baskerville attended Oxford and received his M.D. there in 1611. He became a Fellow of the Royal College of Physicians in 1614. More than a famous and brilliant doctor, Baskerville demonstrated his talent for philosophy when he was chosen to expound before James I upon the monarch's visit to the university. He became physician-in-ordinary to James and to Charles I, who knighted him in 1636. Besides his royal responsibilities, Sir Simon could number more than one hundred influential patients and was noted for his great wealth. He was buried at St. Paul's in 1641.[57]

An inventor as well as a physician, Thomas Grent became a physician-in-ordinary to James I. After obtaining an M.D. from Oxford, the London Fellows voted him into the College of Physicians in 1623; he also served as physician to St. Thomas's Hospital, the Southwark infirmary for the poor of London. He does not seem to have continued royal service under Charles I. Despite his many patents and his annuity, Thomas Grent died in poverty in 1649. His comrades in the College of Physicians voted his widow a moiety of the profits from the second edition of the *London Pharmacopoeia*.[58]

Sir Matthew Lister, a Fellow of the College of Physicians from 1607, was from the same distinguished Yorkshire medical family as Elizabeth's doctor, Edward Lister. He received his M.D. from Basel and had it incorporated at Oxford in 1605 and Cambridge in 1608; the Fellows of the College of Physicians accepted him in 1607. He served as physician to James' queen, and later as physician-in-ordinary to Charles I, who raised him to the rank of knight in 1636; Lister was also associated with the household of the remarkable diarist Anne Clifford, Countess of Pembroke. Lister's fifty pages of recipes, written mostly in Latin with a sort of code, can be found among the Sloane Manuscripts.[59] Since he provides a key to the code (aurum is a dot-centered circle, aqua is an inverted pyramid) and sometimes lapses into English (recommending a plaster of egg and honey for a woman's sore breast), one wonders how camouflaged the remedies were meant to be. Matthew Lister died in 1656 at the age of ninety-two.[60]

William Butler may not have been an official appointee to the Jacobean medical household, but he was called in on occasion for special advice, for example at the time in 1614 when James fell from his horse while hunting at Newmarket.[61] Evidently, despite extensive study at Cambridge, Butler never obtained a medical doctorate, but had a license to practice physic there. John Aubrey called him "the greatest Physitian of his time."[62] A rival of Mayerne's, he was considered an early Paracelsian, but even Paracelsus might have blanched at Butler's radical therapies. With his apothecary, John Crane, Butler would surprise his patients in order to provoke a bodily response, for instance, by throwing a man with ague into the river to cure him. He received a special dispensation to visit his London patients, though he was never a member of the College of Physicians despite intercession from Lord Burghley. Butler's bracer for febrile ague patients called for a pint of biritite poached with a pint of new milk; patients were told to add brown sugar before drinking.[63] A lifelong bachelor, Butler left his considerable estate in 1618 to Caius College.

Perhaps the most serious medical crisis to confront Jacobean physicians was the sickness and death from typhoid fever of the brilliantly promising heir to the throne, eighteen-year-old Henry, Prince of Wales.[64] His contemporaries revered him as a paragon of princely virtue, skilled in both martial arts and social graces. On November 6, 1612, after an illness of two weeks, he died. The usual source of typhoid fever is contamination in water and milk or from the unwashed hands of food servers; the symptoms of the disease are vague, and even today clinical testing is often necessary for certain identification. In Stuart England the disease had neither been identified nor named, so Prince Henry's death gave rise to considerable speculation, including a faint hint of foul play. Some of the Prince's doctors bemoaned his enthusiasm for swimming in the river after a full meal or walking in a moonlit rain; others noted that Henry had continual headaches and occasional nosebleeds. He complained on October 13 of "a great looseness, his belly opening twenty-five times, avoiding a great deal of choller, flegme and putrefied matter."[65] Feeling better, Henry returned to normal palace business for the next few days. Busy with festive arrangements for his sister Elizabeth's marriage to Frederick, Elector of the Palatinate, the Prince of Wales played vigorous tennis with the Count of Nassau, ate heartily, and even listened to two sermons on Sunday, October 25. By that afternoon, however, he was very ill and took to his bed, distressed by high fever and great thirst. Even a single candlelight hurt his sensitive eyes.

Dr. Richard Palmer attended the Prince and during the crisis William Butler was called in, with the king himself directing the efforts of physicians as they labored at the bedside. Seeking to alleviate Henry's fever and thirst, the doctors administered cooling cordials and a julep made of unicorn's horn, powdered pearl, and the "bone of a stag's heart."[66] However, Theodore Mayerne bore the heaviest responsibility for the Prince of Wales's demise. Sent for by James and put in charge of the case, Mayerne was later accused of poisoning the youth, but he accepted plenty of conflicting advice from the other doctors. In seeking to cure him, Henry's physicians merely increased the young man's suffering. Throughout his illness, Prince Henry was not only repeatedly bled, but his head was shaved and cupping glasses applied to draw out superfluous blood from his pate. By November 3 he was delirious and convulsing violently. Dr. Atkins was consulted and pronounced that the prince suffered from "a corrupt putrid fever, the seat whereof was under the liver."[67] On the eleventh day of the prince's ordeal, a cloven cock was applied to the soles of his feet and newly killed pigeons were spread over his body. Various other remedies were frantically tried, including Raleigh's cordial, which the queen had used successfully against fever.[68] After Henry's death, Dr. Butler specifically castigated Mayerne's handling of the case, censuring him for giving Henry a purge of senna and rhubarb the day after he fell ill, causing dispersal of the disease throughout the prince's body. The autopsy exculpated Mayerne and all the other physicians, citing as the cause of death "fever maligne, by reason of the putrefaction of diverse humours gathered together of a long time before."[69]

Mayerne's enemies tried to sully his reputation further by connecting him to the September 1613 death in the Tower of prominent courtier Sir Thomas Overbury. The crown had jailed Overbury on the charge that he had refused a royal appointment, but it was his objection to the impending marriage of James's darling, Viscount Rochester (later Earl of Somerset), to Lady Frances Howard that precipitated his incarceration.[70] While several doctors visited the imprisoned Overbury, Mayerne saw him most often and was Rochester's regular physician. Examiners attributed Overbury's death to a mercury enema, one of Mayerne's choice restorative remedies. Although Mayerne and his apothecary, Paul de Loubell, were consequently absolved of all responsibility for Overbury's death and the Somersets were tried and convicted of murder in the case, one historian believes that "Overbury should be included among the innumerable casualties of seventeenth-century medicine."[71]

Other Jacobean royal doctors included John Macelo (Maccolo or McKulio) and John Hammond. Macelo, who hailed from Edinburgh, was elected a Fellow of the College of Physicians without an examination, surely in deference to the king's pleasure. Author of *Iatria Chymica* in 1622, the year of his death, Macelo was a continentally trained Paracelsian whose M.D. came from the University of Franeker, West Friesland.[72] London-born Hammond, the son of a Chancery master and Chancellor of the London diocese, received an M.D. from Cambridge before being appointed physician to the king and Prince Henry. He gave James a pot of green ginger for the Christmas-New Year holidays in 1606.[73] The French physician René Chartrier has been mentioned as a Jacobean royal doctor. His wife was the elder sister of the famed Parisian midwife, Louise Bourgeois. One historian lists three other doctors as physicians to James I, but it is likely that local practitioners were also consulted while the king was in their vicinity; a Dr. John Sherwood attended Queen Anne when she was at Bath in 1615.[74]

The king occasionally put pressure on the College of Physicians to let in men to his liking, such as Thomas Ridgely, a Cambridge M.D. not sufficiently respectful of the medical profession for the Fellows. John Aubrey quotes "Old Ridgely" as saying that people might be better off if the art of physic had not been invented.[75] Though Ridgely was not a royal doctor, in 1621 James petitioned for him to be admitted into the College; Ridgely had been waiting, as a candidate for the College, since 1617. The Fellows replied that they currently had no room for Ridgely and reminded the king that their statutes were set up to protect the public and the profession, presumably from mavericks like Dr. Ridgely; nevertheless, they admitted him in 1622.[76]

The alchemist Arthur Dee, eldest son of the famed magus, styled himself a physician, though he had no medical degree. Despite that handicap, Dee practiced medicine in Manchester for several years until 1605 when he relocated to London, his position as a liveryman assured by John Dee's gifts to the Mercers' Company. In April 1606 Arthur Dee incurred the prolonged enmity of the College of Physicians by advertising his medical prowess at the Sign of the Elephant and Castle in Fleet Street, adjacent to an apothecary's establishment. Though lacking a license from the College, Dee had posted a list of panaceas that he guaranteed would cure many diseases. Despite the Fellows' intention to crack down on empirics like Dee, many men evaded the College's injunctions. Dee was summoned on numerous occasions for the next decade to appear before the Fellows on charges of illegal practice.[77] Despite his trouble with the College, in 1614 Arthur Dee was named physician to the proposed hospital at the Charterhouse, though he never took up the post. He practiced in London by royal prerogative, probably through the influence of Dr. Mayerne, and by May 1615 he was Queen Anne's physician.[78] His father had turned down invitations to visit the Russian court, but in 1621 Arthur Dee went to Russia for fourteen years and tended Tsar Michael on James I's recommendation.

Queen Anne, who had converted to Roman Catholicism sometime before coming to England, became estranged from the king and lived apart from him after 1606, though she periodically accompanied him on progresses throughout the country.[79] In 1611 she took sick and was in constant ill health for several years. James objected to the influence of the priests whom she kept by her and their insistence that she must cease to attend Anglican services, but when it was clear that she was dying, the royal relationship mellowed and the king visited her at least twice a week during the last few months of her life. Though she appeared to be improving, the queen had "developed a serious form of dropsy" and died on March 2, 1619.[80] Along with Drs. Mayerne and Matthew Lister, John Raven, Suffolk-born and educated at Trinity College, Cambridge, tended Anne at the time of her death. In 1629 the College of Physicians, which had made Raven a Fellow in 1616, probably the time of his appointment to the queen, investigated and indicted him. In 1636 he left London for Suffolk to escape the plague, but he died there that same year.[81]

Some of James' royal surgeons, like William Gooderus and Christopher Frederick, were holdovers from Elizabethan times; others, like Gilbert Primrose, James brought with him from Edinburgh in 1603. James inherited Gooderus as serjeant-surgeon in 1603; Frederick was James's sergeant-surgeon from 1609 to 1623 and twice Master of the Barber-Surgeons, though he did not work harmoniously with the Court of Assistants. Ironically, it was at Frederick the Court of Aldermen pointedly directed a motion in 1605 that nonnatives be denied entry into the livery or mastership of a company.[82] During his tenure, Frederick treated the king for a broken collarbone, renal stones, and hemorrhoids.[83] Primrose, as sergeant-surgeon to the king, had to deal in an individual way with the xenophobia that flared in London following the accession of a foreigner to the throne. In 1605, "Prymerose" petitioned the Barber-Surgeons' Company that his assistant, Cezar Scultinge, a Dutchman, be admitted to the guild without charge as a courtesy to the king's servants. Scultinge, who was also an aide to Master Naismith, Mayerne's surgeon, passed the Company examination on surgical skill without difficulty, but had to pay a four-shilling fee.[84]

Known for his special skills "in the generation of women," and reputed to be competent during childbirth, James Blackbourne applied to and was admitted to the Barber-Surgeons' Company in 1611. He paid £10 for an examination and treated the examiners to dinner.[85] Blackbourne identified himself as a surgeon in the queen's household in February 1615 according to the College of Physicians' Annals. No name, however, is more closely associated with obstetrics than that of Chamberlen. William Chamberlen, paterfamilias of the family, fled to Amsterdam as a Huguenot refugee around 1550; he is credited with inventing the iron forceps. Because of his association with alchemy, William Chamberlen left Holland and took up residence in England. The Chamberlen family's introduction to royal medicine started with William's son, Peter Chamberlen the Elder (d. 1631), accoucheur and surgeon to Queen Anne.[86] In 1605, the queen gave birth to Princess Mary, the first royal child born in England since Jane Seymour delivered Edward VI; in late 1606 another daughter, Sophia, was born at Greenwich. Alice Dennis was the queen's midwife on both occasions, but Chamberlen attended, too. Sophia died on the day of her birth and two-year-old Mary followed her in death the next autumn after a month-long fever.

Although there would be no more babies for Queen Anne, Chamberlen stayed in her favor and in her service. As he was continuously at odds with the College of Physicians for not confining himself to his surgical specialty, her influence helped him survive. In 1609 the Fellows of the College summoned him, charged him with malpractice for giving a certain medicine, and fined him 40 shillings; in 1612 they sentenced him to a term of incarceration in Newgate prison. Thomas Chamberlen, Peter's cousin and Master of the Mercers' Company, interceded and the queen demanded Peter's release. Peter's brother, Peter the Younger (d. 1626), was also a surgeon to the queen and a member of the Barber-Surgeons' Company. Peter the Younger tried to mitigate the College of Physicians' disrespect for him by seeking admission to the organization, but since he lacked a medical degree the Fellows wanted no part of him. Like his older brother, he practiced as a man-midwife, but it was Peter the Younger who tried to organize the London midwives into an association in 1616.

The battle over midwives often pitted the Chamberlens against the College of Physicians. The Fellows agreed with the Chamberlens that the women should be incorporated into an association of their own. The College Annals for February 1617 indicate that each midwife would be certified for membership by medical examination in the College before being admitted to the association by the Bishop of London, who could investigate her moral rectitude.[87] Proponents calculated that lessons in anatomy and parturition by an appointed Fellow would surely benefit these ignorant women. However, Peter Chamberlen the Younger angered the College by asserting that only he and his brother excelled enough in midwifery to be called in as outside experts for those lessons. It is likely that the Chamberlens had already invented a device to aid in delivery, the short obstetrical forceps. Peter the Younger's son, called Peter III, obtained an M.D. from Padua in 1619 and joined the family fracas. Though he had his degree incorporated at both Oxford (1620) and Cambridge (1621), the College of Physicians only reluctantly accepted him in 1628 with the warning that he needed "to alter his style of clothing from that more like the dress worn by the very gay young men at court: that he would not be [fully] admitted until he accustomed himself to the decent habits of the Fellows and wore quiet garments."[88] Given that attitude toward Chamberlen, it is not surprising that the Fellows took the part of the London midwives in their 1634 squabble with him, sending on the midwives' petition against Chamberlen to the Bishop of London; and when the College was asked in 1647 to comment on Chamberlen's advocacy before Parliament of the salubrious effects of public baths, the Fellows equivocated.[89]

The early Stuarts employed a host of household druggists. George Shiers, granted a reversion by Queen Elizabeth herself, was an apprentice to Hugh Morgan during Gloriana's last years. He then served James I through his entire reign, first as yeoman apothecary, when in September 1603 he made perfumes for the entire royal family at a cost of £210. Two months later he became first apothecary at £40 per year plus bouche and diet; the following year Shiers was made household apothecary, required to provide medicines for palace servants. An additional £60 per year was allocated to him for those responsibilities. In 1605 Shiers accepted the post of serjeant of the Confectionary. Despite his multiple apothecary titles, Shiers had no London shop and abstained from activity in the Apothecaries' Society, opting for membership in the Grocers' Company. As part of the ongoing dispute between the two associations, he was named with ten other grocers in a 1622 Star Chamber suit, charged with trying to disgrace the Apothecaries' Society and overthrow its charter; the suit was dismissed. Shiers bought properties in various parts of England including Yorkshire, Hampshire and Dover.[90]

Likewise, Elizabeth's yeoman apothecary, William Weston, was retained by King James for service to Prince Henry from 1604 to 1607 at £20 per annum. He was succeeded in that position at the same terms by Ralph Clayton, whose bills for supplies for 1608 topped £120. After Henry's death, Clayton held no further post under the Stuarts, but was still collecting his yearly salary until 1625, the year he died. A bachelor, Clayton left an inheritance to his nephews and money for poor relief in St. Bride's parish.[91]

The remarkably long-lived and fecund Gideon de Laune was apothecary to the king and queen for most of James's reign. Born in Reims in 1565, de Laune was the son of William de Laune, a Protestant pastor and physician who had settled in London with his family. Gideon de Laune was a member of the Grocers' Company before the apothecaries formed their own association, a move he strongly supported; de Laune became a founding member of the Court of Assistants, the governing body of the Apothecaries' Society, and Master in 1627 and 1637. He married a Chamberlen daughter. While his royal service ended with the death of James I, he grew rich in his dotage from the sale of de Laune's Pill, a secret nostrum made from a purgative gourd, colocynth. The thousands of pounds he earned enabled him to buy a mansion, two shops, and ten tenements.[92] De Laune was elected alderman for Dowgate ward, but he declined the honor due to his foreign birth; he was naturalized in 1635. His wealth made him an inevitable target for the supplication of Charles I's needy government, made even needier by the king's determination to rule without Parliament. Pressed in 1626 to lend 1,000 marks to the crown (£667), he was owed so much by the end of the Civil War that in 1650 he accepted forfeited estates in lieu of £2,048. He gave many gifts to the Apothecaries' Society in his lifetime, including in 1642 his portrait, which escaped the Great Fire despite the destruction of the company hall he had helped to acquire; the portrait and a bust of de Laune still grace the restored building. Gideon de Laune died in 1659 at the age of ninety-four, having sired thirty-seven children; he bequeathed property, including Sharsted estate in Kent, to his grandson, William.[93]

John Clavie (sometimes mistakenly called Olave), a Scotsman who had a large Scottish clientele in London, handled the apothecary needs of James I, Queen Anne, and Prince Henry at a salary of £40 annually in the first years of the Stuart era. Chosen for his office just three months after James' coronation and already wealthy enough to attain notoriety, Clavie struck a deal with two ambitious apothecaries, John Wolfgang Rumler (Romler, Rumlero) and Rumler's brother-in-law, Lewis Lemire (Lamere).[94] They paid him £5 for his patent as James's apothecary, agreeing to supply all drugs to the court for half the profits and the £40 to which Clavie was entitled. When Clavie died in 1607, Rumler became apothecary-in-ordinary to James I and Lemire to the queen. John Rumler's tenure with the Stuarts was long, probably lasting from service to Anne in Scotland before 1603 until the beginning of the Civil War in 1642. He provided a growing list of medicines as well as powders and perfumes. Rumler may have been instrumental in rousing support for the Apothecaries' Society; his name headed the list of the members of the Court of Assistants in the 1617 association charter. Twice Master of the Apothecaries, Rumler had an office in Whitehall and a shop elsewhere with apprentices; he needed a deputy to help him with his duties to the apothecaries' organization since he had much to do at court. Rumler got caught up in the affair of the Overbury death and testified in 1615 with his brother-in-law, Mayerne's apothecary Paul de Loubell, that Overbury had probably died of consumption. There was talk that de Loubell's son might have administered a clyster of corrosive sublimate, but a jailer, Richard Weston, and another apothecary, James Franklin, were executed for murder. In 1620 Rumler garnered a royal grant for the sole production of mercury sublimate, but the Society of Apothecaries withheld its consent.[95]

John Rumler enjoyed the benefits that access to the font of preference could render, including naturalization in 1610, and during James' reign Rumler usually received payment on time for the stock he required (over £1,000 for the queen alone for the period from 1609 to 1613).[96] In 1610 he was accorded safe conduct to go abroad to procure Rhenish wines, a much sought-after and lucrative license to supplement his royal salary. Like Clavie, Rumler savored living well; when his wife traveled to France in 1624, she was allowed to take with her four servants and plenty of apparel. However, like other apothecaries, Rumler was not always reimbursed in a timely fashion for his pharmaceutical wares; £130 was due him at the time of James I's death in 1625. As part of the royal apothecary's duty, Rumler supervised the embalming of James I's body, which required another £282 in supplies that Rumler claimed he bought. Despite the crown's unpaid bills, constant during the years of Charles I's personal rule, Rumler continued to serve the Stuart household as apothecary for life.

Lewis Lemire, from Flanders but with a patent of denization in 1599, served the Stuarts as a royal apothecary from 1607 to 1635, particularly as apothecary to Queen Anne.[97] At Anne's death in March 1619, Lemire was in charge of embalming her body. Like Rumler, Lemire was named to the Society of Apothecaries' Court of Assistants, but evidently Lemire and Rumler feuded over who got the better of the royal appointments. Lemire challenged Rumler's invoice concerning the preparation of James's body; he asserted that *he* had paid for the supplies used.[98] Despite their feud and the money the government owed him, Lemire also continued his service under Charles I.

Nottingham-born John Parkinson was James I's gardener as well as an apothecary-herbalist who was mentioned in the Apothecaries' charter of 1617. The Committee of Physicians charged with preparing the College pharmacopoeia sought his advice; he told them that if they had listened carefully to the admonitions given them already by apothecaries they would not have so many errors to correct.[99] Friendly with Mayerne, Thomas Johnson, the editor of Gerard's *Herball*, and other botanically minded apothecaries, Parkinson introduced many plants, especially for flower gardens, and during the reign of Charles I published two influential books: *Paradisi in Sole Paradisus Terrestris* (1629) on horticulture and *Theatrum Botanicum* (1640) on materia medica, unique plants, and herbs. He urged the creation of pleasure gardens combining pleasant ornamentation with practical applications, noting that peonies are good for epilepsy, gentian is beneficial to the liver, and canterbury bells make a safe gargle.[100]

King James required more than flowers in his final illness. By the age of fifty, he had already begun to seem old, and after Anne's death in 1619 he fell into a dangerous eight-day sickness during which he voided bladder stones, vomited, and suffered from bilious diarrhea. Though he recovered, he had aged considerably and thenceforth he was frequently ill, as his arthritis and gout became chronic in the damp and sunless winter months. By the autumn of

1624, the king could barely sign his name. In March 1625 while at one of his favorite hunting lodges with Buckingham, he fell ill with a tertian ague, an acute fever that waxed and waned with convulsions every third day. Refusing to obey his doctors, several of whom were present, and impatient for the fever to subside, James prescribed for himself, keeping his febrile hands in cold water and drinking large quantities of beer. Since the king had petulantly denigrated his own physicians, for medicines and plasters Buckingham called in a local practitioner, Dr. John Remington, whose remedies the king had previously used. James seemed to improve and planned to move to Hampton Court. But the fever worsened again and William Harvey, who was in attendance on the king, notified Prince Charles that the king's death was near. Charles arrived in time to hear James's profession of faith and to have a long, private conversation with his dying father. The king then sank rapidly, probably suffering through a stroke and dysentery.[101] King James I lingered for three days before succumbing on March 27, 1625, in his fifty-seventh year. His body was brought to London on April 4 in a bier lined with black velvet, accompanied by guards and heralds. The great architect Inigo Jones, another patient of Dr. Mayerne, designed the hearse for James's fabulous state funeral which took place on May 7.

Upon the death of his father, Charles I ascended the thrones of England and Scotland.[102] His continuation of unpopular Jacobean policy and reliance on inept policy-makers enmeshed his realms in foreign imbroglios, polarized domestic politics, and led to the Civil War. He antagonized Calvinists by appointing an Arminian polemicist, Richard Montagu, as his chaplain in 1625; he made William Laud Bishop of London in 1628 and Archbishop of Canterbury in 1633, provoking the hostility of Puritans. When the House of Commons defied the king's fiscal and church policies, Charles ruled for eleven years without a Parliament, but the resulting lack of funds produced a vacillating foreign policy and led to the exaction of hated taxes. Charles's insistence on religious uniformity led to the ill-advised imposition on Scotland of the English *Book of Common Prayer*, causing armed resistance and forcing him finally to summon a Parliament. Differences between Charles and Parliament over constitutional, economic, and religious issues erupted in warfare between Royalist and Parliamentary troops in 1642.

The shattering of Charles's domain was mirrored in the fractious disintegration of the medical community as empiricism in England increased after 1625. Despite his traditional leanings in most matters, the king probably contributed to disaffection between the crown and the College of Physicians. Like his father, Charles I "created" many medical doctorates at the universities for his friends and supporters; the Fellows were appalled when during a three-month stretch in 1642–43 he made twenty-two men physicians. They also fretted over what they perceived as growing episcopal intrusion into their professional liberties and royal ambivalence to the threat posed to their privileges by the upstart surgeons. Hence, the College deliberately separated itself from the court and by 1635 none of Charles' royal physicians played any role in the College's governance. Moreover, when trouble came, the majority of those Fellows who remained in London to run the College sympathized with Parliament, not the king.[103]

Nonetheless, no one could have envisioned the bloody ending of Charles I's rule when he first donned his crowns. Shortly after his accession, Charles, then twenty-four, married by proxy the sixteen-year-old French princess Henrietta Maria, daughter of Henri IV, who had been assassinated when she was only a baby. As a marital choice for their sovereign, Englishmen would not embrace Henrietta Maria, sister to King Louis XIII; they disliked her Catholicism and the objectionable treaty with her brother which included the royal marriage. Neither was she treated well by the Duke of Buckingham, whose fluctuating policy toward France in 1626 offended her greatly and whose influence led Charles later that year to dismiss her entourage from Whitehall. Buckingham's murder in 1628 eliminated the impediment to the royal couple's happiness and they settled into a romantic relationship that produced nine children, including the future Charles II and James II, all providing job opportunities for palace medical personnel. After the death of Buckingham, however, opponents of Caroline policy focused on the king alone.

Like his father, Charles administered the royal touch, a practice firmly entrenched in the religio-political matrix of the land. Partisans of kingship and of the Anglican Church made belief in the king's miraculous powers integral to their concept of the national heritage. Interrupted only by epidemics or scorching weather, the ceremony, which took place on days announced in advance by proclamation throughout the country, attracted huge crowds. To prevent abuse of king and coin, scrofulous petitioners for the royal touch had to present certificates from their pastors testifying that they had not participated in the ceremony on a previous occasion. In 1633, Charles I had the healing service integrated into the *Book of Common Prayer*, and anyone besides the monarch who touched for the King's Evil was considered guilty of a crime.[104] Adversaries of the royal prerogative and of the established church rejected the convention as spiritually fallacious and philosophically absolutist. During the Civil War, sufferers from scrofula needed their healer and when King Charles was captured crowds of sick people flocked to see him. A Parliamentary committee condemned touching for the King's Evil as mere absurdity, but even after Charles's beheading his relics were said to contain healing power.[105]

The business of household medical staffing commenced with cool regularity. The new king even renewed two of his father's investigations into public health issues: the wholesomeness of tobacco and the validity of witchcraft. Having inherited from King James a dislike for the habit of smoking, Charles I requested that the College of Physicians recount for him the effects of tobacco grown in England and Ireland. In October 1628 the Fellows produced a report stating that domestic tobacco was "hurtfull to men's bodies, falling short of the perfection of other tobaccos that are brought from other more southern parts where it hath natural maturity, vigor, and efficiency," an opinion that Dr. Harvey had a hand in drafting.[106] They said nothing about the habit of smoking in general. In 1633 Charles himself referred to tobacco's impairing health and depraving manners, but since the prosperity of the Virginia plantations was at stake, he condemned only homegrown tobacco.

Dr. Harvey also figured in the examination of the "Lancashire witches" in 1634. Witch-crazes occur in places where unresolved religious divisions cause disquiet and paranoia; Stuart Lancashire was such a place, divided between staunch Puritanism and enduring Catholicism.[107] The testimony of an eleven-year-old boy triggered the case, causing seventeen people to be tried for witchcraft. Four women found guilty were sent by a doubtful John Bridgeman, Bishop of Chester, to London to be inspected for desensitized witch-marks, telltale signs of the devil's own. At the behest of the king, at Surgeons' Hall on July 2, Harvey searched their bodies for callus marks and abnormal blemishes, clearing the women of the charges and paving the way for a royal pardon.[108] Even more than James I in his later years, Charles I sought to mitigate fear of widespread witchcraft by appointing trusted physicians and midwives to conduct interviews with the accused and their supposed victims.[109]

The king's own health was good. Charles seems to have overcome childhood rickets and teenage anemia, the "green sickness," to enjoy vitality in adulthood. Henrietta Maria, though not robust, was like her husband rarely ill; in his detailed notes, Dr. Mayerne logged only minor queenly complaints such as tender gums, styes, insomnia, and cold sores.[110] At least eighteen physicians served Charles I, plus five surgeons, four apothecaries, and a midwife, Margaret Mercer; many were veterans of the Stuart household, but some were new to the royal medical scene. Moreover, Henrietta Maria imported a trio of *médecins* from France including Le Sieur Chartier, who accompanied her to England in 1626.[111]

Charles did not sanction chemical doctors because their ideology was too Protestant for him and their philosophy too Platonist. In 1636 the Caroline Code instituted at Oxford strictly regulated medical studies, requiring students to attend Hippocratic or Galenic lectures for three-quarters of an hour or be fined for their absence.[112] Although his First Physician was initially Dr. Mayerne, Charles subscribed to the medical philosophy of household physician William Harvey, an Aristotelian whose beliefs were closer to his own. In fact, Mayerne had to keep his correspondence with alchemists a secret, while Dr. Harvey had permission to experiment upon fowls' eggs and deer in the royal parks from the king, who on occasion watched him work. During the early years of Charles' reign, when the government determined to tackle certain social problems, the king asked Mayerne to report on plague, a recurring bane in England. To the list of traditional factors causing plague, such as vagrancy and alehouses, Mayerne added the conviction that it was carried by rats. He also advocated the building of new hospitals and the setting up of a supervisory commission of health with authority strong enough to override local jurisdictions.[113]

Gradually, however, Mayerne lost the king's esteem and his proposals on plague were never implemented, though he remained the queen's physician.

She relied fully on him as he delivered her nine children without a miscarriage and saved two of them from serious illnesses; his notes on midwifery, complete with diagrams and commentary, were published posthumously.[114] In 1644 at the king's command, Mayerne attended Henrietta Maria as she gave birth to her last child in the relative safety of Exeter. Regardless, Mayerne had sensed the shift away from his perspective and the diminution of his prestige; in 1634 he responded by once more altering the dedication of his long-delayed publication of Thomas Muffet's book on insects from the king to his friend, Dr. Paddy. Conversely, when Harvey published his great work on the motion of the heart and blood in animals, he dedicated it to Charles, noting that the king in his kingdom is like the heart in the body. In July 1639 Charles made his preference for Harvey official and named him Physician to the Person. When the Civil War broke out, Harvey followed the king to Oxford and worked on his dissections at Merton College while Mayerne stayed in London near Parliament; the House of Commons appointed Mayerne and his Walloon protégé John Colladon to attend the king's children in their father's absence.[115] After the queen's escape to France and Charles's execution, Mayerne tried to save the life of delicate fourteen-year-old Princess Elizabeth, her febrile illness compounded by her father's death, but she died in 1650. As for Mayerne himself, he died in 1655 at the age of eighty-two after drinking bad wine with his friends in a tavern near his home at Charing Cross. He was buried at St. Martin's-in-the-Fields beside his first wife, his mother, and five of his children. Only a daughter, Adriana, survived him. He bequeathed the College of Physicians his extensive library, but it was destroyed in the conflagration that swept London eleven years later.

Harvey was physician to Charles I for fourteen years and traveled at his behest on a diplomatic mission to Emperor Ferdinand at Regensburg in 1636 with Thomas Howard, Earl of Arundel, a sign of the king's admiration.[116] As First Physician after 1642, Harvey accompanied the king on his flight from London to a safe haven in Oxford at the outbreak of hostilities; Parliamentary troopers destroyed his manuscripts on the embryo, left behind in Whitehall. He was present at the first battle of the Civil War, Edgehill, in October 1642, reading a book under a hedge until a bullet whistled by. During the cold night that preceded the fighting, Harvey pulled a corpse over himself for warmth against the bitter temperatures.[117] Because of Harvey's loyalty to Charles, Parliament threatened to replace him at St. Bartholomew's and when Oxford finally surrendered in June 1646, Harvey sought shelter with his brother Eliab in London. Although Harvey was ostensibly a Royalist, his pioneering medical writings reveal something akin to republicanism, but he cloaked his challenges to classical theological and scientific theories in apolitical diplomacy.[118] Nonetheless, Harvey's greatest individual trials lay ahead in the Cromwellian Commonwealth. Under the Oxford Articles of the Interregnum, the Committee for Compounding fined those who had served the Royalist cause one-tenth of their wealth.

Former Stuart doctor Arthur Dee harbored long-lived hopes that one day he would return permanently from the Russian court to his homeland as royal physician to England's monarch. In January 1628, he wrote to Sir John Coke, Charles I's Secretary of State, asserting that he wanted to serve the king and that he would "rather accept of £300 there than £500 a yeare heare. . . ."[119] However, his friend Mayerne counseled him not to antagonize the tsar, whose largesse had enriched and exalted Dee, and not to "risk a doubtful chance" competing for a royal medical post in England. Mayerne noted that the contest for medical appointments had grown fierce even though "six, where formerly were only two, now fill the place and receive the pay." Two more men awaited the death of any of the senior doctors, "expecting to receive a hereditary rank granted to themselves by the diploma of the Lord."[120] Nonetheless, despite the presence of these various rivals, King Charles did request that Dee come back to him. In the summer of 1635 the physician left Russia to take up an appointment in November of that year as Physician Extraordinary, a supernumerary post and not quite the status he coveted. He later practiced in Norwich and published *Chemical Collections* on the "secret hermetick science." Dee recalled for friends playing quoits with plates of gold made by his father through alchemy.[121]

Arthur Johnston, appointed Physician to the Household in July 1639, enjoyed describing himself as a royal doctor. Born in Scotland and educated at Padua, where he received the M.D. in 1610, Johnston became Louis XIII's unlikely poet laureate as a writer of Latin verse. He practiced medicine in Paris and got into a squabble there with fellow poet George Eglisham, probably over their differing views on Arminianism rather than rivalry over their muse. Johnston supported the position of moderate Arminians on issues like predestination and free will. After composing an elegy on the death of James I, Johnston may have looked attractive to Charles I and his ministers. Archbishop Laud in particular saw Johnston's lyrics as an antidote to the poems of George Buchanan, King James' tutor in Scotland and an outspoken opponent of royal absolutism. Johnston wrote a satire called *The Consilium* on the artificial conflict stirred up by Eglisham over Buchanan's literary legacy. By 1637 Johnston was rector of King's College, Aberdeen; he died in 1640.[122]

Besides Harvey, five men served Charles I during the Civil War. Sir Edward Greaves, a 1641 Oxford M.D., traveling doctor to the king, and physician to the Royalist army, also had continental training at Padua and Leiden, two of the finest medical schools in Europe. He practiced at Oxford and published on typhus, receiving much acclaim. *Morbus Epidemius* (or the New Disease), described a malignant, contagious fever that was not the plague though about half of its victims did manifest red skin spots. Greaves speculated that this "febris putrida" might be caused by changeable weather, poor diet, or contagion. He recommended vomiting, purging, and enthusiastic bleeding along with a cocktail containing harts' horn shavings and a posset made of carduus applied to the arms and legs. Greaves also suggested fresh air, sleep, and repose as important to recovery, and a "clove or two of garlick" or wormwood beer as a preventative.[123] In 1645 Charles I made him a baronet; he was the first English physician to be given a hereditary title. He became a traveling physician to the king that same year, served him in captivity, and settled in London. In 1657 Greaves was admitted to the College of Physicians, which drew upon his expertise for its 1661 Harveian Oration.[124] During the Interregnum, Greaves concentrated on private practice in the capital. After the Stuart Restoration, Greaves continued his association with the crown; he was consulted by Charles II, while maintaining his Covent Garden office until his death in 1680.

Greaves's "Medical Receipts" or recipes is a 1670 collection of medications written in Latin and instructions for therapy written in English, evidence of a profession in transition from traditional elitism to one in need of popular support. Put together like a scrapbook, a collage with no apparent organization and many blank pages, "Medical Receipts" includes directions like these for "A Bath or Fomentation": "take one ounce of pomegranate (equal rind and flowers); of red rose leaves, plantayne, horsetayle and shepherd's purse each 1/4 ounce. Cut, bruise and boil in a gallon of water. Strain and add two ounces of honey and alum to make it tart. Put in some brandy or red wine and use with hot woollen cloth over linen."[125]

William Denton, ardent Protestant and anti-Catholic physician-in-ordinary to Charles I from 1636, attended the king in his northern kingdom on an expedition to impose Anglicanism on the Scots in 1639. Denton's daughter married Caroline Secretary of State Sir Edward Nicholas. During the Commonwealth period, Denton practiced in London and Westminster; he also ministered to Charles II before and after the Restoration. Another royal appointee was Samuel Turner whom Charles nominated to succeed Arthur Johnston as Physician to the Household in December 1640 at £40 per year. Edward Dawtry (Deantry), an Oxford M.D., attended Charles I at the Battle of Naseby in 1645, a Royalist defeat that ended the first stage of the Civil War.[126] Like Greaves, Walter Charlton was a traveling doctor to Charles I at Oxford, but since Dr. Harvey was in actual attendance upon the king and since Charlton's protracted career blossomed in the following decade, discussion of him can be deferred.

Some miscellaneous Caroline royal physicians remain obscure; others went on to more notoriety after the Stuart Restoration. Jacobean doctor David Beaton continued in service to the Stuarts, and was named senior physician-in-ordinary to Charles I in 1626. A fellow of the Royal College of Physicians from 1629, the Scotsman's absences from required meetings were noted. Beaton may have been on the road at the behest of the crown, as in 1633 when he and Dr. Harvey traveled during several weeks with Charles from London to the king's belated coronation in Edinburgh, stopping at manor houses along the way. Beaton was traveling with the monarch again when Beaton died suddenly in Berwick in 1639.[127] Another lesser-known individual, Samuel Bispham, whose M.D. was from Leiden, served a dual purpose for Charles: physician-in-ordinary and in 1634 ambassador to the Queen Regent of France. He also represented England to the governments of Genoa, Ferrara, and Venice. Bispham complained that he was not paid for the embassy and spent £7,000 of his own money. His "chemical notions," a handwritten book in the Harleian Miscellany, discusses what materials may be appropriate for distillation, advises on the proper methods of infusion and ebullition, and includes a tasty recipe for cooking a pike in anchovies, lemon, and white wine.[128]

Charles I nominated Alexander Reid as his physician in Scotland. Reid, an Aberdonian M.D. by royal mandate, was known for his "cordial electuarie," a fruity mixture molded into a walnut-size tidbit to be taken with a beverage before and after meals. The mélange consisted of conserves of roses, quince, and various flowers and herbs beaten in a mortar and mixed with "syrup of stechas" to make a soft lozenge.[129] Reid had moved to London by 1634, when he participated in the examination of the Lancashire witches with Harvey. Another physician-in-ordinary in Scotland from 1631 to 1650, Alexander Ramsay, a Basel M.D. and Fellow of the London College of Physicians, was active in the attempt to create a similar college in Edinburgh.[130] Celebrated for his great learning and skills, John Wedderbourne (Witherbourne), a professor at the University of St. Andrews, had his medical credentials incorporated at Oxford in 1646 by letters from the chancellor which represented him as "one of His Majesty's physicians-in-ordinary." He immediately went to Holland as Prince Charles's doctor and was knighted for his service to the Stuarts. After the Restoration, Wedderbourne retired as a national hero.[131] Finally, as a captain in the Royal Army, Martin Llewellyn (Lluelyn) was ejected from Oxford by the visitors appointed by Parliament in 1648. Though not a royal doctor, the following year he comforted Charles I as the king was led to the scaffold. He later received his degree and became physician to Charles II after the Restoration.[132]

The surgeons who tended Charles I included William Clowes, Jr., son of the Elizabethan luminary. Apprenticed to his father, Clowes the Younger completed his training in 1605 and became surgeon to Prince Charles, who made him serjeant-surgeon after his accession; Clowes served him until 1642. Although he was twice Master of the Barber-Surgeons' Company during Charles's rule, at the time of his royal appointment he asked the members if he might be excused from the office of renter warden to which he had recently been elected. He couched his supplication in terms of respect for the king, arguing that since no previous monarch had to share his serjeant-surgeon with the Court of the Barber-Surgeons, neither should Charles I. He also remarked that his fellow liverymen ought "to take notice how the College of Physicians and the Company of Apothecaryes of London have ranked the King's physitians and Apothecaryes [and} thereby guess what place I expect." Consequently, the Company discharged Clowes from his elected post, but ordered that "he shall take place next unto the youngest of our Assistants that hath served the place of Upper Warden."[133]

Miscellaneous Caroline surgeons meriting reference include Richard Pyle, married to Catherine Clowes, who became Charles I's serjeant-surgeon in 1642, succeeding his father-in-law; he also attended the future Charles II and ingratiated himself sufficiently with the Stuart heir to be remembered after the Restoration. Michael Andrews, active in the Barber-Surgeons' Company, was a royal surgeon to Charles I. In 1625 he received a life annuity of £150 as surgeon-in-ordinary, a grant that was honored until his death in 1661. In 1636 Andrews' name was engraved on the door to the Barber-Surgeons' anatomy theatre in tribute to his leadership in the organization.[134] Surgeons Richard Wateson and Richard Wiseman ministered to the king and his family during the Civil War, a precarious assignment given the hazards of combat and the later stigma of Royalist service. Wiseman accompanied Prince Charles throughout the conflict and was taken prisoner at the battle of Worcester. John Bolen discharged Wiseman's surgical duties at court during Wiseman's incarceration at Chester.

Henrietta Maria's personal surgeon was Maurice Aubert; he came with her from France. A Frenchman with a special license from the College of Physicians to administer internal medicines in the treatment of surgical diseases, Aubert was to receive an equipment allowance of £600 and a pension for his services to the queen.[135] But so often in the Caroline household, obligations went unpaid, and Aubert complained bitterly of his distress, his predicament heightened by the Civil War. In 1645, his complaints reached the French government, which, acting on behalf of seven- year-old Louis XIV, tabulated the injustices done to Aubert and ordered the resident French ambassador in London, the Marquis de Sabran, to take care of the surgeon's needs. Not only did Aubert fail to receive the compensation due to him for treating the queen before she fled to the continent, but his London house was pillaged and his belongings confiscated by the Parliamentarians.[136]

Charles I required the services of a barber to care for his hair and beard, but some of the barber's duties paralleled those of the court apothecary. Thomas Caldwell became the king's barber in 1625, compensated with a grant of £1,000 and other perquisites; he became Master of the Barber-Surgeons in 1628. In the convoluted ledgers of the Stuart financial world, Caldwell took over another sum (£300) owed to the king by a certain Richard Harbin in lieu of additional emoluments. As part of his duties, Caldwell bought provisions for Charles's coronation bath. Thomas Davys succeeded Caldwell as the king's barber in 1639.[137]

Charles' apothecaries included holdovers from his father's reign and selections of his own. Joliffe Lownes had been Charles' apothecary while Charles was Prince of Wales. A member of the Grocers' Company who joined the Apothecaries' Society in 1617, Lownes fell victim to an unscrupulous drug supplier, Michael Eason. After tests conducted on the material Eason marketed showed it to be contaminated, Eason was imprisoned until a £100 bond could be paid and the pledge elicited that he would concoct no more medicines.[138] Though Lownes's reputation was besmirched by the incident, Charles retained him as his apothecary when he became king. Lownes died in 1627, and was succeeded by John Rumler, apothecary in the previous reign.

Charles appointed Rumler, still loyal to the Stuarts despite their continued neglect of his bills, to the royal household for life. Though he was to be paid £40 annually plus bouche for his work, Rumler also submitted expenses for supplies, including drugs for the poor servants of the household, and expected prompt compensation. He "compounded and served all sweet waters, perfumes, and other odoriferous things" for the queen, and in 1627 became both her apothecary-in-ordinary and, on Lownes' death, personal apothecary to Charles.[139] Rumler claimed he was owed more than £943 for drugs dispensed to the household from 1628 to 1638. During the Civil War he furnished the king at Oxford with medicines; in 1647 he petitioned Parliament for £1,000 for arrears of bills and debentures. To make matters worse, during the war Rumler lost valuables including plate, medicines, and money when the court moved from Shrewsbury. He died in 1650.[140] As for Rumler's estranged brother-in-law, Lewis Lemire, he, too, persisted in his struggle to recoup the costs he had incurred while in service to the Stuarts. In 1632, the king ordered that Lemire be paid the outstanding sums, but the Treasury did not comply and the apothecary died in 1635 without receiving his due. Lemire's widow Mary was left destitute, obliged twice to petition the government for payment of debts in excess of £1,600. Though she was impoverished by Stuart irresponsibility, she begged (but to no avail) that her nephew, Matthew Bushie, who had served twelve years with Lemire and was the brother of Princess Mary's nurse, be made a royal apothecary.[141]

John Parkinson, James' royal gardener-apothecary, became "Botanicus Regius Primerius" under Charles I sometime before 1640. His *Paradisi in Sole, Paradisus Terrestris*, published in 1629, detailed the creation of a garden: preparing the ground, making compost, designing the layout, and obtaining cuttings. Though many more flowers presented themselves to the Caroline gardener than to his Elizabethan counterpart, Parkinson featured iris, daffodil, rosemary, and lavender in his "virtuous" garden. He dedicated his book to Henrietta Maria, although the queen privately patronized the Plancy family of apothecaries. A Monsieur Plancy came with her to England at the time of her marriage to Charles I, receiving £600 and a pension. His son and successor, Pierre Plancy, was endenizened in 1632, the same year in which he became Henrietta Maria's apothecary. It was to be a long association. During the Interregnum, Pierre Plancy attended Henrietta Maria in France, receiving £200 upon the Stuart Restoration for his extraordinary service to the Queen Mother as well as other subsequent payments. However, the Stuart habit of not settling debts resulted in Plancy's being owed over £700 in 1671 from Henrietta Maria's estate.[142]

Several apothecaries proved themselves staunch Royalists by maintaining their attendance on the king through the Civil War, none more than the Metcalfes of Lincolnshire. Adrian Metcalfe obtained the office of apothecary-in-ordinary through a reversion procured by his father, but had to wait for Rumler to vacate the post before he could claim it. In the meantime, Metcalfe provided the sweet waters and perfumes for the royal household and acted as Charles's apothecary in Scotland in 1641; he was admitted as a free burgess of Aberdeen during that time. Munk states that Adrian Metcalfe received an M.D. in 1645 while at Oxford, but Leslie Matthews attributes the diploma to the Archbishop of London's so-called "Lambeth degree."[143] Like others who had supported the king, Metcalfe was fined one-tenth of his wealth by the Committee for Compounding, in his case nearly £34. Francis Metcalfe, Adrian's elder brother, had to pay over £266, because of another brother's Royalist army service. On top of that, Adrian Metcalfe lost a wagon-load of medicines at Naseby and his offices in Whitehall were plundered.[144]

Another family of pharmacists, the Chases, provided druggists for the Stuarts and leadership of the Apothecaries' Society for a century, beginning with Stephen Chase, who served Charles I. Sometime after taking the livery in 1630, Stephen opened a shop in Covent Garden and received the call to court. The Chases took care of their own. Stephen Chase's wife was a "rocker" of the infant Prince of Wales, and his son, Stephen II, furnished the Court of Chancery with wax, holding a patent worth £360 per year.[145] The elder Chase and John Parkinson planned to grow plants on a plot of land near the tennis courts in St. James' Fields; they advanced £100 to obtain permission to do so, but the Civil War intervened and the plan languished. Stephen Chase's offspring would be more fortunate.

Finally, Thomas Rushworth attended Charles I as apothecary at Oxford from February 1646 to November 1647. Exactly two years later, Rushworth received £30 for "pains and expenses," probably much less than he felt he was due, but more than he might have expected. By then his royal patron had been conclusively beaten on the field of battle by the New Model Army of Oliver Cromwell, tried for treason in London by a special Parliamentary court, and sentenced to death. Charles I was beheaded outside of the Banqueting House on January 30, 1649.

No sooner had the axe fallen than devoted followers and souvenir hunters rushed to dip their handkerchiefs in Charles' blood, to pluck hairs from his scalp and beard, threads from his garments, and chips of wood from the block on which he had laid his head. Special powers of healing would be attributed to these relics, especially to the blood-stained cloths, the same forces that resided in his touch when he was alive. The groans and tears that arose from the crowd at the king's demise marked the beginning of his legacy as a royal martyr and a backlash against regicide. On the very day of his execution, *Eikon Basilike*, containing Charles's reflections on the issues that caused his death, made its appearance in the city.[146] In it, Charles explicitly claimed martyrdom; Royalists already thought of him as a saint and bought up thirty-five editions of the book in one year. After the Stuart Restoration, an addition to the *Book of Common Prayer* officially recognized Charles I as a martyr, commemorating the anniversary of his beheading with a special liturgical service and a day of national fasting and atonement for the killing of a king and the setting up of a republic.[147]

Notes

1. Quoted in Hester Chapman, *The Thistle and the Rose* (New York: Coward, McCann and Geoghegan, 1969), 25.

2. For the tumultuous history of the sixteenth-century Stuarts, see Caroline Bingham, *The Stewart Kingdom of Scotland* (New York: St. Martin's Press, 1974) and *James V, King of Scotland* (London: Collins, 1971); R. L. Mackie, *King James IV of Scotland* (Edinburgh: Oliver and Boyd, 1958); Patricia Hill Buchanan, *Margaret Tudor, Queen of Scots* (Edinburgh: Scottish Academic Press, 1985); Gordon Donaldson, *All the Queen's Men: Power and Politics in Mary Stewart's Scotland* (New York: St. Martin's Press, 1983); Antonia Fraser, *Mary, Queen of Scots* (London: Weidenfeld and Nicolson, 1969); and Keith M. Brown, *Bloodfeud in Scotland, 1573–1625* (Edinburgh: J. Donald, 1986).

3. James I has enjoyed a recent revival of interest by biographers. See, for instance, Irene Carrier, *James VI and I, King of Great Britain* (Cambridge: Cambridge University Press, 1998); Christopher Durston, *James I* (New York: Routledge, 1993); Maurice Lee, *Great Britain's Solomon: James VI and I in His Three Kingdoms* (Urbana: University of Illinois Press, 1990); and Roger Lockyer, *James VI and I* (London: Longman, 1998).

4. Most of James' biographers concur that the callow king and Esmé Stuart became lovers, but warn about the difficulties of defining a person's sexuality in past centuries. See David M. Bergeron, *Royal Family, Royal Lovers: King James of England and Scotland* (Columbia: University of Missouri Press, 1991), 29–31.

5. It was a claim muddied by Henry VIII's will which excluded the offspring of Margaret Tudor from the succession while favoring the descendants of Mary Tudor, the younger royal sister.

6. For more on the first Stuart queen of England, see E. C. Williams, *Anne of Denmark* (Harlow, England: Longmans, 1970). Besides Prince Henry, Anne bore Elizabeth in 1596 and the future King Charles I in 1600.

7. A. W. Beasley, "The Disability of James VI and I," *Seventeenth Century* 10 (1995): 154–56.

8. See John D. Comrie, *History of Scottish Medicine*, 2 vols., 2nd ed. (London: Bailliere, Tindall, and Cox, 1932). The Royal College of Physicians of Edinburgh opened in 1681; of its founding members nearly all had medical degrees from France or the Netherlands. See W. S. Craig, *History of the Royal College of Physicians of Edinburgh* (Oxford: Basil Blackwell, 1976).

9. The works are *Ane Breve Descriptioun of the Pest* (Edinburgh: 1568) and *Ane Brief Descriptioun of the Qualiteis and Effectis of the Well of the Woman Hill Besyde Abirdene* (1580), both reprinted in *Tracts by Dr. Gilbert Skeyne, Mediciner to His Majesty* for members of the Bannatyne Club by James Skene in 1860. For more on Skeyne see "Literary Notes," *British Medical Journal* (1912) 1: 688.

10. Craig, *History of the College Edinburgh*, 682–83. The anonymous author of the previously cited "Literary Notes" (*British Medical Journal*) errs in accepting the notion that Craig "did not live to accompany His Majesty to England." According to the *DNB*, Craig lived until 1620. The writer of "Literary Notes" reported that James Chalmers, an Aberdonian, was James's physician before 1603 (a declaration repeated by Clippingdale), but I can find no other evidence of such an appointment. David Stevenson's history of King's College, Aberdeen, does not mention James Chalmers: Stevenson, *King's College, Aberdeen* (Aberdeen: University of Aberdeen Press, 1990).

11. Some evidence of James's medical household can be gleaned from John Nichols, ed., *The Progresses, Processions, and Magnificent Festivities of King James the First*, 4 vols. (London: J. B. Nichols, 1828). See 1: 151 (Craig and Primrose), 443 (Shiers and Marbeck), 545 (Hammond), 597 (Elvin, Martin, and Olave), 598 (Gooderus); 3: 25 (Butler), 28 (Atkins); 4: 721 (Vulp and

Rumlero), 1031 (Paddy), and 1033 (Hayes). After 1714 only one physician-in-ordinary was named (referred to as the second physician), and in 1847 Scottish physician-in-ordinary appointments ceased altogether: Craig, *History of the College of Edinburgh*, 682. See also Kevin Sharpe, "Faction at the Early Stuart Court," *History Today* 33 (October 1983): 39–47; Linda Levy Peck, *Northampton: Patronage and Policy at the Court of James I* (London: Allen and Unwin, 1982).

12. *Basilikon Doron*, James' essay on kingship, can be found in Johann P. Somerville, ed., *King James VI and I: The Political Writings* (Cambridge: Cambridge University Press, 1994).

13. Bloch, *Royal Touch*, 191–92; Lockyer, *James VI and I*, 202.

14. D. Harris Willson, *King James VI and I* (New York: Henry Holt, 1956), 302.

15. Matthews, *Royal Apothecaries*, 100.

16. Willson, *King James VI and I*, 307–8.

17. Lockyer, *James VI and I*, 20. After a few years on the run, Bothwell fled to Naples where he lived for three decades.

18. Annals of the College of Physicians, vol. 3, folios 16b-17a, LRCP; W.S.C. Copeman, *The Apothecaries of London 1617–1967* (London: Pergamon, 1967), ix. That same month, concerned that illegal practitioners were using the queen's name to get business, the College wrote to Viscount Lisle in protest. See also T. D. Whittet, *Clerks, Bedels, and Chemical Operators of the Society of Apothecaries* (London: Apothecaries' Hall, 1977); Cecil Wall, *The London Apothecaries* (London: Apothecaries' Hall, 1955); and Cecil Wall, H. Charles Cameron and E. Ashworth Underwood, *History of the Worshipful Society of Apothecaries of London* Vol. 1 1617–1815, (London: Oxford University Press, 1963).

19. Copeman, *Apothecaries of London*, 16. See also Harold J. Cook, "Policing the Health of London: The College of Physicians and the Early Stuart Monarchy," *Social History of Medicine* 2 (1989), 1–33.

20. Craig (or Cragg) received his English appointment on May 21, 1603; he earned £160 per year for daily attendance on the king. SL MSS 13/168 f. 78. At the New Year in 1606, Craig gave the king a gift of marzipan. Matthews, *Royal Apothecaries*, 84.

21. Quoted in Clark, *Royal College of Physicians* 1: 193.

22. Munk, *Roll* 1: 170.

23. R. G. Mitchell, "William Harvey and Celtic Medicine," *Scottish Medical Journal* 29 (1984): 251.

24. John Aikin, quoted in Randolph Vigne, "Mayerne and his Successors: Some Huguenot Physicians under the Stuarts," *Journal of the Royal College of Physicians of London* 20/3 (July 1986): 222.

25. Moore, *History of the Study of Medicine*, 106. In a 1615 letter from Paris, Mayerne recounted for the king a conversation he had there with English ambassador Thuring about another woman in James' life: his mother, Mary. He also related Thuring's memories of Queen Elizabeth's death; Add. MSS 32092, f. 224, British Library.

26. Moore, *History of the Study of Medicine*, 105. Some historians have speculated that James suffered from porphyria, the disease associated with George III's madness, but others posit that he suffered from mild cerebral palsy with athetoid features somewhat prominent in addition to spasticity. Lockyer, *James VI and I*, 200. A.W. Beasley asserts that cerebral palsy could account for James' habit of leaning on courtiers and slobbering on them; it might be the reason why contemporary observers and more recent historians have thought him homosexual. "It is at least possible to account, on medical grounds, for his habit of embracing his favorites." Beasley, "Disability of James VI and I," 159–60.

27. Mayerne, quoted in Willson, *King James VI and I*, 378.

28. Lady Anne Clifford quoted in ibid., 191.

29. Kybett, "Henry VIII—A Malnourished King," 25. Mayerne was the only doctor in Jacobean England who used the term "scorbutic," but he failed to grasp the significance of James's apparently immoderate need for fruit: Willson, *King James VI and I*, 336, 378.

30. Theodore Mayerne, *Medicinal Counsels or Advices* (London: N. Ponder, 1677), 36–38. Samuel Clippingdale believed that Shakespeare's depiction of Dr. Butts was meant to offend Mayerne. See "Sir William Butt, M.D.: A Local Link with Shakespeare," 7.

31. Mayerne, quoted in Anne Somerset, *Unnatural Murder: Poison at the Court of James I* (London: Weidenfeld and Nicolson, 1997), 169.

32. Pyarali M. Rattansi, "Paracelsus and the Puritan Revolution," *Ambix* 11 (1963): 24.

33. Moore, *History of the Study of Medicine*, 123. The other two are Francis Glisson and Thomas Sydenham.

34. Munk, *Roll* 1: 164; Dobson, "Royal Dentists," 284.

35. Annals of the College of Physicians, vol. 3, folios 52a, 64a, LRCP.

36. Annals of the College of Physicians, vol. 3, f. 104b, LRCP; Munk, *Roll* 1: 200. Cadyman also tended to Parliamentary leader Francis Russell, Earl of Bedford. For more on Charles's queen, see Robert Gray, *The King's Wife* (London: Secker and Warburg, 1990).

37. Dobson and Walker, *Barbers and Barber-Surgeons*, 139.

38. Munk, *Roll* 1: 100–101.

39. Quoted in Willson, *King James VI and I*, 289.

40. See Kenneth Keele, *William Harvey* (London: Nelson, 1965) and Geoffrey Keynes, *The Life of William Harvey* (Oxford: Clarendon Press, 1966) for biographical information; Gweneth Whitteridge, *William Harvey and the Circulation of the Blood* (London: Macdonald, 1971) for Harvey's most important legacy.

41. Garrison, *Introduction to the History of Medicine*, 246, 248.

42. Herbert R. Spencer, *William Harvey, Obstetric Physician and Gynecologist* (London: Harrison and Sons, 1921), 22–23; J. L. Thornton and Patricia C. Want, "William Harvey, 'Father of British Obstetrics' and His Friend Percival Willughby," *British Journal of Obstetrics and Gynaecology* 85/4 (April 1978): 241–45. Harvey's close friend, Dr. Percival Willughby, publicly cited the grievous practices of midwives and trained his daughter to his own standards: see Adrian Wilson, "Memorial of Eleanor Willughby," in *Women, Science and Medicine 1500–1700*, ed. Lynette Hunter and Sarah Hutton (Stroud, England: Sutton, 1997), 138–77.

43. The full title of his seventy-two page tract is *Exercitatio anatomica de motu cordis et sangionis in animalibus*.

44. Garrison, *Introduction to the History of Medicine*, 246.

45. Keynes, *Life of Harvey*, 137–38; Oliver Lawson-Dick, ed., *Aubrey's Brief Lives* (London: Mandarin, 1992), 131–32.

46. Vorst, a rationalist whose work was more sympathetic to the Church Fathers than was the work of most Protestant theologians of his age, was compelled to retire from Leiden and was condemned by the Synod of Dort.

47. Clippingdale, Medical Court Roll, 1: 47, LRCS. Buckingham was James's last and greatest favorite, and satisfied the king's sexual longing: Bergeron, *Royal Family, Royal Lovers*, 165–66. For a full, balanced biography see Roger Lockyer, *Buckingham* (London: Longman, 1981).

48. Eglisham numbers Lord Hamilton among the duke's earlier victims because Hamilton tried to warn the king of his "bewitchment" and suffered death by a similar poison.

49. Annals of the College of Physicians, vol. 2, f. 126a; Clippingdale, Medical Court Roll, 1: 55, LRCS. Moundeforde, thrice President of the College of Physicians in James's reign, was appointed by the Privy Council to take care of Arabella Stuart, the king's cousin, who was imprisoned in the Tower in 1611 for marrying against the king's wishes. When she died there in 1615, the College of Physicians was asked to supervise an autopsy; they reported that she died of a lingering sickness, "a growing oachexy," exacerbated by refusal to accept medical help. Annals of the College of Physicians, vol. 3, f. 22a, LRCP.

50. Atkins, quoted in Charles Carlton, *Charles I*, 2nd ed. (London: Routledge, 1995), 2. Rickets, not identified until 1620, was prevalent in the British Isles and was known as "the English disease." Associated with diet deficiency and lack of sunlight, besides weak joints, rickets manifests itself in a large head, somewhat flattened in back; both Charles and his brother Henry were depicted in early portraits with this rachitic characteristic. Pauline Gregg, *King Charles I* (Berkeley: University of California Press, 1981), 11.

51. C. R. B. Barrett, *History of the Society of the Apothecaries of London* (London: E. Stock, 1905), xix.

52. Annals of the College of Physicians, vol. 2, f. 82a, LRCP.

53. Ibid.

54. Munk, *Roll* 1: 149.

55. Annals of the College of Physicians, vol. 2, folios 131a-b, LRCP.

56. Munk, *Roll* 1: 149.

57. Ibid., 1: 158.

58. Ibid., 1: 184; Clippingdale, Medical Court Roll, 1: 50b, LRCS.

59. SL MSS 3426, folios 29–72b, British Library.

60. Clippingdale, Medical Court Roll, 1: 65, LRCS.

61. Butler is listed as surgeon to James I in Nichols, *Progresses of Queen Elizabeth* 3: 25.

62. Lawson-Dick, *Aubrey's Brief Lives*, 48. Vivian Nutton calls Butler "a pragmatic Galenist of the old school . . . [who] shows no acquaintance with or liking for Paracelsus and his medicine." Jeffrey Boss demurs. For their debate, see Vivian Nutton, "Dr. Butler Revisited," *Medical History* 22 (1978): 417–30.

63. SL MSS 1087, British Library. The manuscript contains more than six hundred recipes with a partial index, but only the ague drink is specifically attributed to Butler. According to the *DNB*, an ale was later named for him.

64. Not all historians subscribe to the typhoid diagnosis. G.P.V. Akrigg describes a half-year decline in the prince's health: see his *Jacobean Pageant or the Court of James I* (London: Hamish Hamilton, 1962), 133–34. For what might have been, see Roy Strong, *Henry, Prince of Wales, and England's Lost Renaissance* (New York: Thames and Hudson, 1986).

65. Charles Cornwallis, "The Life and Death of Our Late Most Incomparable and Heroique Prince Henry, Prince of Wales," in *Somers Tracts* 13 vols., rev., ed. Walter Scott (New York: AMS, 1965) 2: 233. I wish to acknowledge an unpublished paper by Donald Pierce on Prince Henry's death, which the author graciously provided.

66. Mayerne's account quoted in Akrigg, *Jacobean Pageant*, 134. Akrigg notes that King James, afraid of death, had left Whitehall Palace for Theobalds; Queen Anne had already withdrawn to Denmark House.

67. Cornwallis, "Life and Death of Prince Henry," 239.

68. Raleigh's cordial contained a riot of highly-detailed ingredients including "all three natural families—animal, vegetable, and mineral." It consists of harts' horn (slain between August 15 and September 20), to reduce corruption in humors; oriental bezoar (from the intestines of Persian or American ruminants), good for digestion and combating poison or plague; musk (from the belly of a rutting goat); the heart and liver of vipers; pearls; ambergris; ten roots including angelica, birthwort, fraxinella, carline, gentium, viruna, tormentil, valerian, and zedoary; six plants including marjoram and mint; flowers such as those of mace, clove, saffron, and marigold; fruits and berries; sassafras and wood bark; sugar and wine; and minerals such as oriental bole, coral, unicorn mineral, gold, and sealed earth. Mix together and drink! Nicolas LeFevre, *Discourse upon Sir Walter Rawleigh's Great Cordial* (London: J. F., 1664).

69. Some, including his brother, thought Henry was the victim of poisoned grapes. See John H. Jesse, *Memoirs of the Court of England during the Reign of the Stuarts*, 4 vols. (London: R. Bentley, 1840) 1: 171; Gregg, *King Charles I*, 453, n. 4.

70. Rochester's rise from Robert Carr, lowly Scottish page in the royal household, to titled favorite originated in the king's sexual vulnerability to attractive lotharios. Made Earl of Somerset in November 1615, he was soon succeeded in James's affections by Buckingham; Bergeron, *Royal Family, Royal Lovers*, 87.

71. Somerset, *Unnatural Murder*, 171. Somerset notes that besides the concoctions administered to Overbury by physicians other than Mayerne, Sir Thomas imbibed a patent medicine, *aurum potabile*.

72. Annals of the College of Physicians, vol. 3, f. 46b, LRCP; Munk, *Roll* 1: 179.

73. Nichols, *Progresses of James I* 1: 545, note 3; Munk, *Roll* 1: 147.

74. Wilhelm Treue calls Chartrier James I's personal physician, in his undocumented *Doctor at Court*, trans. by Frances Fawcett (London: Weidenfeld and Nicolson, 1958). Nichols lists Doctors

Martin, Elvin, and Sir Edward Radcliffe, "sworn servant and physician to King James I": Nichols, *Progresses of James I* 1: 597, 3: 49, n. 4.

75. Lawson-Dick, *Aubrey's Brief Lives*, 50. Ridgely lived to be an octogenarian.

76. Annals of the College of Physicians, vol. 3, f. 44b, LRCP; Munk, *Roll* 1: 180.

77. John H. Appleby, "Some of Arthur Dee's Associations before Visiting Russia Clarified, including Two Letters from Sir Theodore Mayerne," *Ambix* 26 (1979): 2. Along with Arthur Dee, the Annals list several "doctors" and apothecaries who flouted the College's jurisdiction: Annals of the College of Physicians, vol. 3, f. 11a, LRCP. C.J.S. Thompson lists Arthur Dee as a "quacksalver": see his undocumented *Quacks of Old London* (Philadelphia: J. B. Lippincott, 1929).

78. Appleby, "Some of Arthur Dee's Associations," 5.

79. Separations, indifference, and lack of communication characterize the marriage of James and Anne. After 1607 little remained of the husband-wife relationship, especially as the king turned his attentions to Robert Carr: Bergeron, *Royal Family, Royal Lovers*, 90–91.

80. Willson, *King James VI and I*, 403. The king was at Newmarket at the time of her demise.

81. Munk, 1: *Roll* 108.

82. The motion was rescinded later that year. Repertories of the Court of Aldermen 27, f. 117, Corporation of London Library, London.

83. Young, *Annals*, 551.

84. Ibid., 326. Master Naismith, Nesmith, and Neste Smith are various spellings of the surgeon's name.

85. Ibid., 330–31.

86. "A Huguenot Surgeon," *Proceedings of the Huguenot Society of London* 17 (1942–43): 70–71. Anne of Denmark bore seven children and endured three miscarriages. Only two of her offspring, Charles and Elizabeth, survived her.

87. Annals of the College of Physicians, vol. 3, f. 27a, LRCP. The Annals are at variance with historian Herbert Spencer's assertion that the College felt that incorporation of the midwives "was neither necessary or convenient:" Herbert R. Spencer, *History of British Midwifery 1650–1800* (London: J. Bale, 1927), iii.

88. Annals of the College of Physicians, vol. 3, f. 83b, LRCP. Nichols calls a Mr. Hayes surgeon to James I, but I have found no collaborative evidence of this; Nichols, *Progresses of James I* 4: 1033.

89. Annals of the College of Physicians, vol. 3, folios 144a-145a; vol. 4, f. 15b, LRCP; Peter Chamberlen, *A Voice in Rhama* (London: William Bentley, 1646). In the pamphlet, Chamberlen identifies himself as "one of His Majesty's physicians extraordinary."

90. Matthews, *Royal Apothecaries*, 78, 86.

91. Ibid., 84–87.

92. Ibid., 98–100.

93. See F.N.L. Poynter, "Gideon de Laune and his Family Circle," *The Wellcome History of Medicine Library Publications Lecture Series*, no. 2 (London: Wellcome Medical Library, 1965). One of de Laune's daughters married Peter Chamberlen the Younger.

94. Clavie kept £40 in gold in his desk, £30 in his study, and £22 in a trunk at court where he had a laboratory. Clavie's will also records an accumulation of outstanding debts to be collected. Matthews, *Royal Apothecaries*, 88, 91.

95. Ibid., 92–94. Nichols lists a John Vulp as apothecary to James I, but I can find no evidence of a royal appointment; Nichols, *Progresses of James I* 4: 721, note 1.

96. Matthews identifies a Dr. Scovenus as Anne's physician during this period and records his certifying Rumler's bill, but Scovenus' name does not appear in Munk, Young, or Clippingdale; Matthews, *Royal Apothecaries*, 92.

97. Two procedures enabled aliens to take English nationality: endenization by Letters Patent under the Great Seal or naturalization by an Act of Parliament of 1609, the latter forbidden to anyone who had not taken Communion according to the rite of the Established church.

98. Matthews, *Royal Apothecaries*, 90.

99. Ibid., 92.

100. See John Parkinson, *Garden of Pleasant Flowers* ed. Alfred Hyatt, (London: T. N. Foulis,

1904). Unfortunately, Parkinson's handwritten observations are burned and illegible: SL MSS 2346, folios 187–91, British Library.

101. Willson, *King James VI and I*, 446–47.

102. The scholarly pendulum on Charles I's merits as a king has recently swung with vigor. Compare the pro-Caroline, revisionist studies by Conrad Russell and Kevin Sharpe with the more negative, traditional assessments of L. J. Reeves and Peter Donald. For all its psychological framework, Charles Carlton's *Charles I* contains virtually nothing on medicine and refers to Sir Theodore Mayerne as Thomas (11). See Russell, *Parliaments and English Politics 1621–1629* (Oxford: Oxford University Press, 1979); Sharpe, *The Personal Rule of Charles I* (New Haven, Conn.: Yale University Press, 1992); Reeves, *Charles I and the Road to Personal Rule* (Cambridge: Cambridge University Press, 1989); Donald, *An Uncounselled King: Charles I and the Scottish Troubles 1637–1641* (Cambridge: Cambridge University Press, 1990); and Carlton, *Charles I*.

103. William Joseph Birken, "The Royal College of Physicians of London and Its Support of the Parliamentary Cause in the English Civil War," *Journal of British Studies*, 23 (1983); 50–56. Birken lists Mayerne, Cadyman, Bethune (Beaton), Craig, Grent, Harvey, Lister, and Ramsay as Caroline physicians in the College, but shows that for Mayerne, Craig, and Ramsay even their fidelity to the king was not inevitable.

104. In October 1637, the College, upon a complaint from serjeant-surgeon Clowes, examined James Leverett, a gardener, who claimed to cure the King's Evil. Clowes's list of charges included blaspheming the king's powers. Leverett readily agreed that he had cured some people, and healed his own wrenched thumb, dislocated by surgeons one night. The College pronounced him a deceiver of credulous people: Annals of the College of Physicians, vol. 3, folios 175a-183a, LRCP.

105. Bloch, *Royal Touch*, 208, 210.

106. Quoted in Keynes, *Life of Harvey*, 186.

107. J. D. Marshall, *Lancashire* (London: David and Charles, 1974), 34–43.

108. Also signing the report were several midwives and surgeons including Alexander Reid (Read, Rheedes), William Clowes, James and Aurelia Molins, Richard Wateson, Alexander Baker, and Amis Willuby: Keynes, *Life of Harvey*, 210.

109. Annals of the College of Physicians, vol. 3, f. 83b, LRCP; Keynes, *Life of Harvey*, 188; Sharpe, *Personal Rule of Charles I*, 245–46; and Thornton and Want, "Harvey and Willughby," 243.

110. Moore, *History of the Study of Medicine*, 106. Peter Chamberlen the Elder attended Henrietta Maria when she delivered a dead child at Greenwich in 1628; Dr. Peter Chamberlen took over his uncle's obstetrical duties and aided the queen two years later at the birth of the future Charles II: J. Dewhurst, *Royal Confinements*, 5.

111. Chartier received £1500 for equipment and a pension, as part of the marriage settlement: Matthews, *Royal Apothecaries*, 122. Another French import was Anthony de Choqueux, sent by Henrietta's mother in 1634 to look after her daughter. David Echlin, M.D. Montpellier, became the queen's physician in 1637. See Graham Martin, "Prince Rupert and the Surgeons," *History Today* 40 (December 1990): 40; and R. W. Innes Smith, *English-Speaking Students at the University of Leyden* (Edinburgh: Oliver and Boyd, 1932), xvi.

112. Phyllis Allen, "Medical Education in Seventeenth-Century London," *Journal of the History of Medicine and Allied Sciences* 1 (1946): 119–21. Pro-Galenic statutes dating from 1570 governed Cambridge; no anatomy was required until 1646.

113. Sharpe, *Personal Rule of Charles I*, 622.

114. In *The Compleat Midwife's Practice Enlarged*, ed. John Pechey, 5th ed. (London: H. Rhodes, 1698), Mayerne revealed his "rare secrets." Calling the penis "the yard," Mayerne noted that there exists great diversity in penile size, "little men being, for the most part, best provided." The "yard" enters "the privy member through a great chink."

115. Trevor-Roper, "Paracelsian Movement," 179–80; Clippingdale, Medical Court Roll, 1: 69, LRCS. Some have asserted that Mayerne, as a foreigner, showed less loyalty to Charles than did Harvey: see Vigne, 223. Though Harvey was in actual attendance upon Charles I at Oxford, Walter Charlton, a recent Oxford M.D., received an appointment as the king's physician in 1643.

When Oxford surrendered to Parliament, Harvey returned to London and resumed his private medical practice.

116. Keynes, *Life of Harvey*, 229–63.

117. Antonia Fraser, *Cromwell* (New York: Dell, 1973), 122.

118. See Alan Shepard, "'O seditious citizen of the physicall Common-Wealth!': Harvey's Royalism and His Autopsy of Old Parr," *University of Toronto Quarterly* 65 (1996): 482–506. Shepard says that Harvey's stress on royalism was only a pretense.

119. Dee, quoted in Appleby, "Some of Arthur Dee's Associations," 8.

120. Mayerne, quoted in ibid., 5–6.

121. Maple, *Magic, Medicine and Quackery*, 84; Lawson-Dick, *Aubrey's Brief Lives*, 90.

122. William Johnston, *Bibliography and Portraits of Arthur Johnston, M.D., Physician to James I and Charles I* (Aberdeen: privately printed, 1896). Clippingdale errs in suggesting that Johnston may have merely described himself as a royal physician, but Johnston is not even listed in Munk: Clippingdale, Medical Court Roll 1: 47, LRCS. See also Stevenson, *King's College, Aberdeen*, 97.

123. Sir Edward Greaves, *Morbus Epidemius* (Oxford: L. Lichfield, 1643), 15.

124. SL MSS 302, British Library. The lectures were meant to commemorate the benefactors of the College and exhort the Fellows to search out and study the secrets of nature by experiment.

125. SL MSS 51, British Library.

126. Clippingdale, Medical Court Roll, 1: 69, LRCS. Harold Cook lists Edmund Smith as a physician-in-ordinary to Charles I during the war, but Smith's entry in Munk contains no such claim; Samuel Turner, however, who was a royal physician, is not included in Munk at all. See Harold J. Cook, *The Decline of the Old Medical Regime in Stuart London* (Ithaca, N.Y.: Cornell University Press, 1986), 282; Munk, *Roll* 1: 190.

127. Mitchell, "Harvey and Celtic Medicine," 253; Munk, *Roll* 1: 197.

128. Harleian Miscellany 6940, British Library, London. See Clippingdale, Medical Court Roll, 1: 63b, LRCS. Bispham does not appear in Munk.

129. SL MSS 1087, f. 61. The folio contains a prescription of Mayerne's.

130. Craig, *History of the College of Edinburgh*, 47, 683; Ramsay was not designated a principal physician.

131. Munk, *Roll* 1: 251; Clippingdale, Medical Court Roll, 1: 66, LRCS.

132. Munk, *Roll* 1: 275.

133. Clowes's letter and the Company response are quoted in D'Arcy Power, "Serjeant Surgeons of England," 83.

134. Young, *Annals*, 8, 127, 134, 215. Young identified a letter dated 1625 from Sir James Fullerton, chief of the King's Bedchamber, to Secretary Edward Conway granting Andrews the annuity. Dobson and Walker list Thomas Marston as sergeant- surgeon to the forces of Charles I in 1637, but I can find no corroborating evidence, even in Young: Dobson and Walker, *Barbers and Barber-Surgeons*, 137.

135. Annals of the College of Physicians, vol. 3, f. 92b, LRCP; Munk, *Roll* 1: 197.

136. Add. MSS 5461 f. 170, British Library. The marquis had married an English lady and lived in London; his son was Lewis Sabran, a Jesuit chaplain to James II.

137. Young, *Annals*, 8, 19, 127–28.

138. Matthews, *Royal Apothecaries*, 89.

139. Quoted from the State Papers in Wall, Cameron, and Underwood, *Society of Apothecaries* 1: 94. As Henrietta Maria's apothecary-in-ordinary, Rumler was entitled to "diet" or 6s. 8d. per day. Matthews, *Royal Apothecaries*, 95.

140. Matthews, *Royal Apothecaries*, 96–98.

141. Ibid., 91.

142. Ibid., 122. Louise and Elizabeth Plancy were dressers to the Queen Mother.

143. Munk, *Roll* 1: 255; Matthews, *Royal Apothecaries*, 116. The archbishop had the prerogative from 1512 onward to issue medical licenses from his residence at Lambeth Palace. The fee in the mid-seventeenth century for a Lambeth degree was thirty shillings; Cook, *Decline of the Old Medical Regime*, 45.

144. Matthews, *Royal Apothecaries*, 101–2.

145. Ibid., 103–4, 130. Providing wax to the courts for sealing documents was a major undertaking; the position of "Chafe-wax" to the Great Seal of England included a wax house located at the end of Westminster Hall.

146. For more see Philip A. Knachel, ed., *Eikon Basilikon: The Portraiture of His Sacred Majesty in His Solitude and Sufferings* (Ithaca, N.Y.: Cornell University Press, 1966).

147. The Roman Catholic Church practices canonization, acknowledging the saint as an intercessor with God; Anglican commemoration allows for the "saint" to serve as an exemplar. For more on the memorialization of Charles I, see Byron S. Stewart, "The Cult of the Royal Martyr," *Church History* 38 (1969): 175–87.

Chapter 5

The Medical Staff of the Interregnum (1649–60)

The revolution that killed the king, abolished the monarchy, and inaugurated a Commonwealth had been accomplished by a small group of men. Between 1649 and 1653, a remnant of the Long Parliament, the Rump, relied on the army to shield it from its enemies while trying to reform society and the church. Oliver Cromwell helped the nascent republic to survive by suppressing opposition to it and then forcibly dissolving the Rump in April 1653. His "Barebones" Parliament, composed of 140 pious men (like Praisegod Barebones) selected by Cromwell, broke down in discord after sitting for only six months. The dissolution of this nominated legislature in December 1653 led to the setting up of a Protectorate in which executive authority was vested in Cromwell, the Lord Protector, and a Council of State. In 1657, with political instability increasing the appeal of monarchy, constitutional traditionalists offered Cromwell the crown. He declined the title of king but accepted the right to nominate his successor. Following his death in 1658, his son Richard presided for a while over a lackluster government that hastened the return of the Stuarts. In eleven years venerated institutions had been toppled like dominoes only to be returned to play; vulnerable men, even learned doctors, felt similarly toyed with by the erratic, perilous fortune of politics.

The minutes of the College of Physicians for 1649 are terse. Examining and handling disputes with unlicensed practitioners dominate the records. There is no reference to war, regicide, or the establishment of a new government under the aegis of Oliver Cromwell, only a brief mention of thanks to Alderman Stephen Eastwick for defending the College privileges before the militia of London in a tax dispute.[1] The two medically-related guilds were also cautiously muted in their response to the outcome of the Civil War. The execution of King Charles I went unrecorded by the Clerk of the Apothecaries' Society, only meriting an order replacing the royal arms at the society's hall with those of the Commonwealth, and the Barber-Surgeons revised their oath to delete allegiance to the king and his successors.[2] Given the widespread consequences of the change in authority that occurred in mid-seventeenth-century Britain, one might expect to find similar alterations in other aspects of English life, including medicine. All three medical associations evidently anticipated some repercussions from the new regime, none more than the College of Physicians. Surprisingly, however, it was left largely unmolested by England's new leadership, despite the widespread feeling that the institution was corrupt, because many of its key members, including some of Cromwell's doctors, were not Royalists at all and had supported Parliament in the Civil War. Though not politically aloof, whenever the organization seemed to be in jeopardy from chiliastic zealots, its leaders prudently opted for expediency, lowered the College's profile, and relied upon its friends in government.[3]

Nonetheless, the Fellows' recorded reticence in 1649 masks the metamorphosis in medicine that had begun earlier but which accelerated during the Interregnum, an evangelical struggle for ideological and jurisdictional control mirroring the struggle in society at large. R. S. Roberts asserts that during the Civil War, the practice of medicine burgeoned for the first time since 1512, becoming a testing ground for new concepts and organizational strategies, free from the dominion and extra-judicial discipline of the College.[4] Republican herbalist Nicholas Culpeper, who had been wounded fighting for Parliament, translated without authorization the *London Pharmacopoeia* of the College of Physicians from recondite, popish Latin into English in 1649, opining that the compilation should benefit the common man and that no one should restrict such knowledge. Needless to say, the Fellows were furious with Culpeper. Like Paracelsus, Culpeper foresaw an educated lay populace well-enough informed to practice a largely preventive medicine and to cure simple ailments. Culpeper was not alone. In a 1653 letter addressed to Cromwell, Samuel Hering urged that divines, physicians, and lawyers should all be state-salaried officials, not monopolists dependent on fees paid by the people. In Hering's view, the Royal College of Physicians held such a monopoly. Others called for a new democratic system of public health inspired by natural magic, Paracelsian alchemy, and chemical remedies. Opposition to medical elitism buttressed the key Puritan confidence in a priesthood of all believers, and a long tradition existed, even among royal doctors like Henrician healer Andrew Boorde, of appealing to ordinary men to cure themselves. As Culpeper noted, "all the nation are already physicians."[5]

The Puritan Revolution promised to its adherents a period of opportunity when God would disclose through science the direction to a new paradise on earth. Puritans were likewise sympathetic to a more scientific approach in medicine, their views apodictically counter to traditionalists and their tolerance meager for those still smitten with the power of priest-physicians.[6] Fellows in the College of Physicians, having just achieved a sort of tacit compromise by allying chemical therapy to the Galenic system, split anew over classical traditions versus experimental chemical medicine. More than recipes were involved. Radicals like Noah Biggs accused the Galenists in the College of outright antipathy toward the Commonwealth. In his 1651 tract, *The Vanity of the Craft of Physick,* Biggs argued for Parliamentary revision of university medical curricula in order to overhaul the "Palace Royal" of the profession and plans were discussed to establish a rival College of Medicine in London. The College of Physicians set up a laboratory and appointed an official chemist to parry the charge that it arrogantly rejected chemical therapy.[7]

During the revolutionary years of the Civil War and Interregnum, Paracelsian-influenced medicine ripened into a lively doctrinal issue, spurred by the appearance in England of ten of Paracelsus's works in translation for the first time. Moreover, a torrent of vernacular literature championing Christian Hermeticism and experimental medicine appeared at the end of the Civil War. Periodicals devoted to medical issues, such as *Mercury Medicus* (1647) and *Mercurius Insanus Insanissimus* (1648) appeared in London, imitations of continental publications.[8] To counter the tenacious bloc of Galenists at Oxford, Cromwell appointed several reforming physicians to the faculty, including anatomist Thomas Willis and his research assistant Richard Lower, both later celebrities in the London medical world and family doctors to the restored Stuarts. Although medical education in England still lagged far behind continental standards, forcing a large percentage of students to learn iatrochemistry abroad, the students simply had their university degrees incorporated at Oxford or Cambridge later.[9] Beyond the medical arena, Paracelsian dissension from Galenism made for nice allusions in sermons. After 1650, the conflict grew even more overt as chemical doctors denounced Galenists in print, challenging their knowledge of the latest therapies and adding a new name to the pantheon of theoretical medicine, Jan Baptista van Helmont, pioneer chemist and mystic.[10]

Brussels-born van Helmont studied philosophy at Louvain and earned an M.D. there in 1599. During the several years of travel and research that followed, he was sought out by the leaders of ecclesiastical and secular courts as a physician and an adept. Drawn into the weapon-salve controversy in 1621, van Helmont insisted that his Roman Catholicism did not prevent him from endorsing the magic of sympathetic healing and he praised Paracelsus for his disclosure of natural magnetism. Van Helmont's enemies cited heretical elements in his propositions and brought his work to the attention of the Inquisition, which condemned van Helmont for heresy and magic. Chief among the charges brought against him was his support for Paracelsus and chemical philosophy. In 1634 he was arrested and his books seized. After displaying abject contrition, van Helmont won his release and spent his final years writing on fevers, plague, and the errors of ignorant doctors who adhered to humoral pathology. Van Helmont died in 1644, but his son collected his papers and had them printed in 1648 as *Ortis Medicinae*. Medical historian Allan Debus calls van Helmont's oeuvre "among the most influential medical and scientific publications of the seventeenth century."[11]

Van Helmont's iatric and chemical theories posed a threat to existing medical practices as well as to religious and collegiate doctrines. He considered the ancients heathens, chiding Aristotle and Galen for their unwarranted conclusions and lamenting that medicine had been cultivated by enemies of Christianity—Greeks, Arabs, and Jews.[12] He rejected the doctrine of humors and bloodletting altogether, insisting that only through chemistry could the nature of medicine be understood. At the same time, van Helmont rejected the metaphysical basis of Paracelsianism. Concurrently castigated or embraced across continental Europe, Helmontianism was promulgated in England by Robert Boyle. Ignoring the strictures of his conservative professors at Oxford, Boyle engaged in experimental science, eventually playing a large part in the English acceptance of Helmontian chemistry through his analysis of corpuscular theory. Although Boyle found fault with some aspects of van Helmont's work, he influenced a second generation of Helmontian disciples, many of whom were thrilled by the frontal assault on Galenism.[13] More chemical books were published in translation in the 1650s than in the entire preceding century; Paracelsian-Helmontian interpreters produced most of the new renderings of foreign medical authors' work, coloring themes with their biases.

Walter Charlton, a staunch Royalist, would hardly seem to be among those keen to challenge supremacy of any sort, but he ended up impugning both Galenism and its Helmontian critics. Following his graduation from Oxford with an M. D. in 1643, he had been appointed physician extraordinary to Charles I, then sequestered at Oxford. With the execution of the king, Charlton was named physician to the Stuart court in exile, but without pay or duties. Perhaps because he received no remuneration, he remained in London, publishing ten books in the next decade.[14] By 1650, Charlton openly claimed commitment to the doctrines of van Helmont, effected the first English translations of his work, and wrote an original study of chemical philosophy. If reason was fallible, he argued, faith was not; Paracelsian and Helmontian iatrochemistry, set within an intensely religious vision, could be an alternative to Aristotelian thought.[15] But a counterattack against him, perhaps emanating from unhappy conservatives, may have caused him to reconsider his position on van Helmont, especially since his convictions jeopardized his ability to practice medicine at all. In 1652 Charlton, still only a licentiate of the College of Physicians, felt compelled to defend before the Fellows his treatment of a pregnant woman whose husband charged him with causing his wife's miscarriage and death. The Fellows decided that Charlton was not guilty of malpractice. By 1654, however, Charlton recanted his belief in Helmontianism, calling it "hare-brained and contentious," adopting *avant garde* atomism, fashionable among Royalist intellectuals. He especially ridiculed the more magical elements of Helmontian theory.[16] Charlton praised the College of Physicians as "Solomon's House" for promoting research and intellectual interchange, including, presumably, the discussions that caused him to reconsider his former ideas.[17] Notwithstanding that accolade, in 1655 when Charlton was proposed as a Fellow, the motion to admit him was tabled since there were objections to his candidacy.[18] Suspicions about his doctrinal choices in medicine persisted within the profession even after the Stuart Restoration and, despite his subsequent aulic duties under Charles II and membership in the prestigious Royal Society, Charlton did not become a Fellow of the College of Physicians until 1676.

As the dogmatic, politically tinged contest over theory played itself out among the established doctors, a simultaneous battle for control of the medical profession raged in London between the handful of licensed regular physicians and the increasing numbers of popularly successful healers. More than a theoretical squabble, the competition for medical supremacy in England involved maintenance of the historically discrete functions of physicians, surgeons and apothecaries, as well as the suppression of medical irregulars. Although the Apothecaries' Society, situated in a Puritan London parish, generally followed the Parliamentary penchant of the city, this aspect of the medical controversy had less to do with ideology and more to do with numbers. There plainly were not enough licensed physicians to handle the needs of London's burgeoning population. During the Interregnum, half a million residents of the capital had access to an estimated ninety-two licensed physicians; most could not pay these doctors' prices even if there had been more of doctors available.[19] While the poor received care free at St. Bartholomew's or St. Thomas's hospitals if they had been born in a London parish, the middle class needed affordable doctoring, too.

Because the College of Physicians deliberately kept down its membership and limited the quantity of licensed doctors available in the metropolis, Londoners patronized the lower echelons of the barber surgeons, neighborhood apothecaries, and midwives. Notorious quacksalvers took over an increasing percentage of cases, in part because they were willing to employ any technique or material available for the treatment of patients, but also because they charged less and were more accessible than their university-educated counterparts.[20] College leaders feared the rise of "empirics" and worried that their own members "should be dashed upon some infamous rock with great loss, and be as sport to the winds."[21] They had reason to worry. Around 1656 a nucleus of organized opposition to the Fellows articulated the need for an alternative society to protect the needs of unlicensed practitioners, a "College of Graduate Physicians." Although the proposal did not bear fruit during the Interregnum, the idea was resurrected in the next decade at the time of the great plague. In summary, both medical contests, theoretical and territorial, were waged to attract the ever-increasing numbers of patients seeking professional health care.

These simultaneous competitions for medical dominance intensified at midpoint in the seventeenth century and intersected over the discovery and importation of new drugs from overseas. Paracelsus and his followers had insisted that the protean regimen laid down by the learned Galenists was unnecessary since diseases reveal themselves through fairly constant symptoms. Unfamiliar maladies, seemingly new disorders, befuddled traditionalists and lent credence to their challengers; moreover, recognizable sicknesses like leprosy were on the rise.[22] Ignoring "common simples," Galenists administered complex mixtures containing a great number of ingredients, figuring one of the ingredients might help. Chemical physicians, however, insisted that once a disease was diagnosed, exact countermeasures could be prescribed: a "specific" cure for a specific illness. Much to the dismay of the Fellows in the College of Physicians, apothecaries and medical irregulars led the way, using New World and Asian substances in their search for these specifics. East Indiamen brought opiates and other palliatives to London; apothecaries happily dispensed them to patients less tolerant of pain than ever before. Antimony cups made from Mexican wood were soon covering hopeful Englishmen's tumors and wounds. Something of a backlash ensued against "medicines [that] the rob'd Indies enrich us with" in favor of homely remedies proper to each climate. However, by the time of the Stuart Restoration, a standard pharmaceutical primer in London used by most medical men listed 240 "exotic" drugs, a harbinger of increased medicine importation to come.[23]

Besides tobacco, advanced by some for use as an enema and for goutish patients, and ipecacuanha, originally prescribed for dysentery, cinchona, the first great specific, had the most profound impact on pharmaceutics. Malaria remained one of the most common and serious ailments in Europe during the seventeenth century. Although usually associated with more tropical climates, malarial fevers are not uncommon in colder zones, due to the prolonged incubation period for the disease. In rating the frequency of health complaints among Tudor Englishmen, historian Paul Slack has ranked ague (malaria) at the top of the list.[24] Symptoms included fever, vomiting, diarrhea, sweating, weakness, and thirst, ending in delirium, cramps, and convulsions. Despite improvements in sanitation and the drainage of swamps under Charles I, the southeast of England persisted as a malarial trouble spot. Summer and autumnal infections caused ague outbreaks each spring, and the resultant fever could be debilitating, recurrent, and even fatal.[25] Throughout the battle for medical supremacy, both sides freely prescribed for their ague patients a myriad of combination medicaments to be administered in the hopes that one or more of the ingredients consumed might reduce the patient's discomfort. Quacks and charlatans offered irregular fever remedies outside the professional sanctions of the physicians, surgeons, and apothecaries regulated by guild control. Wives in countless households followed more prosaic treatments for their families: confinement in a closed room followed by doses of coltsfoot, comfrey, or pills made from tar and elecampane. A favorite domestic cure was a decoction of snails, taken from the shells, pounded and boiled in milk, and sweetened with sugar or candied eryngo; earthworms cut into small pieces were sometimes added to the mixture. For the most part, however, expert remedies for ague were founded in traditional Galenism, including bleeding and cupping for relief.[26]

Therefore, the introduction into Britain of a controversial new substance that had distinctive anti-febrile properties posed singular challenges to the medical establishment and precipitated a new age of pharmaceutical empiricism. Jesuits' bark, or cinchona as it was later called, originated in the sunny climate of the tropical mountain regions of Peru. Quinine, a bitter alkaloid in the bark, became the cornerstone of chemotherapy. According to legend, the bark was named cinchona for the Countess of Chinchon, second wife of the Spanish viceroy in Peru, but misspelled by the Swedish botanist and taxonomist Linnaeus. It was said she was cured of a fever in the 1630s by a Jesuit made familiar with its antithermic properties by a village cacique some thirty years earlier.[27] Early writers about cinchona asserted that the bark's curative powers were unknown to the indigenous population of the Peruvian Andes, as no evidence of its use had been found in Indian records, nor in the reports of such early Spanish explorers as Pizarro. Clearly, however, if the Jesuits learned of the bark through a chieftain, the Indians already knew about it; medical historians now believe the properties of the bark were very familiar to indigenous people who confided their knowledge to the Jesuits in the sixteenth century.[28]

By 1635 the bark was available in Alcala de Henares, near Madrid, transported there either by the Count of Chinchon or an unknown Jesuit. It soon surfaced in the pharmacopoeia of Cardinal Juan de Lugo, the Rome-based Attorney General of the Society of Jesus. The Spanish Cardinal, himself a fever sufferer, introduced news of the bark at a gathering of Jesuit provincial fathers in Rome in 1649, and his optimism sparked hopes that it and other medicinal plants of the New World would be proof of divine approval.[29] De Lugo asked Gabriel Fonseca, physician to Pope Innocent X, to test the febrifuge, and it was soon being distributed free to the poor from the doctor's house as well as through the Pharmacy of the Collegio Romano and the Hospital Spirito Santo. Regular shipments began arriving from Peru, and the drug was written up by Pietro Paolo Puccerini, apothecary to the Pharmacy of the Collegio Romano, in his 1649 *Schedula Romana*.[30] In that same year, Louis XIV took cinchona, at about the same time that the drug was selling in Seville for $100 per pound.[31] By 1650, Jesuits' bark was a popular remedy in Rome.

The bark challenged a fundamental Galenic belief in the inherent fermenting action of the blood and made traditional heroic measures unnecessary. Early proponents of cinchona argued that it checked fermentation, thereby rendering bleeding and cupping not only unwarranted but unwise. It is not surprising that Galenic physicians objected to the bark, but intense condemnation of cinchona came from other sources as well. John Chifflet, physician to Archduke Leopold of Austria, denounced the drug as unsatisfactory and dangerous when it failed to cure the Archduke's week-long fever in 1652.[32] Renatus Moreau at the Sorbonne, Louis XIV's doctor, no doubt humiliated when the bark was administered without his advice, further denigrated the medicine.[33] When the bark proved useless against a plague epidemic in 1655, it fell into disuse on the continent.

Since the substance was associated with the Jesuits, the medical controversy surrounding its use escalated in Protestant countries. Regardless, it was tried in England by 1654. That year Dr. John Metford of Northampton gave the bark its first test when he used it successfully to treat a pregnant woman suffering from a quartan fever.[34] Given such environmental conditions as proximity to shallow lagoons in the marshy ground upstream from the city's western perimeter, malarial fevers were a constant feature of life in London. James Thompson subsequently advertised the bark's antipyretic properties in a 1658 edition of *Mercurius Politicus*, noting that one could obtain it at the Black Spotted Eagle in Old Bailey or from Mr. John Crook, bookseller, at the Sign of the Ship in St. Paul's Churchyard.[35]

Two well-known London doctors, Robert Brady and Thomas Willis, the latter a Cromwellian faculty appointee at Oxford, prescribed Peruvian bark by 1660, but the man most closely associated with popularizing the drug in England was Robert Talbor. The son of a registrar to the Bishop of Ely and grandson of a registrar at Cambridge University, Talbor apprenticed to Cambridge apothecary Peter Dent, in whose service he probably first came to value Jesuits' bark. Even before attaining fame as London's most fashionable quacksalver, Talbor practiced curing fevers with an undisclosed remedy in marshy Essex, which he deliberately chose as a testing ground for cinchona because it was "near the seaside where agues are epidemical diseases."[36] He is credited with reviving use of the bark in Europe and upsetting English physicians, who were appalled that a great febrifugal specific had been discovered by "uncivilized people," promulgated by the Jesuits, and revived by a "debauched apothecary's apprentice." Talbor advised mixing powdered bark with anise and parsley, steeping it in claret, and avoiding other drugs while ingesting cinchona. Talbor took direct aim at Galenists when he warned that "it is a mistake in physick to make a hodge podge of a great many ingredients."[37] Though primarily associated with fever cases, cinchona was used in seventeenth-century Britain to stimulate patients' appetites. Physicians also prescribed it to prevent hemorrhage and diarrhea, for which it is completely unsuited. Aware of the possible deleterious side effects of quinine, Talbor catalogued convulsions, seizures, and constipation as potential consequences.[38] Regardless, the drug's impact on ague was phenomenal and the bark became an integral part of the new pharmacy. Ironically, Oliver Cromwell, ridiculed by his enemies as "King of the Fens" because of his opposition to Caroline drainage projects, perished during a virulent 1658 malaria epidemic; after the Restoration Charles II pointedly made the feverologist Talbor his physician-in-ordinary.

Although coffee had been known to Europeans since the beginning of the seventeenth century, it was not in general use in England before about 1650. Sir Francis Bacon wrote in 1624 that the Turks drank coffee because it "comforteth the brain, and heart, and helpeth digestion."[39] A coffee house opened in Oxford in 1655 and soon Londoners quaffed the beverage at establishments throughout the city. Ale-house keepers feared that coffee drinking would spoil their trade and petitioned the Lord Mayor for relief. Dr. Harvey often drank coffee, having been introduced to it by his brothers, merchants in the Levant Company. Harvey definitely paid much attention to the potential medicinal properties of coffee, particularly its beneficial effects on dyspepsia. Some physicians promoted an electuary made of coffee powder, butter, and honey for "the stone" and for gout; Harvey may have used coffee for his own painful gout.[40]

Further light may be shed on this transitional time in medicine by examining the careers of those individuals who served as official medical men during the Interregnum. Though the Commonwealth vested supreme authority in the House of Commons, the Cromwellian Protectorate was really a monarchical government and many of the resources of a potentate were bestowed on the person of Oliver Cromwell.[41] He took over palaces, parks, and other royal appurtenances including a court with a household and a staff of doctors who functioned as both the state's and the Protector's physicians. The court remained the magnetic pole for ambitious professional men of all kinds.

At the same time, the triad of patrimony, patronage, and purchase that had assured royal preferment at court fell victim to Cromwellian reform. For one thing, there were no more wasteful Scottish appointments after the passage in late 1653 of the Instrument of Government, which assimilated the northern kingdom into a unified Commonwealth. Moreover, Cromwell insisted, with some success, that Republican office-seekers be loyal to the ideals of the regime. Royalists like Charles I's surgeon Richard Wateson fell on hard times in the wake of their patron's downfall; Wateson was declared "a papist and delinquent" on a loan, and his property was seized by Cromwell.[42] Changes in state medical personnel could be expected to reflect shifting partisan fortunes, but one can also discern the influence of Cromwell's particular political iconoclasm on the already fragile predicament of the seventeenth-century medical majority. Cromwell's predilection for innovative physicians who supported his agenda ultimately enhanced their status within the profession[43]

Fittingly, Oliver Cromwell disdained touching for the King's Evil and the supernatural privileges of royalty in general. During the years of the Commonwealth and Protectorate, there was no miraculous princely healing by anyone in Great Britain. For his own health needs, two full decades before he took the reins of power in England, Cromwell sought out the best-known proponent of chemical medicine in the country, Theodore Mayerne, ironically a royal doctor, too[44] Dr. Mayerne examined Cromwell in London in September 1628, six months after the future Lord Protector's election to Parliament. Cromwell had been purposefully drinking the medicinal waters of Wellingborough in Northamptonshire, but still suffered from stomach ache and persistent pain on his left side; Mayerne may have prescribed rue, a common remedy for stitch in the side. Dr. Mayerne remarked that Cromwell's skin was dry and withered, but his principal observation focused on his patient's extreme melancholy, a diagnosis made by Cromwell's hometown doctor and echoed by later physicians. When Cromwell was only twenty-four, Dr. Simcott of Huntingdon described him as "very splentic and often thought that he was about to die."[45] Cromwell himself must have felt sufficiently concerned about his chronic moodiness to consult Mayerne, the capital's leading doctor. Antonia Fraser suggests that Cromwell suffered a sort of nervous breakdown, perhaps as part of the "darkness" Puritans believed enveloped the spirit before true conversion, and was periodically handicapped throughout his adult life by extreme mental stress.[46]

There was nothing new about melancholia. Hippocrates characterized it as prolonged and fearful depression; Galen added symptoms of flatulence and digestive disturbances due to an excess of black bile, the morose humor, thereby marking melancholia as a cold, dry disease of the brain and abdomen. When

Oliver Cromwell displayed symptoms of melancholia in the mid-seventeenth century, the traditional heroic remedies of Galenic medicine, though challenged in anatomy and cardiovascular physiology, were still being applied for nervous disorders. Remedies purged the body of bilious excess. Harsh enemas and clysters provoked defecation; plants like sea onion relieved stoppages of the liver and spleen. Other physicians applied less drastic remedies. Apples were thought to exhilarate the mind and prevent melancholy; for despondency, apothecaries made lozenges called "pleres archoniticon" from spices, coral, musk, camphor, and peppermint water.[47] Not until the 1660s, when Thomas Willis turned the application of chemical explanations for disease to neuro-psychiatric conditions, was black bile challenged as the cause of melancholia.[48]

Like a few of his regal predecessors, Oliver Cromwell was something of a hypochondriac, whose fever would increase when he was told that his pulse was irregular.[49] According to his family doctor, Cromwell self-prescribed mithridate, a compound for poison smeared on leather and used as a plaster to ward off the plague, and in so doing healed his acned face. From the age of thirty-two to thirty-seven, Cromwell lived in St. Ives and complained frequently of sore throat; he attended church services with a piece of red flannel wrapped around his neck.[50] He was genuinely sick in 1649 in Ireland, possibly with malaria, the first onslaught of the disease that would dog him later. By 1655 his health had deteriorated markedly, exacerbated by the illnesses of his wife and his favorite daughter, Elizabeth Claypool. Cromwell suffered through bladder troubles including agonizing stones that caused him to run about in an agitated way; he also endured gout, and a boil on his chest in early 1656 required lancing by his surgeon. That spring he escaped serious injury en route to a friend's estate at Wimbledon when his coach plunged from the Lambeth ferry into the Thames. Rumors circulated that Cromwell's hands trembled and his eyes were often tear-filled; some speculated that he had lost his mind.[51]

His physicians treated the Lord Protector for ague with cinchona and myroxylon, another popular bark of the time, but one with unpleasant side effects. An infusion of the bark and maize was used for colds and pimples, but myroxylon (vernacular name balsamo) can itself precipitate fever and delirium; some nineteenth-century historians speculated that it might have contributed to Cromwell's death. Septicaemia, caused by infected kidneys and bladder, seems a more plausible cause.[52] Still, despite excruciating pain from "the stone," he persisted. The final blow to Cromwell's health came with the death of his beloved daughter Elizabeth in early August 1658. She had endured months of agonized decline, probably due to uterine or intestinal cancer. Just a few weeks later, when Cromwell developed a spiking fever and back pain, the state physicians diagnosed a "bastard tertian ague"; the Protector expired September 3, 1658.[53]

Although the Commonwealth and Protectorate era was brief in years, at least four physicians and three surgeons served Cromwell. George Bate (Bates) of Buckinghamshire demonstrated a resilience that must be testimony either to an extraordinary bedside manner or to breathtaking political agility. At age fifteen, he began his studies at New College, Oxford, where he was one of the college clerks. In a sequence that forecast his later shifts in allegiance, Bate transferred to Queen's College and then to St. Edmund's, where he received his arts and his Bachelor of Medicine degrees in 1629, the latter giving him license to practice around Oxford. In 1637 the university awarded him a doctorate in medicine. Bate soon migrated to London where the College of Physicians received him as a Fellow in 1640. Early observers labeled him a Puritan, but he evidenced strong enough Royalist sympathies when Charles I's court was at Oxford to be made a physician-in-ordinary to the king.[54] Bate is best-known for his published defense of Charles I in the king's confrontation with Parliament. *The Regall Apology*, written in English, was first published in Paris and London in 1648. Using the pseudonym Theodorus Veridicus, Bate turned his original account into an expanded Latin work, *Elenchus Motuum Nuperorum in Anglia*; the first part, covering the king's relationship with Parliament, appeared in Paris in 1649 and in Frankfurt and Edinburgh in 1650. An English version, *A Compendious Narrative of the Late Troubles in England*, was printed in London in 1652.

Bate's earlier loyalties to the king did not prevent him, as physician to the Charterhouse in 1643, from ministering to Oliver Cromwell, then General of the Parliamentary Army. One historian labels Bate a "staunch government supporter" in the College of Physicians, part of a "powerful and influential caucus" sympathetic to Cromwell.[55] Bate worked with Francis Glisson and Assuerus Regimorter on rickets, resulting in the 1650 publication of *De Rachitude*. In 1651 Bate and Lawrence Wright, already physician-in-ordinary and Bate's senior by twenty years, doctored Cromwell when he fell dangerously ill in Edinburgh. Cromwell designated Bate his chief physician in 1653.[56] For the next five years, Bate attended the Lord Protector and his family, including Cromwell's son Richard and his daughter, Elizabeth. At the Restoration, Bate was appointed physician to Charles II on June 20, 1660; some claimed that this appointment was made because rumors circulated that Bate had hastened Cromwell's death with a lethal medication. However, Bate evaded responsibility by detailing the symptoms of the Protector's fatal illness and the results of the autopsy.[57]

Jonathan Goddard, physician-in-chief to the Parliamentary army, emerged as one of the more celebrated iatric men of the Interregnum. Born in 1617 at Greenwich, Goddard matriculated at Oxford, but left the university without taking a degree. After traveling on the continent for some time, he returned to England to study at Cambridge, receiving his M.D. in 1643. He was made a Fellow the College of Physicians in 1646, delivering the prestigious Gulstonian lectures there in 1648. His political identification with the Commonwealth was strong. Goddard accompanied Oliver Cromwell to Ireland in 1649, nursed him through a bout of low malarial fever, and went on to Scotland with him the following year. Goddard returned to London with Cromwell after the Battle of Worcester in September 1651, shortly before being chosen warden of Merton College, Oxford.[58] Since Cromwell was chancellor of Oxford University, he appointed Goddard in 1652 to deal with grants and dispensations at the institution in Cromwell's absence. As warden of Merton, Goddard sat in the Barebones Parliament called by Cromwell in the summer of 1653 and that same year he was a member of the Council of State. Therefore, Dr. Goddard was an important member of the government when it surrendered power to Cromwell as Lord Protector in December. He sat on a number of committees including one on the care of lunatics. Goddard simultaneously enjoyed a professorship in physic from 1655 at Gresham College in London. As long as Cromwell was in control, Goddard's political star continued to rise.

The return of the Stuarts diminished Goddard's status in government, for Charles II removed him from his wardenship, appointing in his stead Edward Reynolds, the king's chaplain. Undeterred by this setback, Goddard left Oxford, but retained his post on the faculty of Gresham College. There, he participated in meetings with six of his colleagues that helped to set up the Royal Society for the Advancement of Natural Science, which he served as a member of its first board. Dr. Goddard published extensively on such diverse matters as observing chameleons and making wine from sugar cane, and is said to have fashioned the first English telescope. Despite Goddard's widespread fame as a chemist and inventor, Charles II never honored Goddard with a medical appointment, doubtless because of his political affiliation.

Goddard served on the governing board of the College of Physicians from 1660 to 1672, demonstrating remarkable professional longevity and leadership on a key College issue: the activities of insolent, aggressive apothecaries. Goddard, a fierce opponent of the London druggists, wrote two vitriolic treatises against them, *A Discourse Concerning Physick and the Many Abuses thereof by Apothecaries* (1668) and *A Discourse Setting Forth the Unhappy Condition of the Practice of Physic in London* (1670). In the latter tract, Goddard bemoaned the divisions within medicine and denied that he wanted to ruin apothecaries. Goddard affirmed, however, that physicians should be most familiar with medicines and ought to be able to offer cheaper and better drugs to their patients than the apothecaries did. At the very least, physicians could offer some vigorous competition to shop-keeping druggists. Goddard died in 1675, the victim of an apoplectic fit that his eponymous drops could not cure.[59]

Cromwell named John Bathurst, whose father was a Sussex doctor, as another protectoral physician. Bathurst received his arts degrees from Pembroke College, Cambridge, and acquired an M.D. there in 1637. The College of Physicians welcomed him as a member that same year and his degree was incorporated at Oxford in 1642. Bathurst made a reputation for himself tending to sick seamen of the fleet after Robert Blake's prolonged engagement with the Dutch in February 1653 and again in 1658. Representing Richmond, Yorkshire, in the Protector's second Parliament, and in the 1658 Parliament summoned by Richard Cromwell, Bathurst was numbered among the "court party" within

Parliament.[60] Besides his duties to the Lord Protector, Dr. Bathurst simultaneously was the physician of the Royalist Fanshawe family. Sir Richard Fanshawe was captured at the Battle of Worcester (1651) and detained at Whitehall Palace. Dr. Bathurst probably saved his patient's life, though not with pills or plasters. It was Bathurst's medical certificate verifying Fanshawe's illness that enabled his patient to win release from Whitehall and to retire to private life, overruling the orders of Sir Henry Vane the Younger, a leading member of the Commonwealth council of state.[61] Dr. Bathurst amassed a sizable fortune in private practice, enjoying an annual income of £2,000. Bathurst's 1656 letter to a colleague, Dr. S. Bare, discussing a mutual patient, Mr. Crosby, was written half in English, half in Latin, illustrating the ambivalence some Cromwellian physicians felt toward revealing the secrets of their trade. Given the fact that Bathurst's father and son were doctors, he may have felt compelled to guard some of the cachet of his family's profession.[62] John Bathurst passed away in 1659 at age fifty-two.

Lawrence Wright, a native of Essex from Puritan stock, was the fourth physician-in-ordinary to Oliver Cromwell. He received his B.A. and M.A. degrees at Emmanuel College, Cambridge, but then traveled abroad for further training at the famed medical schools of Leiden and Padua, receiving an M.D. from the latter. By the middle of the seventeenth century, Leiden had some claim to primacy among continental medical schools and it attracted many sons of prosperous Englishmen and Scotsmen with professional ambitions. Following the usual procedures, Wright had his Padua degree incorporated at Cambridge in 1618 and became a Fellow of the College of Physicians in 1622, serving as censor in 1628 and 1638, as well as consiliarius from 1647 to 1657, bridging the gap between monarchy and commonwealth. He was Cromwell's physician-in-ordinary before 1651 and his brother, Nathaniel Wright, was a navy commissioner. Besides his responsibilities to the Lord Protector, with whom "he was reputed to be in particular favor," Lawrence Wright was physician to the Charterhouse from 1624 to 1643 and its governor in 1652; he was also on the Board of Physicians in 1656 when it recommended the establishment of a College of Physicians in Edinburgh.[63] Wright succumbed to a quartan ague in 1657; his son, Henry, was made a baronet by the Lord Protector for his work on the trade commission of the Council of State.[64]

Besides these appointees, Clippingdale lists Thomas Sydenham as a Cromwellian doctor, perhaps because of his military service on the Parliamentary side in the Civil War, but there does not appear to be corroborating evidence that he received any government appointment.[65] Nonetheless, Sydenham's influence on medicine during the period was profound and deserves mention. A clinician who studied at Montpellier, Sydenham created a tripartite medical method: describing the disease before him, determining the praxis or remedy, and using that specific treatment. Taking careful notes on measles, he seemed to perceive more than his peers. He wrote monographs on febrile disorders, dysentery, and syphilis, turning his fellow physicians' attention toward particular diseases and the necessity of proper diagnosis. He told his pupil Hans Sloane to "go to the bedside; it is there alone you can learn disease." Sydenham learned about one ailment through painful personal experience, writing a masterful treatise on gout, an affliction from which he himself suffered. "Gout," he wrote, "rarely attacks fools!"[66] Reinterpreting Hippocrates' conception of pestilence, Sydenham began to ferret out the idea of contagion.[67]

However, Sydenham, like many of his peers, did not abandon Galenic methods altogether, advocating bleeding, especially for epidemic fevers and apoplexy. The standard advice was to bleed the sufferer enough to fill a pint basin, although some physicians argued that the first bleeding ought to continue until the patient fainted. After the initial venesection, sufferers were regularly bled to syncope, yielding 104 ounces of blood in four days, 210 ounces in six. The public approved bleeding for medical reasons. Diarists John Evelyn and Samuel Pepys both recorded their being bled, Pepys regularly, as a preventive measure. Samuel Pepys noted that he paid five shillings in 1662 to a surgeon for withdrawing two cups of his blood, "I being exceedingly full of blood."[68] Evelyn remarked that Dr. Harvey himself advocated that "all young people should be let blood," and many physicians felt that if you were not bled periodically, "you would explode like a gun shot off."[69] But Sydenham did not acknowledge the implications of Harveian circulation nor did he even refer to it in his works. As a Puritan, he rejected the need for post-mortems. He dosed his patients vigorously with a canary wine bracer for smallpox, then blamed overtreatment by doctors for the disease's spread. He prescribed "the divine gift" of liquid opium for pain and dispensed Peruvian cinchona for fever, albeit prudently, thereby popularizing use of the bark.[70]

Two men served during the Cromwellian period as serjeant-surgeons to the Lord Protector: Thomas Trapham and Edward Arris. Licensed to practice surgery by Oxford University in 1633, Trapham put his services at the disposal of the Parliamentary Army in 1642. His notoriety emanates not so much from his surgical skills as from his callous comment to confederates after embalming and recapitating the body of Charles I: "I sewed on the head of a goose."[71] Later, in *Elenchus Motuum*, the pragmatic Bate referred to Trapham as "a rascally quack physician" who might have promulgated infamies about the dead king were it not for the presence of "an honest physician," himself. Despite this episode, perhaps because of it, in May 1549 Trapham was created surgeon to the General of the Parliamentary Army. He attended Cromwell in 1651 at the Battle of Worcester. After the Restoration, unlike the nimble Bate, Trapham was unable to shake off the taint of his partisanship and he retired to Abingdon, Berkshire, practicing his profession for two more decades. Charles II had him removed from the Abingdon town council in 1663 and Trapham's wife, Elizabeth, was fined for religious nonconformity. Trapham lived until 1683, saying no more for posterity, and leaving all his worldly goods to his widow. His son and namesake, a Leiden and Caen graduate, was killed in an earthquake on a 1692 expedition to Jamaica.[72]

Edward Arris, Cromwell's serjeant-surgeon in 1651, had a distinguished career, culminating in his election as Master of the Barber Surgeons that same year. Arris came from a family dedicated to medicine; his father was a surgeon and so was his son. Arris gave £510 to fund a series of lectures to his surgical brethren on muscles; he died in 1676. More interesting is the career of Edward Moleyns (Molins, Mullins, Moulins, or Molines), scion of a surgical family and the leading lithotomist of his day.[73] Like his father before him and his son after him, Moleyns held the offices of surgeon and "surgeon for the stone" at St. Bartholomew's and St. Thomas' hospitals. He lost those posts because of his outspoken political views and service to King Charles. While he was away from London with the army in the Civil War, the House of Commons ordered his dismissal and nominated a successor. But the directors of St. Thomas' hospital preferred to appoint Thomas Hollier, "surgeon for scald heads" there since 1638. The position stayed connected with the Moleyns family, however, as Hollier had been apprenticed to Edward Moleyns' father and was married to Edward Moleyns' niece.[74]

Even admirers like famed Caroline surgeon Richard Wiseman, who called Edward Moleyns "an excellent operator," thought him something of a hothead, and the Barber Surgeons' Court fined him for using bad language in refusing to accept its jurisdiction in a case involving him and another surgeon, a Mr. Coppinger.[75] Licensed for two decades by the College of Physicians to administer internal medicines in surgical diseases, in 1655 Moleyns was called in by Bate and other doctors when their treatment of Cromwell's gallstones proved ineffective. Because of his Royalist sentiments, Moleyns thought he ought to refuse any reward for curing a regicide, but the Lord Protector asked him to accept £1000 in the name of King Charles.[76] Edward Moleyns survived the Interregnum with his conscience intact. The Restoration allowed him to reclaim his appointments at the two royal hospitals, but in October 1660 Moleyns broke his ankle and the fracture became infected. Surgeons with less skill than Moleyns amputated the leg and he perished within a week; his elder son, James, succeeded him at St. Thomas and went on to become surgeon-in-ordinary to Charles II and James II.[77]

One other Interregnum surgeon of note is Christopher Irvine, surgeon from 1653 to General George Monck, Commander-in-Chief in Scotland, an appointment Irvine kept until 1660. In 1655 Irvine translated a work by Martin Blochwich called *Anatomie of the Elder,* advocating homely remedies rather "than the most renowned exoticks." Nature, Blochwich insisted, provided each climate with the medicinal materials appropriate to the ailments of that region. Especially worthwhile is the elder tree (boor tree) and all of its components: berries, buds, leaves, and bark. The book, using Galenic terms, tells how to make various powders, conserves, and syrups to be used for fevers and ear troubles, as diuretics, for jaundice and scurvy, and for menstrual disorders. Regarding the latter, a problem that translator Irvine is not likely to have encountered often as an army surgeon, a "defect in the monthly terms proceeds from a tough humor, closing the orifices of the histerick veins." The treatment is to "open the belly and disburden it of that putrid filth; give them the wine of the berries which looseneth the belly and maketh thin the blood and gross humors."[78]

An ardent Royalist, Irvine himself wrote *Medicina Magnetica*, published in Edinburgh in 1656 and dedicated to Monck. Subtitled "A Rare and Wonderful Art of Curing by Sympathy," the work discarded Galenic parlance to endorse "natural magick," brought about by the soul working outside the body. All bodies produce "corporeal beams," Irvine said, and even excrement retains a portion of the body's vital spirits. Accordingly, one should be careful of the feces of diseased people and not let an enemy obtain one's own. Who knew "what violent pains are procured by a kindled coal with spirit of wine or aquavite put into those excrements?"[79] Irvine contended that to cure by sympathy the physician must be schooled in astrology, medicine, and botany. He also exalted the magnetic cure of disease such as jaundice, and described the transplantation of magnets impregnated with "the true mummey of Paracelsus" mingled with "fat earth."[80] Coupled with his advocacy of these ideas, however, Irvine subscribed to traditional therapies like phlebotomies and purges. Irvine's career continued to flourish after the Stuart Restoration.

Despite their growing prominence in the nascent medical marketplace, records for apothecaries attached to the Commonwealth government or to the Lord Protector are hard to come by. Leslie Matthews intentionally omits Republican apothecaries from his monograph on royal appointees and Roy Sherwood, while reciting the virtues of Cromwell's doctors and surgeons, overlooks court druggists in his examination of the Interregnum medical staff. Sherwood does not include "apothecary" as a category within the protectoral court, but acknowledges that all of the more essential of the numerous subdepartments of a royal household persisted in Cromwell's.[81] The Household Index and the Establishment Books in the Royal Archives contain no references to medical staff between the two Charles Stuarts, and Sainty and Bucholz's *Officials of the Royal Household 1660–1837* takes up its cataloging after the Restoration. Even Clippingdale, usually eager to include even the most peripheral on his "Medical Court Roll," lists no Cromwellian apothecaries. Finally, the Worshipful Society of Apothecaries of London itself has no record of any apothecaries who served the state during the Interregnum.[82] However, because it was customary for a physician to work continually with the same apothecary, one might assume that Jack Shipton, who made medicines for George Bate's patients for twenty years, performed similar duties for the Commonwealth and Protectorate courts.

Though not perhaps for his pharmaceutical prowess, Richard Cromwell employed Thomas Clarges, an apothecary by training, in the waning days of the Protectorate. Clarges had apprenticed to an Oxford druggist-optician sometime before 1634, but he moved to London and started another apprenticeship in the London Merchant Taylors' Company, becoming a freeman of that company in 1641. To the displeasure of the Apothecaries' Society, Clarges became the apothecary of Dr. Thomas Cadyman, former physician to Queen Henrietta Maria. He was classified as an "unlawful worker" in 1642 and prohibited from setting up shop within the precincts of the company. Clarges worked out the difficulties with the Apothecaries' Society, paid a fine, and joined the association. By 1652, after examination by the College of Physicians, he was promoted to the apothecaries' livery. Clarges continued to work for Cadyman's widow and took several apprentices, one of whom, Richard Whittles, Charles II would make apothecary-general to his new standing army.

In 1656, Clarges became a Member of Parliament; he held a series of seats in the House of Commons until his death including those representing Westminster, Southwark, and Oxford University. Clarges took dispatches in 1659 from Richard Cromwell to General Monck in Scotland, where Clarges at that time held a Parliamentary seat, but he served as an envoy rather than a medical man and owed his prominence to the marriage of his sister to Monck in 1654 rather than to his own standing as an apothecary. Clarges acted as Monck's correspondent in London and was his liaison with army officers there. After Monck marched to the capital, Clarges was rewarded with the posts of Commissary-General of the Musters and Clerk of the Hanaper (chancery recorder).[83] In May 1660 Clarges, along with Dr. Samuel Barrow, relayed to Charles Stuart at Breda the invitation of Parliament to return to England, and was immediately knighted by Charles. Clarges remained active in politics after the Restoration and became a member of the Irish Privy Council; Pepys periodically wrote of him in his diary. Oxford University conferred an honorary doctorate of medicine on Clarges in January 1689, a felicitous award considering his humble beginnings as an apothecary's apprentice. Sir Thomas Clarges left a large amount of land and property when he died in 1695.[84]

A better guess as to who might have fulfilled some of the pharmaceutical needs of the republican government is Nicholas Culpeper, physician manqué and renowned herbalist. No less an authority than F.N.L. Poynter, former librarian at the Wellcome Institute in London, has called Culpeper "a figure of outstanding importance, for he had a greater influence on medical practice in England between 1650 and 1750 than either Harvey or Syndenham."[85] Born in London in 1616, the posthumous son of a rector, Culpeper studied at Cambridge and was considered a bright scholar, probably intended for the church, but the accidental death of his fiancée by lightning on her way to their elopement rendezvous blighted his further studies. Culpeper later blamed a restricted patrimony for his early departure from the university.[86] He apprenticed himself to three London apothecaries, but from about 1640 he had his own shop in Spitalfields and read about medicine. He married and had seven children, only one of whom survived childhood. Aroused by the poverty of his clients, Culpeper supplied them with low-cost plant medicines. The monopoly of the College Fellows, it seemed to Culpeper, put treatment beyond the reach of the indigent. He fumed that in Italy all physicians, whatever their reputation, had to administer to everyone, rich or poor, and that their fees were limited to the equivalent of about twenty cents.[87]

A zealous Puritan, Culpeper identified with the Parliamentary party from the time of its earliest objections to Charles I's personal rule; his short service in the Civil War ended when in 1643 he received a musket-shot wound in the chest.[88] A desire to communicate better with his clients, whom he saw at a rate of about forty per day, prompted his decision to publish a herbal in 1649, the same year in which his translation of the *London Pharmacopoeia* appeared. Culpeper deemed the Latin herbals of John Gerard and John Parkinson too esoteric and too dependent on foreign flora. His *Complete Herbal* used the common appellations of plants; moreover, Culpeper often told his clients where in the nearby countryside they could collect the appropriate vegetation. He never recommended more than one plant medicine if only one was needed. Professor of Pharmacognosy E. J. Shallard calls Culpeper's *Herbal* "a poor man's dispensatory" and, despite the price and standard of literacy needed to absorb its contents, the book proved hugely popular.[89]

Culpeper also composed a two-volume *Directory for Midwives*, subtitled "A Guide for Women in Their Conception, Bearing, and Suckling Their Children," published in London by Peter Cole in 1651. Culpeper's biographer suggests that the apothecary was motivated by his own wife's inability to have children, her health undermined by progressive kidney disease.[90] Culpeper did not believe in the movement of men into midwifery, disdaining the Chamberlens as "she physicians." He explicitly admonished his readers of the midwifery manual not to "call for help of a man-midwife, which is a disparagent, not only to yourselves but also to your profession." Written in a plain and simple style, and dedicated not to a notable patron but "to the matron," Culpeper's book deals less with the art of delivery, with which he could not have had much experience, than with preventive measures like cleanliness, diet, and exercise. He hoped to widen the education of the midwife to include anatomy, prenatal care, and infant health. To broaden his own knowledge, Culpeper attended the anatomical lectures at the Barber Surgeons' Company and made his own observations of dogs. Culpeper's *Midwifery* was reprinted seventeen times, the last edition appearing in 1777, and had a great impact on early English obstetrics.

Astrology guided much of Culpeper's thinking and he averred that the destruction of the monarchy could be deduced from an eclipse of the sun in March 1652.[91] Culpeper's *Herbal* was based in astrology, as was his entire understanding of medicine. An earlier work, *Semiotica Uranica or An Astrological Judgment of Diseases*, helped the reader decide which planet was responsible for a patient's illness and which body parts were affected. Treatment would be based on the use of plants governed by the heavenly bodies in opposition to the ones associated with particular parts of the body. However, Culpeper subscribed to the notion that some diseases could be cured by celestial sympathy, chosen by the planet associated with the disease to cure one of its own.

Meanwhile, Culpeper's old wound tortured him and he developed tuberculosis. Writing at a furious pace and withdrawing from the physical rigors of his practice, he penned an explanation in English of *Galen's Art of Physick* for those who insisted on adhering to the doctrines of the ancients. Culpeper did not ignore Galenism altogether; he coauthored treatises on blood-letting, cupping, and scarifying, and the ailments that could be cured using those techniques. He dabbled in alchemy, too, writing a discourse on *aurum potabile*, "necessary to the study of hermetick philosophy," published posthumously by the radical printer Peter Cole in 1656. Cole tried to refute the idea that Culpeper was exclusively Paracelsian, being persuaded that he had mellowed toward Galenism in his infirmity.[92] It is possible that Culpeper had some role in providing medicines to Commonwealth leaders, but other apothecaries must have also ministered to the protectoral courts of Oliver and Richard Cromwell. Nicholas Culpeper died in 1654, shortly after writing an ephemeris for the year, noting another great eclipse of the sun on August 2.

According to *Mercurius Politicus*, at Oliver Cromwell's death his physicians and surgeons disemboweled and embalmed the Lord Protector's body. Dr. Bate had kept watch over Cromwell the night before he died; he also conducted the official autopsy. Long after the post-mortem, Bate related a problem with the embalming procedure: "Though the bowels were taken out and his body filled with spices," putrid matter "purged and wrought through all." Despite the corpse being wrapped in a four-layer shroud and confined in two coffins of lead and wood, the stench was so offensive that the sarcophagus had to be interred in Westminster Abbey before a state funeral could be held.[93] Bate and Goddard walked together in the Protector's memorial procession. The corruption of Cromwell's reeking corpse reported by Dr. Bate seemed significant to Englishmen after 1660. They dug up Cromwell's body, dragged it to Tyburn, and beheaded it.

Richard Cromwell, Lord Protector by succession, displayed little aptitude for statecraft, but for six months his father ruled from the grave. Following trouble with the army, Richard Cromwell was dismissed by the recalled Rump of the Long Parliament.[94] The confusion following his downfall led most people to endorse restoration of the Stuarts. General Monck dissolved Parliament and discreetly advised Charles Stuart about the constitutional guarantees necessary to make his return acceptable. A Convention Parliament voted for the exiled king's recall and he landed in May 1660 to an enthusiastic reception. By the time of Charles II's coronation, the outcome of both medical contests, theoretical and jurisdictional, had been decided in favor of the new guard—the continentally trained, Paracelsian-Helmontian empiricists and the popularly supported "irregulars" who practiced medicine in London outside the control of the Royal College of Physicians.[95] Though the College of Physicians hailed Charles II, likening him to a phoenix and decrying the seditious "tribunes and ill-conditioned scoundrels" who had damaged the kingdom, the College had already lost its authoritative position at the apex of the English medicine. The new king was himself a devotee of chemical experimentation and analysis. He intended to play a major role in shaping the medical community for decades to come and his court appointments would reflect his theoretical orientation.

Notes

1. Eastwick, a girdler who died in 1675, represented Dowgate and Bridge wards in his civic career. Annals of the College of Physicians, vol. 4, f. 29b, LRCP; Alfred Beaven, *Aldermen of the City of London* 2 vols. (London: Eden Fisher, 1913), 1: 60, 141. Harold J. Cook has written the best account of the College's travails in the seventeenth century, *The Decline of the Old Medical Regime in Stuart London*.

2. See Penelope Hunting, *A History of the Society of Apothecaries*, (London: Society of Apothecaries, 1998), 61; Young, *Annals*, 142.

3. See Lindsay Sharp, "The Royal College of Physicians and Interregnum Politics," *Medical History* 19 (1975): 107–28. Birken makes a strong claim that the College was an enthusiastic ally of Parliament during the Civil War and beyond: see "The College and Its Support of Parliament," 58–62. Christopher Hill insists that "most apothecaries supported Parliament in the Civil War [while] physicians supported the King," but had that been the case, drastic reforms would surely have been imposed: Christopher Hill, *Change and Continuity in Seventeenth-Century England* (New Haven, Conn.: Yale University Press, 1991), 159.

4. R. S. Roberts, "The Personnel and Practice of Medicine in Tudor-Stuart England, Part 2: London," *Medical History* 8 (1964): 228. This is a variation on the thesis associated with R. K. Merton, linking Puritanism with the rise of modern science. See R. K. Merton, *Science, Technology and Society in Seventeenth Century England* (New York: H. Fertig, 1970).

5. Culpeper quoted in Hill, *Change and Continuity*, 160. See also Andrew Wear, "Puritan Perceptions of Illness in Seventeenth-Century England," in *Patients and Practitioners*, ed. Roy Porter (Cambridge: Cambridge University Press, 1985), 55–59; F.N.L Poynter, "Nicholas Culpeper and the Paracelsians," in *Science, Medicine and Society in the Renaissance*, ed. Allen G. Debus, 2 vols. (New York: Science History Publications, 1972), 1: 201–20; and Charles Webster, "English Medical Reformers of the Puritan Revolution: A Background to the Society for Chymical Physitians," *Ambix* 14 (1967): 16–41.

6. Webster, *The Great Instauration: Science, Medicine and Reform in England 1626–1660*, xvi, 127; Andrew Wear, "Puritan Perceptions of Illness," 60.

7. Hill, *Continuity and Change*, 164; Sharp, "The College and Interregnum Politics," 109; Trevor-Roper, "Paracelsian Movement," 188; and Allen G. Debus, "Paracelsian Medicine," in *Medicine in Seventeenth-Century England*, ed. Allen G. Debus (Berkeley: University of California Press, 1974), 38. Biggs also chided Paracelsians who championed astral influences in medicine.

8. Fielding H. Garrison, "The Medical and Scientific Periodicals of the Seventeenth and Eighteenth Centuries," *Bulletin of the Institute of the History of Medicine* 2/8 (October 1934): 293.

9. Allen, "Medical Education in Seventeenth-Century England," 127–30.

10. Debus, *English Paracelsians*, 176, 181; Rattansi, "Paracelsus and the Puritan Revolution," 24. For more on Helmont, see Walter Pagel, *From Paracelsus to Van Helmont*, ed. Marianne Winder (London: Variorum Reprints, 1986).

11. Debus, *The Chemical Philosophy*, 2: 303–4, 310–11.

12. Ibid., 2: 359.

13. See Antonio Clericuzio, "From van Helmont to Boyle: A Study of the Transmission of Hemontian Chemical and Medical Theories in Seventeenth-Century England," *British Journal for the History of Science* 26 (1993): 303–35.

14. Cook calls Charlton's *Darkness of Atheism Refuted by the Light of Nature* (1652) and *Physiologia*

Epicuro-Gassendo-Charletoniana (1654), both of which were tracts supporting anomism, his most important works during this period. Cook, *Decline of the Old Medical Regime*, 119.

15. Rattansi, "Paracelsus and the Puritan Revolution," 28: See Nina Rattner Gelbart, "The Intellectual Development of Walter Charlton," *Ambix* 18/3 (1971): 149–68.

16. Rattansi, "Paracelsus and the Puritan Revolution," 30; Sharp, "The College and Interregnum Politics," 117. Charlton was accused of atheism, his usefulness to the College gone. By contrast chemical therapy seemed tame. Hugh Trevor-Roper asserts that van Helmont rid Paracelsianism of its explosive content and that by 1654 a more conservative Cromwell detached the study of chemistry from millenarian and revolutionary ideology: Trevor-Roper, "Paracelsian Movement," 191, 193. "Weapon-salve" is an example Rattansi gives of the Helmontian principles that Charlton rejected.

17. Walter Charlton, *Immortality of the Human Soul* (London: W. Wilson, 1657), introduction. Charlton examined the differences in man's brains from animals: SL MSS 698, folios 74–87, British Library.

18. Even though Charlton had been a royal doctor and entitled to customary respect, the College began to close ranks against radicals, empirics, and the unlicensed. See Annals of the College of Physicians, 4: folios 20b, 22a-22b, 24b, 26b, 41a, and 53b, LRCP.

19. Rattansi, "The Helmontian-Galenist Controversy in Restoration England," 6.

20. Pelling and Webster, "Medical Practitioners," 182. Paul Slack asserts that "Paracelsian remedies were as acceptable as any others to readers of popular medical tracts" around 1600: see Slack, *The Impact of Plague in Tudor and Stuart England*, 149–99.

21. Registrar George Ent, quoted in Annals of the College of Physicians, vol. 4, f. 68b, LRCP. Though some have reported that Oliver Cromwell was a member of the Society of Apothecaries, its Archivist, Dee Cook, assures me that he was not.

22. See Lloyd G. Stevenson, "New Diseases in the Seventeenth Century," *Bulletin for the History of Medicine* 39 (1965): 1–21; Creighton, *A History of Epidemics in Britain*, 1: 532–33.

23. Martin Blochwich, *Anatomie of the Elder* (London: 1655); Pelling and Webster, "Medical Practitioners," 178; and Geoffrey Holmes, *Augustan England: Professions, State and Society 1680–1730* (London: George Allen and Unwin, 1982), 185.

24. Paul Slack, "Mirrors of Health and the Treasures of Poor Men," in *Health, Medicine and Mortality in the Sixteenth Century* ed. Charles Webster (Cambridge: Cambridge University Press, 1979), 263.

25. Hackett, *Malaria in Europe*, 31, 88, 161. See also M. Dobson, "Marsh Fever," *Journal of Historical Geography* 6 (1980): 357–89.

26. Hole, *The English Housewife in the Seventeenth Century*, 88–89; Roger A. Hambridge, "Empirocomany, or an Infatuation in Favour of Empiricism or Quackery," in *Literature and Science and Medicine*, ed. Serge Soupel and Roger A. Hambridge, (Los Angeles: UCLA, 1982), 70.

27. Friedrich A. Fluckiger, *The Cinchona Barks* (Philadelphia: Blakiston, 1884), 82. For centuries, the Countess was credited with introducing the remedy into Spain and Italy upon her return to Europe. Though some recent works continue to perpetuate this story, the charming myth was effectively disproved in 1941 by A. W. Haggis. There is no evidence that the Countess, who died in Colombia before even reaching Europe, was ever attacked by intermittent fevers; in fact, the diary of her husband indicates that it was he who was feverish sporadically from 1631 to 1638 and was bled for his ailments. See A. W. Haggis, "Fundamental Errors in the Early History of Cinchona", *Bulletin of the History of Medicine* 11 (1942): 568–87.

28. Jaime Jaramillo-Arango, *The Conquest of Malaria* (London: Heinemann, 1950), 31. Jaramillo-Arango argues that as early as 1378 the disease was rampant in the armies of the Pachacutec, who used the bark macerated in fermented maize wine. Etymological investigation reveals that aboriginals called the tree "quina quina," or "bark of barks" in the Quichuan language, indicating, through the use of the double name, a plant with medical qualities.

29. Duran-Reynals, *The Fever-Bark Tree*, 38. See also Rohde's chapter on "Herbals of the New World," *Old English Herbals*, 120–41.

30. Jaramillo-Arango, *Conquest of Malaria*, 37, 45, 73.

31. A French expedition brought Joseph de Jussieu to Peru in 1735 to study the fever-bark tree. His descriptions prompted Linnaeus to name the drug "cinchona," and to embellish the myth about its transmission to Europe.

32. Creighton, *Epidemics* 2: 320.

33. Jaramillo-Arango, *Conquest of Malaria*, 78.

34. John Metford, Observations et Curationes Northamptontae, SL MSS 2812, British Library.

35. Creighton, *Epidemics*, 2: 320.

36. Robert Talbor, *Pyretologia: A Rational Account of the Causes and Cures of Agues* (London: R. Clavel, 1672), 27.

37. Gideon Harvey, *The Conclave of Physicians* (London: James Partridge, 1683), 165; George Baker, "Observations on the Late Intermittent Fevers," *Medical Transactions* 3 (1785): 213; Robert Talbor, *The English Remedy* (London: J Wallis, 1682), 29.

38. Talbor, *Pyretologia*, 44.

39. Francis Bacon, *Sylva Sylvarum* (London: n.p. 1627), 191.

40. Keynes, *Life of Harvey*, 407–8. Among Dr. Harvey's bequests to his brother Eliab was his "coffey pot."

41. Biographies of Cromwell include Christopher Hill, *God's Englishman* (New York: Harper, 1972); Antonia Fraser, *Cromwell* (New York: Dell, 1973); and Barry Coward, *Oliver Cromwell* (London: Longman, 1991. For more on Cromwell's perquisites, see Roy Sherwood, *The Court of Oliver Cromwell* (London: Croom Helm, 1977).

42. Quoted in Young, *Annals*, 139. Wateson had taken out a loan of £1,200 on the security of sealed bonds, which were confiscated by Cromwell.

43. G. E. Aylmer lists a number of physicians, more than a few educated in Scotland or the Netherlands, whose public service during the Interregnum was administrative or nonmedical, suggesting "more than a random association between medicine and the puritan-parliamentarian-republican cause:" see Aylmer, *The State's Servants: The Civil Service of the English Republic 1649–1660* (London: Routledge and Kegan Paul, 1973), 277.

44. Besides tending Cromwell, Mayerne and his protégé John Colladon, a fellow Huguenot, cared for other patients among King Charles's enemies. Both ministered to John Pym, leader of the Parliamentary opposition, and both signed Pym's post-mortem report certifying that he had succumbed to an "impostume in the bowel." See Vigne, "Mayerne and His Successors," 224.

45. Quoted in Treue, *Doctor at Court*, 21.

46. Fraser, *Cromwell*, 55–60.

47. Archer, *Everyman His Own Doctor*, 34; Leslie Matthews, "The Day Book of the Court Apothecary," *Medical History* 22 (1978): Appendix II, 171.

48. See Stanley W. Jackson, "Melancholia and the Waning of the Humoral Theory," *Journal of the History of Medicine* 32 (1978): 367–76.

49. Jesse, *Memoirs of the Court of England* 2: 118.

50. Fraser, *Cromwell*, 56; Treue, *Doctor at Court*, 21.

51. Fraser, *Cromwell*, 662–63. Elizabeth Cromwell, Oliver's wife, survived until 1672.

52. Fraser, *Cromwell*, 771; Fraser misspells the name of the bark as "myroxlyon."

53. L. J. Bruce-Chwatt, "George Bate—Cromwell's Devious Physician," *Journal of the Royal College of Physicians of London* 17/2 (1983): 144.

54. George C. Peachey, "Thomas Trapham—Cromwell's Surgeon—and Others," *Proceedings of the Royal Society of Medicine* 24 (1931): 1442.

55. Sharp, "The College and Interregnum Politics," 116. The others include Jonathan Goddard, Ralph Bathurst, Thomas Coxe, Daniel Whistler, and Thomas Wharton.

56. In 1656, he was part of the Board of Physicians that recommended the establishment of a College of Physicians in Edinburgh: Craig, *History of the College of Edinburgh*, 48.

57. Peachey, "Thomas Trapham," 1443. Using solely circumstantial evidence, H. F. McMains claims that Dr. Bate, in conspiracy with Thomas Clarges, poisoned Oliver Cromwell with mercury

and antimony: see H. F. McMains, *The Death of Oliver Cromwell* (Lexington: University Press of Kentucky, 2000), 108–20.

58. Doctors Claudius Fenwick and Samuel Barrow were left in charge of tending to the army in Scotland after Goddard's departure; in 1654 Barrow remained the sole physician in this position. See A. L. Wyman, "Samuel Barrow, M.D., Physician to Charles II and Admirer of John Milton," *Medical History* 18 (1974): 335–39. In 1659 General Monck promoted Barrow to the post of Judge Advocate, an important legal office.

59. Munk, *Roll* 1: 240.

60. Sherwood, *Court of Cromwell*, 111.

61. Fanshawe made good use of his "retirement," producing an English translation of Luis de Camoen's *The Lusiads*, and later serving in the government of Charles II. Sir Henry Vane was executed as a regicide in 1662. Ronald Hutton, *Charles II* (Oxford: Clarendon Press, 1989), 122, 170.

62. Add. MSS 46378 B, f. 10, British Library.

63. Craig, *History of the College of Edinburgh*, 48.

64. Munk, *Roll* 1: 169–70.

65. Clippingdale, Medical Court Roll, 1: 75. However, Sydenham's apothecary, Daniel Malthus, was a royal apothecary. G. E. Aylmer names Dr. Joseph Waterhouse, brother of Cromwell's steward, Nathaniel Waterhouse, a protectoral physician along with Bathurst, Wright, and Trapham, but I can find no collaborative primary or secondary evidence; Munk lists a Thomas Waterhouse, an honorary Fellow of the College from 1669, who practiced in Exeter. See Aylmer's *The State's Servants*, 276.

66. Quoted in George Newman, "Thomas Sydenham, Reformer of English Medicine," *Interpreters of Nature* (Freeport, N.Y.: Books for Libraries, 1968), 29. See also Henry E. Sigerist, *The Great Doctors* (New York: Norton, 1933).

67. L. J. Rather demolishes the notion that Sydenham deserves to be called "the English Hippocrates": see Rather, "Pathology at Mid-Century," in *Medicine in Seventeenth-Century England*, ed. Allen G. Debus (Berkeley: University of California Press, 1974), 103.

68. Robert Latham, ed., *The Illustrated Pepys* (Berkeley: University of California Press, 1978), 39.

69. J. L. Turk and Elizabeth Allen, "Bleeding and Cupping," *Annals of the Royal College of Surgeons* 65/2 (March 1983): 128; E. S. de Beer, ed., *The Diary of John Evelyn*, 6 vols. (Oxford: Clarendon Press, 1955) 4: 425; Clemens, "Notes," 315.

70. Garrison, *Introduction to the History of Medicine*, 271; Creighton, *Epidemics* 2: 321. Alfred White Franklin, "Clinical Medicine," in *Medicine in Seventeenth-Century England*, ed. Allen G. Debus (Berkeley: University of California Press, 1974), 136.

71. Clippingdale, Medical Court Roll, 1: 78, LRCS.

72. Peachey, "Thomas Trapham," 1448; Munk, *Roll* 1: 345.

73. Munk (*Roll* 1: 193) errs saying it was James Moleyns who treated Cromwell. Edward's father, James, died in 1639; Edward's son, also James, became surgeon to the Stuart household in 1680 and surgeon-in-ordinary to James II in 1685. He trephined the skull of Prince Rupert, a Stuart cousin, in 1667. See G.C.R. Morris, "Which Molins Treated Cromwell for the Stone and Did Not Prescribe for Pepys?" *Medical History* 26 (1982): 429–35; Graham Martin, "Prince Rupert and the Surgeons," *History Today* 40 (December 1990): 41.

74. G.C.R. Morris, "A Portrait of Thomas Hollier, Pepys's Surgeon," *Annals of the Royal College of Surgeons of England* 61 (1979): 224.

75. Martin, "Prince Rupert and the Surgeons," 41; Young, *Annals*, 27.

76. Annals of the College of Physicians, vol. 3, f. 166a, LRCP; Munk, *Roll* 1: 193. Peachey adds that Moleyns asked for a drink after working on Cromwell, was taken to the wine cellar, and toasted the health of Charles Stuart: Peachey, "Thomas Trapham," 1442.

77. Morris, "Portrait of Hollier," 226.

78. Blochwich, *Anatomie of the Elder*, 170. The book is dedicated to Alexander Pennycuil, surgeon to General Bannier of the "Scotch" army.

79. Christopher Irvine, *Medicina Magnetica* (Edinburgh: n.p., 1656), 83.

80. Ibid., 70.

81. Sherwood, *Court of Cromwell*, 35, 168–73.

82. I thank Dee Cook, Archivist to the Society of Apothecaries, for her efforts to locate any clues to the identity of the Cromwellian appointees. Like earlier works, the most recent history of the guild contains no reference to personnel who served on the Interregnum staff: see Hunting, *History of the Apothecaries*, 57–62. No Cromwellian barbers are on record either.

83. The hanaper (or hamper) was a wickerwork box in which fees paid on common law writs were kept. The office of Clerk of the Hanaper was abolished in 1852.

84. Hunting, *History of Apothecaries*, 59; T. D. Whittet, "Sir Thomas Clarges, Apothecary and Envoy," *Journal of the Royal Society of Medicine*, 81 (1988): 464–67. Whittet states that Clarges died the equivalent of a multimillionaire in modern reckoning.

85. F.N.L. Poynter, "Nicholas Culpeper and His Books," *Journal of the History of Medicine* 17 (1962): 153.

86. Rohde, 164. Rohde is not a friendly source: she calls Culpeper "infamous," his work "a travesty," and his politics "Roundhead."

87. Poynter, "Culpeper and His Books," 157.

88. Poynter, "Culpeper and the Paracelsians," 201; George Edward Trease, *Pharmacy in History* (London: Balliere, Tindall and Cox, 1964), 118, 128.

89. David Potterton, ed., *Culpeper's Color Herbal*, foreword by E. J. Shellard (New York: Sterling Publishing, 1983), 6.

90. Olav Thulesius, *Nicholas Culpeper* (New York: St. Martin's Press, 1992), 78–79. Thulesius emphasizes Culpeper's interest in astrology, witchcraft, and alchemy.

91. Nicholas Culpeper, *Catastrophe Magnatum or the Fall of Monarchie* (London: Vere and Brooke, 1652).

92. Poynter, "Culpeper and the Paracelsians," 202. Poynter agrees with Cole that Culpeper tempered his views and that he did author alchemical works.

93. George Bate, *Elenchus Motuum Nuperorum in Anglia: A Short Historical Account of the Rise and Progress of the Late Troubles in England* (London: A. Swalle, 1683), Part II: 236. A funeral of great pomp did follow the hurried entombment.

94. He escaped to France, returning in 1680 and spending the rest of his life in untroubled seclusion. He passed away in 1712.

95. Rattansi, "Helmontian-Galenist Controversy," 1.

Chapter 6

Doctors to the Restored Stuarts (1660–88)

The end of the English republic coincided with the end of the Stuart dynasty's exile. Charles II, recalled by the Convention Parliament and acknowledged king before arriving in Britain, was welcomed with unrestrained public rejoicing as he returned to London in triumph. It had been a long journey home for the son of an executed potentate. After his father's beheading in 1649, Charles was crowned at Scone by the Scots and proclaimed king of Ireland. In 1651, just twenty-one, he invaded England at the head of a Scottish army, but lost to Cromwell's forces at Worcester. Disguised by supporters, Charles luckily escaped detection and fled to the continent, where he lived for nine years in exile. He dwelled for a while in Paris, Cologne, The Hague, Brussels, and Bruges, in the last-mentioned location as a pensioner of Spain. He hoped to foment a Royalist rising on his behalf and contemplated invading England, but as time passed and Spanish funds dwindled, that hope diminished, too. When a restoration of the monarchy became possible, Charles and his advisers made contact with those in power, negotiated wisely, and produced the Declaration of Breda, a document containing the concessions that smoothed the way for Charles's return to England. Two medical men mediated with Charles as agents for General Monck: Samuel Barrow, a physician and advocate general to the army, and Thomas Clarges, an apothecary. Charles enjoyed a raucous reception in England in late May 1660. Taking up residence in Whitehall Palace, he spent the next two months accepting the congratulations of foreign ambassadors, local government representatives, and individual aristocrats. The king rewarded Barrow in August 1660 with an appointment as physician-in-ordinary at £100 per annum, the customary twelve shillings a day in board wages, and one horse-livery a year.[1] Before long, however, the unsettled constitutional and religious issues reemerged to bedevil the Stuarts.

Charles II, a stranger to most of the country, astutely revived the royal touching ceremony, thrilling his subjects and reminding skeptics of the ineffable privilege of a king. Presumably, he assumed that he had the marvelous ability to heal from the moment of his father's death, as his subjects indubitably believed. Preachers, writers, even physicians and scientists touted the amazing potency of the imperial gift. Some even thought that the king, the nation's first physician, could cure diseases like the French pox, scurvy, rickets, and strumas.[2] Charles performed the hereditary miracle in exile, touching scrofulous followers ferried to the temporary court in the Low Countries by enterprising merchants. Since the Stuart purse was empty, Charles distributed silver touchpieces instead of gold, but the passionate feeling imparted by the ritual was the same. Popular belief in the supernatural remedy for the King's Evil, a remedy denied its victims for so long, furnished Charles Stuart with a weapon of wonder. Richard Wiseman, Charles's surgeon on the continent, witnessed the touching of multitudes of believers and reported that inexplicable cures resulted from the Stuart touch, enhancing Charles' mystique throughout Britain. While only just recognized as sovereign by Parliament and still at Breda, Charles presided over a somber healing liturgy. Only a few days after arriving in England, he touched six hundred persons in one sitting; he subsequently touched throngs for the King's Evil every Friday in the Banqueting House at Whitehall. Wiseman kept meticulous track of the numbers attending these solemnities in the King's Register of Healing. From May 1660 to September 1664 the king touched twenty-three thousand persons; thousands more came to see him in subsequent years, perhaps as many as one hundred thousand, seemingly "half the nation," during his twenty-five-year reign.[3]

Despite his affinity for the magic of the touching ceremony and the conscientious way in which he carried out the royal rite, Charles II relished science and medicine. He became the founding force, the "Fundator," behind the famous Royal Society, although not its financial benefactor, and made science fashionable.[4] Springing from meetings of scientists, physicians, and philosophers dating to 1645, the Royal Society was formally organized in 1660 and adopted its first charter two years later. It became only the second commissioned learned society in the capital, albeit not the professional group that it is today. A haphazard quality permeated early member selection: initial Fellows included Christopher Wren, Samuel Pepys, and Isaac Newton, but nearly half of the members were noblemen, courtiers, or dilettantes like John Evelyn, drawn to the Society more for political reasons than for science. About 16 percent of the British Fellows elected between 1660 and 1700 were medical practitioners, but several well-known London physicians stayed away altogether, uninterested in the amateurs' activities. Even with the appointment in 1662 of Robert Hooke as Curator of Experiments, the Society remained "a place of report rather than a research institute."[5] Fellows told one another about deadly poisons, looked at natural curiosities like sharks' teeth, and took part in demonstrations of a kind of camera obscura. Topics raised at initial meetings included some subjects in which the king was interested: oysters, weather, and beer; the Duke of Buckingham promised to bring in a unicorn's horn, regarded as a medical panacea.

According to one of his many biographers, where science and medicine were concerned, Charles II became an esteemed leader of post-Restoration society.[6] Given the Caroline predilection for scientific thought and inquiry, it is not surprising that the king had an impact on the scholarly and practical aspects of medicine. The Convention Parliament left the important work of forming a new administration to him. He made most of his early medical appointments in deference to the standards of legitimacy, endorsing the claims of those who had obtained those offices, or the reversion of them, under Charles I. He culled medical men from his father's court and appointed others on whom he had relied in exile. Though some of the most celebrated physicians in the kingdom tended to the needs of the Caroline court, the king, like his subjects, had no qualms about supporting unconventional empirics if their remedies worked. As Roy Porter has noted, the free market system encouraged empirics; Charles II and the public demanded "whatever systems, therapies and drugs were on offer."[7] After the Restoration, the demand for and supply of medical literature accelerated the development of an already vibrant marketplace for the healing arts. In no small part, the triumph of the medical entrepreneur was due to the publication of popular books of home remedies, herbals, and wellness regimes that purported to demystify diagnosis and cure.[8] By selling printed matter that enabled every man to become his own doctor, as the title of one publication by royal doctor John Archer proposed, London bookmen undermined the legal monopoly of the traditional medical establishment and assured the victory of its challengers.[9] Competition for the patient's money had never been greater than it was after 1660, and by the end of the Stuart era the medical establishment had been turned upside down.[10]

Charles II's doctors faced formidable tasks, which extended beyond tending to the routine maladies of the household. The first decade of the new king's reign included war with the Dutch, bubonic plague, and an urban fire of epic proportions; one hundred thousand may have succumbed in 1665 during the last major outbreak of plague in Britain.[11] Moreover, after an initial honeymoon period of goodwill with Parliament and the people, Charles II incurred the constant wrath of his subjects, who disagreed with his insistence on formal episcopacy in the church, dissented from his friendship with Louis XIV and the French international agenda, and objected to the probable succession of Charles's Roman Catholic brother, James, Duke of York.[12] The fury of these antagonists aroused them to partisan organization, a campaign to exclude James from the throne, and an eventual revolution, called "glorious" by its proponents, against James II in 1688. The public health calamities and political crises produced ethical problems for the royal doctors as titular leaders of their profession and swayed the king toward medical reform. During his momentous twenty-five year reign, Charles II required the presence in England of no fewer than thirty-six attending physicians, five of them appointed in June 1660, three botanical or chemical physicians, nineteen surgeons. and four apothecaries. He appointed six Scottish doctors and a surgeon-apothecary for service north of the border, since the Restoration brought back the northern kingdom's native monarchy and national independence. In addition to these medicos, five "irregulars" could be found plying their nostrums on the king.

Prior to the Restoration, eleven members of the Royal College of Physicians divulged their political proclivities by ministering to Charles in exile throughout Europe. None was more important to him than John Hinton, Henrietta

Maria's London-born physician and a Royalist in the Civil War. Hinton promoted a petition for peace submitted to the Long Parliament, testifying before the House of Commons, but when peace efforts failed, he sided with the king on the field of battle. Hinton's M.D. was from Leiden, but after he marched with the Charles I's army, Oxford incorporated his degree in 1642 and the king made him Prince Charles's physician-in-ordinary. He gloried in his service to the sovereign, attending the king at Edgehill and then recruiting additional troops from Oxford. Hinton boasted that he dissuaded Prince Charles from "foolish bravery" that would have gotten him captured.[13] Reputedly skilled as an accoucheur, Hinton attended the birth of the Princess Henrietta in June 1644 at Exeter and afterward helped the queen flee to Cornwall and then to France. After the death of Charles I, Dr. Hinton ministered to Charles II at his migrant court on the continent but, when Hinton traveled to London to encourage the Stuart cause, he was seized and imprisoned. Hinton was rewarded after the Restoration for his dutiful and loyal actions with an English appointment as Physician to the Person and a knighthood.[14]

Charles' own health appears to have been excellent from infancy to about fifty years of age; his childhood diseases had been routinely treated with purgatives and drinks of chicken broth, rhubarb, and senna.[15] The king generally displayed vitality as an adult; he played tennis, danced, walked and swam long distances, and he rode a winning horse at Newmarket at age fifty-four. Though Charles sired no offspring with his wife, he had at least fourteen illegitimate children, whom Privy Councillor George Savile, Marquis of Halifax, said "were the effects of good health and a good constitution." The king survived smallpox at twenty, the occasional fever, and a serious bout of malaria in 1679 for which he demanded cinchona. James Stuart was likewise the patient of a variety of royal practitioners from his days as heir presumptive to his own postrevolutionary exile in France. Though generally robust, James suffered at critical times in his life from violent nosebleeds, which kept him inactive for days and which his doctors treated as psychosomatic. He probably suffered from syphilis, a disease that mimics the symptoms of many others, which he passed on to his first wife and elder daughters.[16] The Stuart siblings had many doctors in common and, when James came to the throne, he continued the appointments of the entire staff in Scotland.

Charles II's inaugural First Physician in England was Alexander Fraizer (Frasier), a faithful Royalist begrudgingly said by famed diarist Samuel Pepys to have unequaled influence with the monarch: "He can do what he please with the king in spite of any man, and upon the same with the Prince."[17] The Scottish-born Fraizer studied medicine at Montpellier, receiving his M.D. in 1635; he became a Fellow of the College of Physicians in 1641. A trusted political adviser whose wife was a dresser to Charles's Portuguese queen, Catherine of Braganza, Fraizer had a long relationship with the Stuarts, dating back to his attendance on Charles at the Battle of Worcester and in exile in France. He connived in secret with inept Caroline supporters in Scotland, but Charles forgave him his political miscues and his purported hard-drinking because of the excellence of his medicine.[18] Besides being a natural schemer, Fraizer was a skilled practitioner, able to deliver a courtesan's baby and cure its father of venereal disease with equal dexterity.[19] His royal patients did not always pull through, however. He attended the king's second brother, twenty-year-old Henry, Duke of Gloucester, fatally stricken with smallpox in September 1660. In December the virus attacked Charles's sister Mary, aged twenty-nine, Princess Royal of Great Britain and Princess Dowager of the Netherlands, who perished just as quickly as Gloucester despite Fraizer's best efforts, begging King Charles to act as guardian to her son. The doctor also ministered to James's doomed infant sons, the Dukes of Cambridge and Kendal, in 1667.

Fraizer was more fortunate with his diagnosis and treatment of Prince Rupert, the king's cousin and Royalist Commander-in-Chief during the early stage of the Civil War. Later, while a mercenary for France in its intermittent conflict with the Spanish Netherlands, Rupert withstood a minor scalp wound from a pistol ball. He lived with the wound for seventeen years, but after the Stuart Restoration, while acting as Admiral of the Fleet in 1664, Rupert was hit on the head by a block from the rigging. An extradural abscess developed and would not heal, necessitating surgery. As First Physician, Dr. Fraizer supervised the successful trephining of the prince's skull by James Moleyns in 1667.[20] Following the surgery, the prince was bled and clystered, cupped and scarified on the shoulders, all standard practices after cranial operations. Rupert made a rapid recovery and lived another fifteen years, dying in 1682 at the age of sixty-two. Dr. Fraizer himself died in 1681, but not before arranging for the appointment of his son, Charles, as physician-in-ordinary to the king in August 1677 and the granting of a medical degree from Cambridge to Charles Fraizer by royal mandate in 1678.[21]

Stuart royal doctors were sometimes connected to the decisive political events of the day, such as the "Popish Plot" of the late 1670s, a fictitious Catholic conspiracy invented by a deranged Protestant clergyman, Titus Oates. Fear of a papal resurgence in England pole-axed the kingdom and spawned Country or Whig party opposition to the succession of the Duke of York.[22] Emotions ran high; one of Charles II's own doctors, William Denton, wrote an anti-Catholic tirade in support of Parliamentary attempts to remove the dangers associated with Catholic recusants and admonished the king as God's vice-regent on earth to maintain and preserve the Anglican religion in its purity.[23] Dr. Alexander Fraizer's role in the Popish Plot was peripheral; he had an unpleasant run-in with a casualty of Oates' dementia, Sir Edmund Berry Godfrey. Godfrey established a prosperous wood-mongering business in the Strand, which led to his appointment as justice of the peace for Westminster. Though King Charles rewarded Godfrey's diligent maintenance of domestic order during the plague with a knighthood in 1666, in that same year Godfrey promoted the "Irish stroker," Valentine Greatrakes, the most prominent occult healer of the seventeenth century.

Greatrakes, who had served in Cromwell's army, claimed to be able to cure the King's Evil by divine intercession.[24] After building up notoriety in Ireland

and expanding his repertoire to include ague and other diseases, Greatrakes came to England to try to cure the headaches of Anne, Viscountess Conway. Championed by some of the leading intellectuals of the day, including Robert Boyle and John Wilkins, Greatrakes aided scores of sick Londoners who besieged his lodgings. He failed, however, in a demonstration before Charles II and his physicians and quickly returned to Ireland. The king often fostered the careers of charlatans or quacksalvers who claimed to cure with home remedies, but Greatrakes was something utterly different. Godfrey's public support for a man, and a Cromwellian antimonarchist at that, who claimed to have an anointed sovereign's healing capacity, cannot have endeared him to King Charles.[25]

In 1669 Godfrey personally ran afoul of the court, specifically of Alexander Fraizer. Fraizer owed Godfrey's business £30 for firewood, so Godfrey had his bailiffs arrest the doctor. Furious at what he regarded as a breach of his prerogative, the king directed that the bailiffs be whipped and that Judge Godfrey be detained in the porter's lodge at Whitehall. Pepys, no friend of Fraizer's but a supporter of Godfrey, reported that the judge refused to eat, asserting that the law was on his side. Godfrey was released after six days and returned to his prosperous and happy life. Nearly a decade later, in September 1678 Titus Oates swore depositions before Godfrey attesting to a cabal to assassinate the king, massacre Protestants, and place Charles's Roman Catholic brother on the throne. As public frenzy over the plot grew, Godfrey presciently feared for his own safety. He was found slain on October 17; the murder was never solved, but suspicion centered on several Roman Catholics associated with the Caroline court.[26] Alexander Fraizer was never embroiled in the Godfrey matter, but another Stuart royal doctor, Sir George Wakeman faced real danger; unlike Fraizer's, Wakeman's position was central.

Wakeman, physician-in-ordinary to Queen Catherine, was a zealous Roman Catholic and a staunch Royalist, imprisoned during the Interregnum for plotting against the Protector.[27] In 1661 Charles II made him a baronet, Wakeman of Beckford, and he enjoyed a reputation as the most accomplished Catholic physician in England. Titus Oates implicated Wakeman specifically and the queen by inference in testimony accusing the doctor of conniving to poison Charles II and his bastard son, James, Duke of Monmouth, so that the Duke of York might seize power. Oates swore that Wakeman was given £15,000 by certain Jesuits to kill the king.[28] The doctor's friends stood by him during the ordeal, which Whigs hoped to use to undermine the queen. Along with three Benedictine monks, Dr. Wakeman was indicted for high treason at the Old Bailey on July 18, 1679, and tried by Lord Chief Justice William Scroggs. Wakeman took an active part in his own defense, calling witnesses and examining those who gave evidence against him. Although a jury found all the accused not guilty, the verdict was wildly unpopular and broadsides openly denounced Scroggs for taking bribes. A "Pope-burning" procession through the city included representations of the murdered Godfrey and a Jesuits' bark-bearing Wakeman, "the Pope's doctor."[29] No wonder that Wakeman swiftly went abroad for his own safety, and he remained there until sometime before 1685 when he returned to London to give what must have been satisfying evidence against Oates, on trial himself for perjury.

Another of Charles II's First Physicians was the egregious George Bate, erstwhile doctor to Oliver Cromwell during the Interregnum, and, as shown in Chapter Five, no stranger himself to political imbroglios. The king designated Bate Physician to the Person in June 1660, but when the Duke of Gloucester fell ill in September, Bate assisted Dr. Alexander Fraizer in caring for the young man.[30] Bate wrote a report to Princess Mary's secretary on her brother's rapid deterioration and death. He and Fraizer administered cordials as the pox spread and "ripened," and they thought that Gloucester was out of danger when his pulse suddenly weakened and his breathing became labored. Evidently criticism of the royal doctors' treatment of Henry was circulating. Bate thought it was propagated by former Stuart family physician John Colladon, but he denied the rumor that the prince had been bled every day. Dr. Bate diagnosed a humor gone to the head and noted that he "had never seen so fast a deterioration in a patient in twenty years of practice." During the autopsy, examiners found the corpse's lungs filled with blood, which Bate asserted was consistent with smallpox but which the attending surgeons thought might have resulted from probing the jugular vein.[31]

Despite his failure to save Gloucester, Bate cemented his position with the Stuarts, and reassured those who brooded about his chameleon-like allegiance, by publishing a second part of *Elenchus Motuum* in 1661, dealing with the years 1649–59, a diatribe against those who contrived to "murder our late pious and sacred soveraigne, King Charles I." Bate's contemporary, Baldwin Hamey, threw doubt on Bate's authorship of *Elenchus Motuum*; others credited Charles II's chief adviser, Edward Hyde, Earl of Clarendon, with providing materials used in the work.[32] Nonetheless, Robert Pugh, a captain in the king's army, certainly thought Bate was the writer, and assailed him in an attack on the book, *Elenchus Elenchi: sive Animadversiones in Georgii Batei*, published in Paris in 1664.

Dr. Bate became one of the earliest fellows of the Royal Society and lectured on anatomy in 1666 at the College of Physicians. A posthumous collection of his prescriptions is available as *Pharmacopoeia Bateana*, edited by his longtime apothecary, Jack Shipton, and printed in 1688. Bate's remedies encompassed medicinal waters, spirits, oils, salts, electuaries, and infusions like *rosa solis*, which Bate vouched was good for the heart and liver. William Salmon published a second edition, one thousand pages in length, in 1694; it contained some recipes of Bate's Royal Society colleague and fellow Cromwellian physician Jonathan Goddard, including his eponymous volatile drops for fainting and apoplexy, made of a rather macabre mixture of ammonia, harts' horn, dried viper, and oil in which was marinated the skull of a hanged man.[33] Bequeathing a sizable estate including tenements in London to his three children, George Bate succumbed to the "French pox" in 1668, having weathered more political storms than most men in public life.

Besides Drs. Fraizer, Hinton, and Bate, two other physicians received June 1660 appointments as Physician to the Person: William Quartermaine and John Baber. Quartermaine, born in Buckinghamshire around 1630, held an M.D. from Pembroke College, Oxford, received in 1657. Dr. Quartermaine must have been with Charles in exile, for he was surely a passenger on one of the flotilla of ships accompanying the king from the Netherlands to England; Pepys mentions dining with Quartermaine and other physicians during the Channel crossing.[34] Quartermaine ranked second among the Caroline royal physicians. Admitted as a Fellow of the College of Physicians in 1661, Quartermaine was also an early participant in the activities of the Royal Society. He was clearly in His Majesty's good graces. A warrant from Charles II to Caroline Attorney General Geoffrey Palmer in June 1660 granted "our trusty and well-beloved Dr. William Quartermain, one of our physicians-in-ordinary," the right to convey spring water from Hyde Park through underground pipes to Westminster. The grant was good for ninety-nine years to Quartermaine and to his assignees. In an addendum, the warrant granted to Quartermaine "all singular sums of money due him yet unpaid," hinting at the recurrent irregularity of Stuart disbursements to his employees.[35] Quartermaine invested in "sea-worked" land and may have lost whatever money he might have made from the Hyde Park springs venture in the other scheme. He died in 1667.[36]

Sir John Baber, ranked third among the physicians to the Person, hailed from Wells where his father, a barrister, had been the town recorder and its representative in Parliament. Young Baber was educated at St. Peter's, Westminster, and Christ Church College, Oxford. After the surrender of Oxford to the New Model Army in April 1646, Baber was ejected from the university by Parliamentary spokesmen there, but commendatory letters from John Lambert, one of Cromwell's most puissant generals and temporary governor of Oxford, got him readmitted. Baber received his undergraduate degree in medicine later in 1646, moved to Leiden for further study, and obtained an M.D. from Angers in 1648; that degree was incorporated by Oxford in 1650. The College of Physicians made Baber a Fellow in 1657. Charles II knighted him in 1660 at the time that he became a royal doctor. Baber's social standing rose as he enjoyed the king's approbation. His first wife died in 1658, but Baber's position at court enabled him in 1674 to find a new bride, Ann Murray, widow of a groom of the chamber under Charles I and herself the daughter of a viscount. After her death, he married another noblewoman, Bridget, Viscountess Kilmorey, in 1680.[37]

Dr. Baber was a Nonconformist and objected in satirical verse to the accession of James II, a Roman Catholic convert, who understandably did not choose to maintain Baber in his medical post. Like many professional men of the time, Baber fancied himself something of a poet, a talent he put to use for the benefit of his politics. The doctor wrote a five-page burlesque upon James' coronation;

using the pseudonym Bavius, he followed that up with another sarcastic poem, this one ten pages in length, praising "the Queen's being delivere'd of a son." In the heyday of earnest tracts and giddy parodies, an anonymous broadside, published "for the London coffee-houses," quickly answered his scorn, calling him a "lamentable and most incorrigible scribbler." No less a writer than playwright Aphra Behn is the likely author of *To the Poet Bavius*, another disparaging response to his satire.[38]

As previously mentioned, Samuel Barrow, General Monck's go-between in the spring of 1660, won a medical appointment from Charles II (though not a knighthood like his fellow mediator, Thomas Clarges). He was still listed as one of the king's doctors in 1679, but probably spent more time in political and legal business than in medicine.[39] Though he does not appear to have had legal credentials, under Charles II Barrow was Advocate General and Judge Marshall of the English army, conducting at least twelve courts martial. Despite his medical background, he did not join the College of Physicians or the staff of any hospital. He started a history of the Civil War, but did not finish it. Barrow died in 1682 and was buried in Fulham church.[40]

At the start of his reign, King Charles nominated two physicians to his sizable household: Tobias Whitaker and Timothy Clarke. Whitaker, identified by the *Dictionary of National Biography* (*DNB*) as a Norwich doctor, may not have had a university degree at all.[41] Admonishing the reader to "listen to your doctor," he produced a fascinating treatise in 1638 called *The Tree of Human Life*, "sold at his [London] shop in Popeshead Ally," an indication that he was well aware of the burgeoning medical marketplace. Drawing upon Aristotle's contraries, Whitaker urged those with a hot and moist temperament to choose a cold and dry diet and vice versa. The publication focused on the therapeutic use of wine and argued that distinct kinds of wine, depending on the needs of one's character, could help bolster good health throughout a lifetime. Wine nourishes above all other aliments; it "corroborates, evacuates, and exhilarates the spirits."[42] Whitaker published a lengthy piece on "the French pest," *An Elenchus of Opinions concerning the Cure of the Small Pox*. Whatever attraction Whitaker's views had for Charles II, Whitaker secured his appointment in June 1660 at £50 per annum and held it for six years until his death.[43]

Timothy Clarke, whose 1652 M.D. was from Balliol College, Oxford, enjoyed some celebrity as an anatomist and, according to his good friend Pepys, dissected two bodies, a male and a female, before the curious sovereign on May 11, 1663. Pepys reported that "the king was highly pleased" with the demonstration. At about the same time, the government commissioned Clarke as physician to "new-raised forces within the kingdom." Pepys evidently valued Clarke's medical advice himself, noting a diuretic beverage of the doctor's made of reduced posset to which was added millet, caraway seeds, and manna, dried sap from a European ash tree, to be "quaffed three times in a half-hour."[44] Clarke was an original member of the Royal Society and became a councillor in the organization. On the death of Quartermaine in 1667, Clarke was appointed

Charles' second physician-in-ordinary, creating a vacancy in the household that Thomas Waldron would fill. The Restoration elevated some in the profession at a cost to others, and in 1663 Clarke complained bitterly to the College of Physicians' comitia, the organization's executive committee, that new men were being advanced by the Fellows ahead of candidates of long standing. Not until 1666 did the College accord Clarke Fellowship and only after the king asked that he be admitted with all courtesies.[45] He became an officer in 1670, but died the following year. As for Worcester-born Waldron, he appears to have been something of a prodigy, receiving his M.D. from Oxford in 1643 at nineteen. He was, however, a candidate for membership in the College of Physicians for a decade before the Fellows made him one of their own in 1665, a snub similar to the one given to Clarke. Waldron's appointment to the royal household predated Charles II's relocation from Hampton Court Palace. Waldron and royal apothecary John Jones petitioned the king in 1671 that they needed remodeled lodgings as a result of that move, the rooms set aside for them being decrepit.[46] Waldron remained on the job until his death in 1677 and was buried in Westminster Abbey.

Besides these physicians, Queen Catherine had a personal doctor, Fernando Mendes da Costa, a Portuguese *converso*, who according to Munk was rewarded in 1669 for treating her at Newcastle for erysipelas. Historian Norma Perry disagrees, saying that it was Antonio Mendes, Fernando's father, who treated Catherine's skin, although acknowledging that Fernando arrived in 1669 and was made body physician to the queen in March 1678. The University of Montpellier had awarded Fernando Mendes a doctorate of medicine in 1666; he had covered his Sephardic origins there by enrolling as a Spaniard, hence escaping the prejudice against Jews. Mendes ministered to Charles on occasion as well and maintained his Catholicity. The queen, Munk has reported, became godmother in 1678 to Mendes' daughter, named Catherine in her honor; Perry argues, however, that there is no baptismal evidence in the chapels royal that a Catherine Mendes ever received that sacrament.[47] James II instructed the College of Physicians to invite Mendes into its Fellowship in 1687, the same day as Hans Sloane, physician to Christ's Hospital and later royal doctor to George II; Mendes was erased from the roll as a Catholic, not as a Jew, after the Glorious Revolution. Though Queen Catherine eventually returned to Portugal in 1692, those on her staff who remained behind were retained and paid by her until her death in 1705. The long-lived Mendes stayed in England and kept up friendly connections and consultations with Fellows of the College of Physicians well into the eighteenth century. In a 1721 letter from his house on Broad Street to Sloane, Mendes thanked him for referring a patient and requested the name of "a good bonesetter—honest and dexterous."[48] Ferdinando Mendes passed away in 1725. Two other physicians are associated with Catherine of Braganza. Cambridge-educated Sir Francis Prujean, President of the College of Physicians from 1650 to 1654, attended the queen once in 1661 when she had spotted fever; he prescribed a soothing cordial for her, developed in his own laboratory. A Padua M. D., Theodore de Vaux, Mayerne's godson and editor, also served Charles and Catherine from the late 1660s, and stayed on after 1685 as physician to Catherine as the Queen Dowager.[49]

Charles Scarburgh (Scarborough) succeeded Bate as First Physician to Charles II, appointed in 1672. Born in London in 1616, Scarburgh attended Caius College, Cambridge, receiving his arts degrees there before the outbreak of the Civil War. His Royalist politics cost him his Caius fellowship, however, so he transferred to Merton College, Oxford, where he met and befriended William Harvey. He worked with Harvey on the generation of animals and obtained an M.D. from Oxford in 1646 by letters from the chancellor of the university. He became a Fellow of the College of Physicians in 1650. Following the Interregnum, Scarburgh's degree was incorporated at Cambridge and he moved to London, quickly catapulted into a position of leadership at the College of Physicians. The Fellows chose him as censor on two occasions, as an elect in 1677, and as consiliarius in 1684. Harvey transferred his Lumleian lectureship to Scarburgh and bequeathed him a velvet gown and surgical instruments. For an honorarium of £10, Scarburgh also gave anatomical lectures at the Barber Surgeons' Hall, where his portrait still hangs. Pepys reported attending one of Scarburgh's lectures in February 1663, and Scarburgh gave him a personal demonstration of the "manner of the disease of the stone and the cutting."[50]

The Sloane Manuscripts contain Scarburgh's notes for one of his orations, an amalgam of traditional and modern theories; he crossed out words and changed parts of the lecture, mixing Latin, Greek, and English. The lecture topic is the head, "tower [of the body and] seat of divinity in us," fittingly ornamented by "hayr." In it, Scarburgh discusses dissecting "dura mater and pia mater," but quotes Galen throughout the piece.[51] A founding Fellow of the Royal Society, Scarburgh loved mathematics and medicine equally. He discoursed on Euclid and trigonometry with the same passion as on muscles. King Charles knighted him in 1669, even before awarding him aulic responsibilities which included attending the Duke of York on the Edinburgh-bound frigate *Gloucester* in 1682. When the ship struck a sandbank off Yarmouth and began to sink, delays in evacuation cost dozens of lives, delays for which the Duke was blamed. Despite this harbinger of misfortunes to come, Scarburgh lingered through the Stuart dynasty as doctor to James after his accession and to Prince George of Denmark, consort of Queen Anne. Scarburgh had political success as well as professional, representing Camelford, Cornwall, in the House of Commons from 1685 to 1687, but he lost his position at court at the Glorious Revolution. Scarburgh accumulated a large library of more than 2,300 pieces, which was purchased at his death in 1694 by Lord Spencer to be added to King William's library at St. James's palace. Unfortunately, the death later that year of Queen Mary, the project's patroness, ended the plan, and the collection was dispersed.[52]

Among Scarburgh's legacies is his eyewitness description of the last illness of Charles II in 1685, written the following year to repudiate any suspicions about what had happened; though First Physician, Scarburgh was only one of twelve doctors in attendance.[53] Until 1679 the king had exhibited remarkable stamina, but shortly after the Wakeman trial, he fell desperately sick, seized with a fever at Windsor. Padua-educated John Micklethwaite, then President of the College of Physicians, was sent for and prescribed cinchona, which revived the royal patient; a grateful Charles knighted Micklethwaite. The king recovered, but not before politicians and courtiers guaranteed the Duke of York the crown over the illegitimate Monmouth. In some ways the king's infirmity had resuscitated James's right of inheritance more effectively than politicking inside and outside of Parliament. Having secured the throne for his brother and captured the renewed allegiance of his subjects, Charles became sick again in 1682; he seemed to recuperate completely, again treated with Jesuits' bark, a remedy preferred by all of the queen's doctors except Dr. Mendes. Charles resumed playing vigorous tennis, rode and hawked as before, and hunted regularly. Then, following a sleepless night on February 1, 1685, he awoke unable to speak, later screamed in agony, and fell unconscious. Scarburgh opined that Charles had had an apoplexy attack, but there was no characteristic facial paralysis.

As his illness beset the king, his physicians bled him sixteen ounces, gave him Goddard's drops and an antispasmodic black cherry julep, then bled him another ten ounces. His head was shaved by veteran royal barber Ralph Foliard and the irritant cantharides, nicknamed "Spanish fly," was applied as a blistering agent.[54] Remarkably, the king revived, but on February 3, he was seized with another attack. In their panic to save the king, the royal doctors administered fifty-eight drugs in a five-day period; they purged, plastered, and scalded him, forcing his mouth open to receive nourishment that would then be deliberately expelled.[55] There was no suspicion of poison then, nor should there be now; indeed, the efforts of the physicians were applauded as courageous and exhaustive. Scarburgh did confirm that the king converted to Roman Catholicism on his deathbed and then bid adieu to his queen, his brother, and his children. Charles II died on February 6, 1685. A post-mortem examination disclosed inordinate amounts of fluid in the ventricles.[56]

After Scarburgh's appointment in 1672, the next medical man to receive Charles II's favor was Thomas Williams, an apothecary by training. A practitioner from Eltham and an honorary or extra-licentiate of the Royal College of Physicians, Williams did not earn his M. D. through conventional study. Instead, the State Papers of 1669 registered a petition from the king for a medical degree from Cambridge to go to the king's apothecary.[57] The following year Williams, who has been labeled a Helmontian, was made chemical physician to the king at forty marks per annum.[58] In 1674 he was created a baron. As a follower of van Helmont, Williams became embroiled in the escalating medical controversy between traditionalists and Helmontians, which intensified after the Restoration and threatened the monopoly of the Royal College of Physicians. So influential with the king were the enigmatic Helmontians that they pressed him for a separate physicians' college of their own in London in 1665. Many politicians, including the Duke of Buckingham, Elias Ashmole, and General Monck, supported the Helmontians' desire for a second institution and for full membership in the Royal Society. The College of Physicians vigorously opposed such proposals, and sought to exploit divisions between the Helmontians and the apothecaries. But the Helmontians, who braved London in 1665 to minister to plague victims while many of the Galenists fled to the countryside, were devastated as a group by the epidemic. Decimated, the Helmontians were left to play only "a brief role as a third party" in the physician-apothecary strife.[59]

Not all of the traditionalists were cowardly and callous, deserting their patients at the time of the great plague. Edward Dawtry (Deantry), who attended Charles I at the Battle of Naseby, plus Peter Barwick, and Thomas Witherley, both among Charles II's physicians, volunteered to attend the sick poor during the epidemic. Witherley, whose M.D. was from Cambridge in 1655, afforded leadership to the College of Physicians at this critical juncture. After his acceptance as a Fellow, he climbed rapidly through the organization's offices, becoming an elect in 1678, censor in 1683, and President from 1684 to 1687, bridging the transition from Charles II to James II.[60] Witherley steered the College through some of its most confident times as it instigated a clean up of the medical marketplace, eliminated its debts, and allied with the rejuvenated Stuart government. By February 1687 the College had a new charter, granting it all its former rights, and obtained from James II a directive to exercise them. As long as King James ruled, the influence of corporations like the College of Physicians would be strong. A royal doctor like Witherley was the perfect leader for the College; likewise, the President of the College was the perfect royal doctor for James.

Edmund King refashioned himself from surgeon to physician with the approval of Charles II. King came to the monarch's attention because of his distinction as an experimental chemist. Gilbert Sheldon, Archbishop of Canterbury, created King a doctor of medicine; Cambridge agreed to incorporate King's doctorate as a university degree in 1671. In response to a request from His Majesty, King prepared a handwritten report in February 1675 on his activities as a physician, emphasizing his familiarity with the circulation of the blood, the pulse, kidneys, and intestines, based on dissections on human and animal cadavers; "the body," he wrote, "consists chiefly of tubes and liquors."[61] Dr. King was sworn in as a physician-in-ordinary in 1676. With a letter from Charles, the College of Physicians accepted King as an honorary Fellow in 1677, enabling him to complete his occupational transformation in London. Despite the fact that his medical degree originated as *honoris causis*, King was respected as a fine anatomist, surgeon, and physician. John Evelyn transcribed King's presentations to other virtuosi at the Royal Society.[62] Immediately upon Charles' attack in 1685, King was sent for and he ordered that the royal patient be bled. Only after Charles regained consciousness did the other royal doctors approve the phlebotomy, a procedure for which the Privy Council voted King £1,000 and for which he was never paid, perhaps because Charles did die.[63] James II nominated Edmund King for a regular Fellowship in the College of Physicians in 1687; after the Glorious Revolution, King spent his old age dissecting brains, purportedly over a hundred of them, until his death at eighty in 1709.

The final appointee as a physician to the Caroline household was Edmund Dickinson (Dickenson), whose chemical and alchemical experiments, like Edmund King's, inspired Charles II. Born in Berkshire, Dickinson studied at Oxford's Merton College, obtaining all of his degrees there; his M.D. came in 1656. Like many medical men of his time, Dickinson's interests were wide-ranging and his energies inexhaustible. He wrote about the Pythian Apollo and the Oracle at Delphi; he argued that the Egyptian Hercules was Joshua, and that Joshua was called Ogmius by the Gauls.[64] Well-known at Oxford for his chemistry and for his many Latin treatises on varied subjects, he treated distinguished patients like Henry Bennet, the Earl of Arlington and Charles's Lord Chamberlain, whom Dickinson cured of a huge hernia with a plaster. When in London, Dickinson worked at the house of his friend, Thomas Willis, the leading English exponent of chemiatry or chemical medicine. Other physicians were suspicious of Dickinson's methods and his belief in universal medicine, but Arlington extolled Dickinson to the king, who made him a royal doctor in February 1677; the College of Physicians admitted him to their Fellowship the same year. King Charles delighted in chemical demonstrations and set up a laboratory in Whitehall so that he and Dickinson could carry out research trials whenever the spirit moved him.[65] Dickinson stayed as a royal doctor under James II until the 1688 revolution, then spent the next nineteen years in study. His book, *Physica vetus et vera,* published in 1702, uses atomic theory mixed with classical and biblical passages, representative of the so-called virtuosi of the Augustan Age in Britain.[66]

The last two physicians to the Person appointed before the Glorious Revolution were Robert Brady and Hugh Chamberlen, both nominated in 1682. Brady was a stalwart Royalist accorded many advantages by the restored Stuarts. In 1660 by royal mandate, he became master of Caius College, Cambridge; simultaneously, *per literas regias*, Cambridge awarded him a medical doctorate, which was essential to his credentials as Professor of Physic. The king also made Brady Keeper of the Records in the Tower, a post in which a partisan appointee might be generous to a ruler's place in history; Brady developed proficiency outside of medicine as an expert on the English constitution. Additionally, Brady represented Cambridge University in Charles's parliaments until 1685. James II extended Brady's designation as physician-in-ordinary.

Hugh Chamberlen the Elder, outspoken like the rest of his clan, drove a new generation of Fellows in the College of Physicians to distraction, so it must have been with a certain glee that Charles made him Physician to the Person. Chamberlen's concerns were always controversial; whether it was Jesuits' bark, prophylactics for plague, organized midwifery, land bank projects, or union with Scotland, Chamberlen espoused them all in print.[67] Chamberlen's family is credited with designing and publicizing a type of obstetrical forceps vastly superior to the hooks formerly used. Hugh's father, Peter Chamberlen III (eldest son of Peter the Younger and the father of fourteen sons), claimed a personal preferment as physician to the royal household at the Restoration since he had ministered to the household of Charles I. His *Humble Petition*, a proposal for public baths and bath-stoves originally published in 1648, was reprinted in 1662 and touted him as "first physician to the royal progeny and to His Most Sacred Majesty." Some credit him with improving the design of the family forceps and he certainly prospered because of them, however, it was Hugh who took the instrument to Paris in 1673 for famed accoucheur François Mauriceau to see. Hugh Chamberlen had translated Mauriceau's book on midwifery into English that same year and that probably gained him entry to the great man-midwife. Unfortunately, in a demonstration of the forceps for Mauriceau on a woman in labor, the patient expired when her womb was perforated.[68]

Hugh Chamberlen had no medical degree until 1689, and then only by *comitiis regiis*. Even though he was a royal doctor, Fellow of the Royal Society, and an acclaimed man-midwife, the College of Physicians refused to admit him until 1694; in fact, the Fellows were asked to consider a complaint against him in 1688 for causing the death of Phoebe Wilmer, a pregnant woman to whom he administered four "vomits," four purges, and three bleedings of eight ounces each. She had miscarried on two previous occasions, so Chamberlen gave her *crocus metallorum* (antimony and nitre) and *extractum rudii*. The latter was a powerful hydragogue, cathartic, and emmenagogue made from black hellebore. Mrs. Wilmer miscarried, experienced horrific diarrhea, and died. The College found Hugh Chamberlen guilty of malpractice and fined him £10.[69] Notwithstanding these incidents, Chamberlen continued in royal service to James II's queen and was summoned to attend her in 1688, but arrived too late.

Besides these physicians to the Person and to the household whose appointments were embodied in Letters Patent under the Great Seal, many other doctors tended to the Stuart brothers on particular occasions or for specific ailments and were not covered by the Lord Chamberlain's warrant. Furthermore, although the monarch had doctors in regular attendance, progresses through the country required local medical men to be on call. Dr. William Ramesey, who lived in Plymouth after 1668 when Munk says he was a physician-in-ordinary, probed just the sort of enigmatic subjects that captivated King Charles. He wrote on Christian astrology, eclipses, and poisons, topics that piqued the curiosity of many men and women, and published on elminthologia, worms in human bodies. Charles II certainly subscribed to the thesis of Ramesey's *The Gentleman's Companion*: a gentleman does not rebel.[70]

Ramesey was but one of the numerous other royal doctors. Clippingdale enumerates Edward Dawtry, Martin Llewellyn, John Colladon, and William

Denton, all veterans of medical service under Charles I, and Peter Barwick as physicians to Charles II in some capacity. These are in addition to the doctors whose service was immediately recognized by the king in 1660 and who held administrative entitlement.[71] Barwick, a Royalist whose brother was Dean of St. Paul's, had known the king since the Battle of Worcester in 1651. A Cambridge M.D., Barwick settled in London, married a rich widow who was a kinswoman of Archbishop Laud, and became a Fellow of the College of Physicians in 1655. He defended Harvey's theories on the circulation of the blood and became famous himself for his treatment of smallpox and fevers. He consulted regularly with other prominent doctors and was particularly taken with "the cortex," another name for Jesuit's bark. Barwick became physician-in-ordinary to Charles II in 1660. He had stature as a humanitarian; he weathered the plague in London and prescribed gratis for the poor. Barwick was an officer of the College of Physicians on multiple occasions during the next three decades before going blind in 1694; he died in 1705.[72]

Clippingdale's "Medical Court Roll" for the reign of Charles II subsequent to the Restoration is encyclopedic. Clippingdale lists thirty-six physicians in all who doctored the king or his household after 1660.[73] A few deserve further discussion because of the distinction of their lives or because their particular careers illuminate important directions in English medicine in the later seventeenth century. For instance, Edward Browne, the well-traveled physician to St. Bartholomew's Hospital and a Caroline royal doctor, was a star in the London medical firmament. The king called him as "learned as any of the College and as well-bred as any at court."[74] Browne's résumé encompassed Fellowship in the Royal Society, Presidency of the College of Physicians, and a large practice including the Earl of Rochester and the Marquis of Dorset among his patients. Working in conference with Dr. de Vaux, Browne used a febrifuge powder, probably cinchona, on an ague patient in January 1664.[75] He embraced laboratory research as intrinsic to good medicine and daily dissected things ranging from bovine legs to turkey hearts; he wrote the pharmacopoeia for St. Bartholomew's and studied botany. Moreover, Browne's irenic professionalism seems unique in the fractious Restoration medical world. Before making his own diagnoses, he deliberately consulted with physicians holding disparate perspectives and with estimable surgeons and apothecaries, always considerate of their views.[76]

Both Walter Needham, "a physician of very great reputation," and Daniel Coxe, M.D. by the king's command, engaged in experiments and promulgated their findings.[77] Needham, doctor to the Lord Chamberlain, physician to the Charterhouse, and a Fellow of the Royal Society, wrote on fetal anatomy and read a paper to his compeers at the Royal Society on his experiments in stopping arterial bleeding. In 1683 Hans Sloane must have asked him to study a report on his wife, for Needham responded by letter to Mrs. Sloane, remarking that he was at too great a distance to examine her, that the mass in her breast did not seem to be cancerous, "though a very troublesome swelling." Needham recommended Mrs. Corbett's plaster, "as long as there is any hopes of dispersing it," along with a poultice Mrs. Sloane could get an apothecary to make. Needham included the poultice recipe in Latin. He advised that if the swelling "breaks," she could apply a common digestive made with "wheat flower, honey, egg yolk, and turpentine to draw and heal it."[78]

Daniel Coxe, appointed to tend the king in 1665, performed several experiments involving that old Stuart bugbear, tobacco. He administered oral doses of tobacco to a young man, who reported on its disagreeable taste, then experienced dizziness and vomiting. Coxe next tried the same dosage out on a cat, who exhibited the same symptoms as the man and then perished in fifteen minutes. He autopsied the animal, which smelled strongly of tobacco oil.[79] Despite his investigations, Coxe is better known for his 1669 harangue against the London apothecaries, *Discourse (about) Physick and Physicians*. In it, Coxe invokes Hippocrates, Galen, and all the greats to berate the error-prone druggists upon whom doctors depended for good medicines. Given the bad feeling between physicians and pharmacists, Coxe argued that doctors themselves ought to be making and disbursing medicaments, not for profit, but in the best interests of their patients. Coxe's like-minded associates in the College of Physicians, including Jonathan Goddard, who feared apothecaries would ruin doctors' practices, embraced this proposal and later created a dispensary controlled by the Fellows.[80]

Even more illustrious than Browne, Needham, and Coxe were colleagues Thomas Willis and Richard Lower, arguably among the most fashionable doctors of their time and research collaborators at Christ Church, Oxford, where Willis was Sedeleian Professor of Natural History. No less a student than John Locke took notes on Willis's 1661–64 lectures and preserved for posterity a glimpse of the university's intellectual vitality.[81] After the Restoration both Willis and Lower settled in London and developed large, affluent practices. Willis, elder of the two by a decade and from a family that fervently supported the Stuarts, helped found the Royal Society. His classification of the cerebral nerves, including the first description of the seventh cranial nerve, is commemorated in the naming of the "circle of Willis," the polygonal meeting of arteries at the base of the brain.[82] Christopher Wren contributed illustrations to Willis's *Cerebri anatome* (1664). Willis felt that the cerebrum was the center of thought and discussed the physiological and pathological problems of the brain. A theorist who was also good at close, clinical observation, Willis diagnosed sweetness of breath and urine in persons suffering from diabetes. He wrote many books exhibiting great ingenuity and learning; among them are works on myasthenia gravis, puerperal fever, typhoid, nervous diseases, hysteria, and paracusis of Willis, the phenomenon of hearing best in a noisy environment.[83] If not the regular physician to the Duke of York and his family, he was surely consulted often; Thomas Willis died in 1675.

Cornish-born Richard Lower assisted Willis in his anatomical research on the nervous system at Oxford, then, after obtaining his M.D. from Christ Church

College in 1665, followed his mentor to London, establishing himself in Covent Garden and catering to a chic clientele. He joined the Royal Society and became a Fellow of the College of Physicians. In 1665, in the presence of Boyle, Lower transfused the blood of one dog to another; he repeated the demonstration before the Royal Society in 1669. He described the ridge across the inner surface of the right atrium (the *tuberculum intervenosum*), since called the tubercle of Lower. His comrades in the College of Physicians referred to him as "the most noted physician in Westminster and London, and asserted [that] no man's name was more cried up at court than his."[84] *Dr. Lower's Receipts*, over one hundred pages of recipes published posthumously, illustrates the range of his treatments. He concocted an eponymous tincture for colic composed of senna, anise, and coriander; for heartburn he devised a milky drink laced with chalk and crabs' eyes. For painful urine, Lower mixed fennel, horseradish, turpentine, and syrup of marshmallows; he invented a salve for "shrunken sinews" that required twelve young swallows boiled with rosemary and lavender in fresh butter.[85]

Dr. Lower was esteemed and celebrated like Willis for his work in physiology, and at Willis' death, Lower inherited his practice. Unlike Willis, however, Lower's politics eventually hurt his career. In 1679, Lower, whose father was a persecuted Quaker, sided with the Whigs in their encouragement of Oates and lost his patrons at court. Politics were also at the root of a quarrel between Lower and Charles Scarburgh in May 1688. As a Whig, Lower disliked the College of Physicians' authoritarian crack-down on unlicensed empirics and apothecaries, but Scarburgh, a Royalist and physician to James II, supported these tactics. Their quarrel may have centered on Scarburgh's treatment that spring of a pregnant Queen Mary, when she was in danger of miscarrying. When Lower passed away in 1691, he left many bequests to charity, including £1,000 to St. Bartholomew's, but not a penny to the College.[86]

Not all appointments as physician, permanent or ad hoc, were given to those in orthodox medical practice. Robert Morison (1620–1683) was better known as a botanist than an anatomist. Nevertheless, the Aberdeen-born Scot rose to prominence as senior physician, "botanic professor," and superintendent of all the royal gardens, named by Charles II in 1669. The Civil War had interrupted Morison's promising early academic career, and he was wounded in battle when the Scottish Covenanters invaded England. Fleeing to France after his recovery, Morison obtained an M. D. from Angers in 1648.[87] Further study under the French king's botanist, Vespasian Robin, enabled Morison to develop his own methods of botanical classification. He was employed by the Duke of Orleans as a supervisor of his gardens at Blois, and through him met Charles before the Restoration. Morison was summoned to England in August 1660, one of the first in a network of medical Scotsmen who served the later Stuarts. He published *Praeludia Botanica* in 1669, and the work garnered him great prestige, though his classification system has subsequently been criticized for failing to acknowledge the work of other botanists and for failing to adhere to his own principles.[88] His salary as king's physician was set at £200 per annum, but his financial security was short-lived. The king had other plans for St. James' Park and ordered Morison in May 1669 to relinquish the Royal Physic Garden with its house and land to John Hawley at the Exchequer.

Needing income, Morison found additional employment in December of the same year as professor of botany at University College, Oxford. The Earl of Danby wanted a physic garden at Oxford and a botanist-professor to supervise it. Morison's medical degree was immediately incorporated at the university, and he gave his first lecture in September 1670, though he spent most of his time in the physic garden reading aloud on herbs and plants.[89] He appeared before the Royal College of Physicians in December 1673 to request a £5 pledge from each member to defer the costs of a "Historia Plantarum Naturalis." The Fellows noted their admiration for the professor, not himself a member of the College of Physicians, and agreed.[90] Morison never lived to see the publication of his work. He died in London in 1683 after fracturing his skull when hit by a coach in the Strand near Charing Cross, and he was buried at St. Martin's-in-the-Fields. Like some other aulic appointees of the Stuarts, Morison had not been promptly paid for his service to the court, and he had written the year before his demise to the Archbishop of Canterbury that he needed the money owed him by the Caroline government. Morison's widow, without a pension to live on, was still trying futilely in 1693 to get what her husband was owed, the sizable sum of £4,400.[91]

Another of the botanical or chemical physicians was Nicolas LeFevre, who shared with Morison a French introduction to Charles II and difficulty in collecting his wages.[92] A graduate of the University of Sedan, LeFevre was appointed by Louis XIV's physician, Antoine Vallot, as demonstrator in chemistry at the Jardin des Plantes in Paris where diarist John Evelyn was his pupil. In 1660 LeFevre published an enormously successful chemistry text. Dedicated to Charles II and the Society of Apothecaries, the book expounded Paracelsian and iatrochemical ideas in a "philosophical" section. The volume, replete with cryptic symbols and numbers, included treatments for colic, rheumatism, palpitations of the heart, and worms. LeFevre suggested using amber for hysteria, chicory and rhubarb as a cholagogic, and a drink of milk and tobacco for asthma.[93]

LeFevre was invited after the Restoration to become the king's professor of chemistry and apothecary-in-ordinary to the household. Though he was to receive £150 as "professor of chymicks," he often had to petition for his salary, even his allowance for laboratory fuel. In addition, because some of his tasks replicated those done by the apothecary to the household, the Board of the Green Cloth reminded LeFevre that John Jones was the official appointee, and that LeFevre's job was a delimited one.[94] Nevertheless, LeFevre was given permission to import wines duty-free for the king's use, perhaps a mollifying award.

One of LeFevre's pharmaceutical specialties was Raleigh's Cordial, which he prepared in September 1662 while Evelyn and the king watched. Not surprisingly, in 1663 he became a Fellow of the Royal Society and in 1664 published a treatise on his favorite remedy. LeFevre argued that the cordial's genius was not only in curing what ailed a sick patient, but in maintaining a state of wellness in the healthy. He reported that the concoction contained all three "natural families," animal, vegetable, and mineral components in thirteen ingredients.[95] LeFevre expired in 1669.

Robert Talbor, famed for his secret ague cure, did not have a medical degree at all, but still enjoyed the king's bounty. The apothecary had gained fame as a feverologist when Charles, "the most inquisitive King in the world [and] the greatest patron of Empirics," sent for him on the recommendation of a courtier in June 1672.[96] During Talbor's visit, he and the king experimented together with cinchona preparations, the dosage of which Talbor seems to have perfected, and fooled the royal doctors as to its composition. A few weeks afterward, Charles appointed Talbor Physician to the Person, gave him an annuity of £100, and later knighted Talbor because the king remembered from his experience with Talbor how to cure his own case of ague.[97] Talbor moved to London and established himself next to Gray's Inn Gate in Holborn; he treated the daughter of Viscount John Mordaunt, Governor of Windsor Castle, and published *Pyretolgia: A Rational Account of the Cause and Cure of Agues* (1672). In May 1678 the king adjured the College of Physicians to leave Talbor unmolested and his practice undisturbed. Purposefully, Talbor bought up "all the quinquina that he could find" in France and England. He enjoyed the benefits of Charles's patronage at home and on the continent, traveling to Spain to cure Queen Marie Louise and to France to triumphantly treat the *dauphine* with quinine wine, as well as relatives of prominent épistolière Madame de Sévigné. Louis XIV purchased Talbor's formula for 3,000 crowns and a life pension.[98] By agreement in 1682, the year after Talbor's death, *The English Remedy* appeared in Paris and London; in it, Talbor summed up a truth about medicine and monopoly: when the bark "was only in the hands of the Jesuits" it was expensive, but the drug became cheaper "as soon as the drogists began to trade in it."[99] Evelyn recorded that the Royal Society experimented with Jesuits' Powder in 1683, by then "so famous for Talbor's curing agues with it," to see if it "would hinder both ebullition and fermentation".[100]

The most controversial of all the Caroline medical appointments were those made to charlatans and mountebanks who caught the king's eye. By definition, a charlatan had a fixed location, while a mountebank traveled from town to town, often escorted by a harlequin-attired servant and a monkey to entertain onlookers. To the chagrin of the College of Physicians, Charles II began licensing mountebanks, giving them permits to travel, perform, and sell from a stage. Armed with royal permission, itinerant quacks brought their theatrical brand of medicine to the people, hawking medicaments at fairs, spas and crossroads.[101] Worse yet, spurning the guidance of the Lord Chamberlain, the king sometimes hired quacks for the court, like the Italian George Moretto and Hamburg citizen Cornelius Tilborg (Tilbury, Tilborne), both of whom became royal doctors. Moretto had a license to travel from April 1665; after impressing Charles II with a demonstration in 1682, Tilborg sold orvietan, a poison antidote, and other unspecified medicines throughout the realm. Though Tilborg had no medical degree, he entitled himself "doctor" in the handbills distributed by his zany before the program. The king made Tilborg a physician-in-ordinary and gave him a gold medal and chain, more payment than some of his regular appointees received.[102]

One final example of the sort of empiric whom Charles II patronized is John Archer, chemical physician-in-ordinary in 1671. The frontispiece of his book, *Every Man His Own Doctor,* identifies the author as a royal doctor. Despite the Paracelsian-tinged title and democratic intent, Archer's book reflects Galenic concepts and categories. He described fever as a "preternatural heat kindled in the heart," which can be cured by "two or three of our vomiting pills."[103] Archer criticized Jesuits' bark as producing too severe sweats; his own cordials were easier on the patient. An advertising quack, Archer was never licensed by the College of Physicians, but thrived in the post-Restoration medical marketplace. He used his publications as promotional advertisements, selling his nostrums between the hours of 11 A.M. and 5 P.M. from an establishment near Charing Cross and his book from his house in Knightsbridge. In 1684, Archer published *Secrets Disclosed of Consumptions*, which included instructions for distinguishing scurvy from venereal disease. Treatment with mercury had become a common therapy for syphilis, but Archer cautioned that it was poisonous.[104] His common-sense exhortation for "piles" included temperance and exercise: "Be not wicked or foolish overmuch, why wilt thou die before thy time?" When dietary moderation failed, Archer called for a "universal cordial called Antonio, made of bezoar, ambergreece, pearl, unicorn's horn and coral."[105] Though his medical specialty allegedly was the fistula, he boasted of three remarkable inventions: the vapor bath, a new type of oven, and a one-horse chariot.

By warrant from the Lord Chamberlain, embodied in Letters Patent under the Great Seal, three serjeant-surgeoncy appointments were made in February 1661 to men with preferment claims: Richard Pyle, Humphrey Painter, and John Knight. They joined the already-appointed Surgeon to the Person, Richard Wiseman, and household surgeon, Thomas Woodhall, both named the previous June. Remuneration for a serjeant-surgeon until 1685 consisted of wages of £80, board wages of £140, and an annuity of £150, making a total of £370. Richard Pyle, concurrently First Principal Surgeon and serjeant-surgeon, claimed the designation from 1642; his entitlement was substantiated in March 1661. Pyle cared for Charles as Prince of Wales in the West of England campaign of 1645–46 and was married to the niece of Charles I's serjeant-surgeon, William Clowes the Younger. Despite his rank and history with the king, petitions in April 1669 make apparent that the emoluments promised him were in arrears.[106] Humphrey Painter, another of Charles II's serjeant-surgeons, was Master of the Barber Surgeons' Company in 1661, but he had long been a member of its livery. The *Annals* show his pledge of £3 in 1638 to the guild's building fund.[107] His and Pyle's career were overshadowed by the third member of the surgeoncy triumvirate.

John Knight made the transition from priest to surgeon, having forsaken a career in the church to become apprenticed to surgeon Edward Moleyns at the age of thirty-nine. A stalwart Royalist, Knight fled to Holland in 1648, attached himself to Charles's court in exile and possibly worked as an agent in the secret service for Edward Hyde, Charles's Lord Chancellor. In his sixtieth year, Knight returned with the king on his voyage from The Hague to Dover; Charles made him serjeant-surgeon the following winter. He was admitted to the Barber Surgeons without fee in 1662 and by the ensuing year was Master of the Company. Caius College granted him an M.D. in 1669 at the king's request.[108] As Surgeon-General to the Royal Forces, Knight was responsible for medicines and the treatment of soldiers during the second Dutch war and served as a member of the Commission for the Sick and Wounded. A handwritten notebook in Latin of Knight's remedies, many of them physicians' prescriptions that he administered, includes clysters, elixirs, and plasters; he especially recommended a millipede emulsion as a diuretic.[109] When two skeletons were uncovered in a chest at the bottom of a deep hole in the Tower, Knight was called in to investigate. He reported that the bones were those of children and that they were intermixed with pieces of velvet, leading to the belief that the murdered nephews of Richard III had finally been found. Perhaps in return for his forensic analysis, he obtained the property of a suicide by a royal grant in 1676 as a gratuity.[110] He died in 1680.

Surgeons to the person received wages of £40, board wages of around £127, and a pension of £150. Richard Wiseman surely earned that income and his reputation as a great surgeon, adept at clinical observation. Fielding Garrison lauded Wiseman "for playing the same part in surgery as Sydenham did in medicine."[111] At the Battle of Worcester before his capture by Cromwell's forces, he treated many soldiers with grievous head injuries, and he devoted a considerable portion of his most important book to head wounds. Dedicated to Charles II and published in 1676, *Severall Chirurgicall Treatises* discusses six hundred of Wiseman's cases and treatments as well as subjects like tumors, ulcers, diseases of the anus, amputations, and fractures. His "design was to help sea-chirurgians, who seldom trouble their cabbins with many books," but civilian surgeons could also benefit from his military training.[112] He wrote a study on gonorrhea in which he described the first external urethrotomy for stricture, which he performed with Edward Moleyns in 1652.

Wiseman's loyalty was praiseworthy, too. He remained steadfast to Charles II through those difficult years in exile, and spent two years in Lambeth prison, the residence of the Archbishop of Canterbury having been put to this use during the Interregnum, for treating an ailing Royalist in the Tower. Even after Wiseman's release, he was subject to so much harassment that he left England and enlisted in the Spanish navy. Charles II brought him back to London where he was rewarded for his faithful service. Wiseman astutely returned the favor; his records of the king's touching ceremonies helped deepen the popularity of His Majesty. Wiseman's biographer asserts that Pyle, Knight, and Painter were jealous of Wiseman's eminence and friendship with the king.[113] Many of his books were used by Samuel Johnson in compiling his famous dictionary. Wiseman was elected to the Barber Surgeons' Court of Assistants in 1664 and became Master of the Company the following year. When Painter expired in 1672, Charles elevated Wiseman to a serjeant-surgeoncy, a post he held until his death in 1676. Richard Wiseman was buried in his parish church, St. Paul's at Covent Garden, lamented by his fellow surgeons.[114]

Surgeons to the Caroline household received wages of £40, board wages of £140, and a pension of £100. The opportunity for advancement through the royal surgical ranks often depended on the death of one's superior. Thomas Woodhall (Woodall), son of the surgeon at St. Bartholomew's Hospital and himself on the staff of St. Thomas's Hospital, was the first appointed in June 1660. Eager to teach anatomy lessons to other medical men, Woodhall dissected the bodies of executed criminals in the hall of the Barber Surgeons' Company. Samuel Pepys related news of Woodhall's death in March 1667, precipitated by a drunken brawl with a Frenchman at Somerset House. According to Pepys the Duke of York planned to obtain Woodhall's place at St. Thomas's for his own patronage purposes.[115] Sackville Whittle filled the vacancy in the household medical staff created by Woodhall's demise.

Whittle was in attendance upon the king at the Newmarket horse-races in 1668. An order signed by Charles's Chancellor of the Exchequer, Baron Ashley, on July 8, 1671, authorized the payment of "£40 by debentures to Whittle by virtue of his majesty's letters of patent," an indication that Whittle's surgeon's salary was overdue.[116] With Wiseman's promotion to serjeant-surgeon, Whittle rose from household surgeon to personal service and a better pension in February 1672. That advancement in turn furthered the career of James Pierce (Pearce), surgeon to the Duke of York and Surgeon-General to the Fleet. Pierce, a close friend of Pepys mentioned often in the famous diary, climbed the aulic ladder when he became surgeon to the household on Whittle's advancement. Pepys recounted Pierce's experiments on and dissections of animals, such as the time in May 1664 when Pierce and Dr. Clarke killed a dog by injecting opium into its hind leg. Pepys remarked that they had trouble "hitting the vein," but the dog finally became unconscious and died. In July 1668 Pierce and Doctors Clarke, Waldron, and Lower dissected the eyes of sheep and oxen to Pepys' "great information."[117] Pierce complained to Pepys of money problems with a London banking house and gossiped with him about matters at court. Despite a reputation as a "clumsy operator," in 1681 he moved into the office of Surgeon to the Person, probably on the death of Sackville Whittle, and in March 1685 James II made him serjeant surgeon.[118] The final Caroline household appointment was made when James Moleyns, scion of the surgical family, was designated surgeon to the household in February 1681. Besides his duties to the Stuarts, Moleyns rendered surgical expertise to St. Thomas's Hospital. Moleyns climbed to personal surgeoncy under James II in March 1685.

Among the extra surgeons-in-ordinary appointed to minister to Charles II was John Browne, a Norwich-born practitioner mentored by Thomas Browne, whose son and John's contemporary, Edward, was a physician to the king. John Browne arrived in London in 1676 after a decade of surgery in Norfolk, and caught Charles's eye with books on muscles and tumors. Using Galenic assumptions, he examined the metaphysical causes of tumors and determined which veins to bleed, how to purge, and what to apply to the poisoned organ. When all else fails, he wrote, apply live pigeons to the parts affected. Browne considered erysipelas to be a tumor requiring plentiful bleeding and a rhubarb electuary; for cancer, unguent of frogs or oil of nightshade was recommended; in the case of pestilential buboes, oysters should extract the toxin.[119] Browne is credited with writing one of the best accounts of the King's Evil, *Adenochoiradelogia*; Browne maintained that besides struma the royal gift of healing worked on new diseases emanating from the sins of the people and could cure nonconformity, too.[120] Besides nominating him as the sovereign's surgeon-in-ordinary, the crown backed Browne for an appointment in surgery at St. Thomas's Hospital in 1683; he served in that capacity until discharged, possibly for political reasons, in 1691.

However, Browne and the rest of the surgical staff may have been forced out by the hospital board of governors for malpractice. William III chose to retain Browne as surgeon, so, although the London hospitals sometimes demonstrated autonomy in their medical judgments, a political explanation for his fall from St. Thomas's seems unlikely.[121] Moreover, Browne was sued in 1687 in the Mayor's Court by a London widow, Susanna Levine, whose broken leg was not tended to as well as she thought appropriate and who did not intend to pay for Browne's ineptitude. Her treatment was bungled, witnesses testified, by Browne's apprentice and her suffering endured for two years, during which time the leg was repeatedly rebroken and reset. Among those testifying for Browne in the Levine case was fellow native of Norwich William Briggs, also dismissed from St. Thomas's and a royal doctor and oculist to William III.[122]

Charles II's royal apothecaries were John Chase and John Jones, the former to the Person and the latter to the household. Although remuneration attached to these offices varied, Chase was to receive salary and board wages totaling £242. For a century the Chases furnished medicines for the court and led their professional association. Chase's father, Stephen, had served Charles I. According to a petition from Stephen's daughter Anne, for their Royalist loyalty both her parents had endured incarceration and molestation during the Civil War. Despite these hardships, Stephen Chase lived to see the Stuarts enthroned again and was able to acquire a manor given by Charles II to one of his mistresses.[123] John Chase filled two great cupboards at Whitehall with medicaments and perfumes; when they overflowed he brought in trunks and chests to his room there. He fabricated the hundreds of fragrant silk bags needed yearly for the bed and table linens of Charles and Catherine. When the king traveled, his apothecary moved, too. Chase often complained that he spent too much of his own money for the royal barbers' aromatic powders, room deodorizing, and wardrobe cleaning, estimating in 1667 that he was owed £6,000 for such expenses. From that petition, one can discern the extent of his duties, from bath preparation to provisions for healing ceremonies. He also embalmed Stuart corpses, including Charles II's aunt, Elizabeth, Queen of Bohemia, in 1661, and twenty-four years later Charles himself, for which service he charged £218. Of course, as was often the case with Stuart officeholders, Chase did not even collect his pledged salary, let alone his supplementary expenditures. He was still petitioning the government in 1688, the year he died, for back wages.[124] For whatever it was worth, he had, however, secured a court preferment for his son, James, second apothecary to James II and Apothecary to the Person in the reign of William and Mary.

Another seasoned apothecary, John Jones, made perfumes and sweet waters for the myriad inhabitants of the Stuart courts from 1661 until 1692. His career exemplifies the advantages of royal service and his tactics reveal his own assertive nature as he strove for available perquisites. Along with Dr. Waldron, he sought better palace rooms in 1671 by petition, his chosen means of furthering his ambition. Jones hoped to become Master of the Society of Apothecaries in 1673, but lost the election; he did, however, sit as a member of its Court of Assistants. In lieu of paying some fines he owed the Society, in 1676 Jones donated a portrait of Charles I to be hung in its hall. Jones wanted to establish his family's claim to court offices as the Chases had done, so in 1677 he convincingly petitioned the Lord Chamberlain that his son, William, should have the reversion of his position after his death. That same year, without paying the usual fees, Jones was awarded a medical doctorate by fiat, the first of its kind, by the Master of the Faculties at Lambeth Palace, a prerogative returned to the Archbishop of Canterbury after the Restoration. According to Jones's Lambeth application, he was an alumnus of Oriel College, Oxford, but there is no proof of his having obtained a degree from there; nonetheless, he now had a license to practice throughout England.[125]

However, Jones still wanted more respect in the medical community and more benefits from his service. He lobbied the Duke of Monmouth in 1678 to force Cambridge University to grant him an honorary M.D. The king agreed to help in the apothecary's quest and wrote a letter to the chancellor of the university extolling Jones' learning and devoted service. Despite the absence of evidence that Jones accomplished his credential objective, his colleagues at future meetings of the Apothecaries' Society referred to him as "Dr. Jones."[126] In 1681, he petitioned for the gift of a canonry at Christ Church, Oxford, for another son, John, the senior proctor at the university. Given all this initiative on Jones's part, it is no surprise that he became very wealthy. Despite his service to James II, after the Revolution of 1688 Jones loaned the Exchequer of William and Mary over £2,300. Deceased in 1693, having accumulated properties in various counties and stock in the Royal African Company, John Jones left cash bequests of over £2000 to his family and substantial monies to charity.[127]

Queen Catherine's druggist was William Rosewell, a strong defender of the apothecaries in their face-off with the College of Physicians. Rosewell had begun his career as personal attendant to Richard Neile, Archbishop of York. A fervent Royalist, "Major" Rosewell failed in 1655 to obtain the apothecary's post at St. Thomas's Hospital in London; in fact, his service to the Stuarts cost him his estate. At the Restoration, however, Rosewell not only secured his claim to the hospital post, but Charles II convincingly recommended him as Master of the Apothecaries' Society, in which Rosewell had been a freeman since 1628. Unfortunately, the queen was no better at paying her servants than was the king. Rosewell had to seek funding from the Treasury Chamber for the perfumes he had made for Catherine's private chapel.[128] Despite his financial worries with the Stuarts, Rosewell zealously represented the apothecaries' best interests for many years in their ongoing struggle with the College of Physicians. Like Jones, he obtained a Lambeth M.D.

Other unorthodox Caroline pharmaceutical commissions went to Moise Charas, Isaac Garnier, and Charles Angibaud, all French exiles who held extraordinary posts. Charas, a Huguenot driven from his homeland by Louis XIV's revocation of the Edict of Nantes, became Charles' apothecary in 1680. Charas was known as the first demonstrator of theriac, a polypharmaceutic preparation used to counter the effects of poisons. Given the prevailing fear of toxins so evident in post-Popish Plot public and private musings, Charas' specialty won him recognition in England and endenization in 1681. A fellow Huguenot, Isaac Garnier, became Charles' apothecary in 1682. Garnier, who brought four sons and a daughter with him from France, was naturalized in 1684 and went on to a long career as a prosperous London druggist. He affiliated with the Apothecaries' Society in 1692 and for many years sat in its Court of Assistants, parlaying his cachet as a royal doctor into a thriving, long-lived metropolitan business. Censors from the College of Physicians in 1724 commended his shop in Pall Mall.

In addition, Garnier reaped occupational preferments for his family; his son and grandson became apothecaries to the army. As for Charles Angibaud, endenizened like Charas in 1681, his pharmaceutical appointment commenced in 1684. He extended his usefulness to the English government under Charles II's successors, becoming Apothecary General to the Army and Military Hospitals in Ireland under William and Mary in 1689. According to the terms of that position, Angibaud was to be paid three pence a day for each wounded soldier and two pence a day for each sick soldier during their hospitalization. His bill for nearly £500 remained unpaid as late as 1711.[129]

The Stuart brothers required a number of medical personnel based in Scotland, and accordingly proved instrumental in the chartering of the Royal College of Physicians in Edinburgh. Of the nine physicians identified in the patent of Charles II creating the college in the northern kingdom, six received appointments as physicians to the monarch. One of the Scottish doctors shared by both kings was the son of the Keeper of the Great Seal for the Privy Council in Scotland under Chancellor John Hay, Earl of Tweeddale. Sir Robert Sibbald (1641–1712), born in Fifeshire of a genteel family, studied in Scotland and on the continent, obtaining an M.D. from Angers.[130] Following his graduation in 1662 he resided a while in London, where he became acquainted with English scholars to whom he was introduced by his relative, Dr. Andrew Balfour. Sibbald was a flexible traditionalist in medicine, more immersed in Scottish antiquarian history and the possibilities of establishing a Royal Society of Scotland.[131] He came to the notice of the Stuarts first as a geographer, botanist, and founding member of a medical-virtuoso club in Edinburgh, which, under the patronage of the Duke of York, became in 1681 the Royal College of Physicians of Edinburgh.[132] In 1682 he was named physician to Charles II on the recommendation of his friend, James Drummond, Duke of Perth, who persuaded the doctor to convert to Roman Catholicism.[133]

Sibbald was elected President of the Edinburgh College in 1684, and during his tenure its pharmacopoeia was compiled. He was influential in the establishment of a medical school at the University in Edinburgh, where in 1685 he became the first professor of medicine. Following the coronation of James II, who retained Sibbald in office as he did all of his brother's physicians, the learned Scot left for London and honorary Fellowship in the London College. Sibbald later wrote that he got sick while in the capital, implying that his illness contributed to his religious confusion.[134] Not surprisingly, Sibbald, long associated with James II (whom he always referred to as James VII), did not support the coming to Britain of William of Orange.

Sibbald renounced his conversion and returned to Scotland to recant openly.[135] Though many of his contemporaries doubted the sincerity of either conversion or renunciation, Sibbald proceeded with his public activities including the donation of a natural history collection to the University of Edinburgh in 1697. Sibbald worked tirelessly and, as it turned out, fruitlessly for the establishment of a Royal Society of Scotland. Though the proposed President of the Society was the Duke of Hamilton, a non-Jacobite, a majority of the proposed membership of the group in Edinburgh sat on opposition benches or sided with the Jacobites in postrevolutionary Scottish Parliaments. One of the suggested councillors of the society was the Earl of Tweeddale, keeping the Sibbald-Hay nexus intact for another generation.[136]

Personal and professional squabbles, as well as the volatile politics of the early eighteenth century, doomed Sibbald's efforts to establish a Royal Society in Scotland, and in frustration he founded the Scottish Society of Antiquaries in 1703. Energetic and productive, he published numerous pamphlets on a variety of topics ranging from natural history to histories of the Picts and of Stirling. Sibbald sustained his London friendships after his departure, as evidenced by his extensive existing correspondence on literary and historical matters. In a June 1696 missive to Sir Hans Sloane, Sibbald thanked the physician for some lapis and told him that he had tried to send Sloane some books and a catalogue of the recently deceased Balfour's memorabilia, but evidently they had gotten lost.[137]

Sibbald's previously mentioned cousin, Andrew Balfour, served as Charles's physician-in-ordinary in Scotland from 1681, and was created a baronet that same year. His medical degree was from Caen in 1661, and later that year Charles chose Balfour to chaperon young John Wilmot, Earl of Rochester, during his foreign travels.[138] Rochester's precocious carousing at Oxford called for avuncular attention; Balfour, respected for his learning, supervised the teenager's three-year Grand Tour. Balfour's sober influence was short-lived, and Rochester returned to his rakish, libertine ways for the rest of his life. Like his relative, Sibbald, Balfour maintained cordial correspondences with renowned London physicians, including Charles Scarburgh. Balfour was worried in 1691 about the condition of Lord Lauderdale, who despite the purgatives given him, still had a bellyache. Balfour and fellow Stuart appointee Dr. Alexander Stevenson, first president of the Royal College of Physicians in Edinburgh and physician to Heriot's Hospital, requested advice from Scarburgh on further treatment.[139] Balfour's *Letters Write (sic) to A Friend* were published posthumously in 1700, and deal conventionally with travels (not, evidently, in the company of Rochester) in London, Paris, and Italy.[140]

Other Scottish appointments made by Charles II and renewed by James II included Christopher Irvine, Thomas Burnet, and David Hay. Irvine, surgeon to Monck's army in Scotland, survived the Interregnum to become surgeon to the Horse Guards, a post he held until 1681. That year, the Scottish Privy Council approved his petition to practice medicine in Edinburgh, of which he was a burgess, without harassment by the new College of Physicians there. The *DNB* says that Irvine taught school before obtaining a medical degree from Edinburgh University, but as there were no medical schools in Scotland in the 1680s, Irvine probably passed an examination given by a group of doctors rather than graduating from a college after taking classes. At any rate, the Scottish Parliament ratified his approved petition in 1685. Clippingdale refers to Irvine as physician-general to Scotland and "historiographer" to Charles II and James II.[141]

Thomas Burnet, knighted by Charles II, typified the Scotsman who went to France to study medicine; he took a degree from Montpellier, still "unswerving" in its Galenic bias.[142] A founding Fellow of the College of Physicians in Edinburgh, Burnet spent much of his time writing Latin works on philosophy and science. His *Thesaurus Medicinal Practical* (London: 1683) is a dictionary intended for professionals; even the preface is in Latin. Burnet, brother of the influential historian and political adviser Bishop Gilbert Burnet, managed to bridge the reigns of all the later Stuart monarchs, serving Charles II, James II, William and Mary, and Anne. Charles II made another doctor, David Hay, a physician-in-ordinary for Scotland in 1672 and he was one of the nine doctors named in the patent creating the College of Physicians in Edinburgh.[143] The surgeon-apothecary in Scotland during the Caroline era was Hugh Brown.

King James VII of Scotland and II of England got off to a splendid start when he inherited the national crowns in 1685.[144] After the pandemonium over the exclusion crisis waned, his accession at age fifty-one had gone smoothly and he promised in his first speech as monarch to preserve the government and eschew arbitrary power. He had experience in leadership positions as Lord High Admiral and seasoning in Scotland. Despite his Catholicism, James II enjoyed strong, objective support and was able to parry the thrust of Monmouth's weakened uprising on behalf of Protestantism in the summer of 1685. In the posthumous Bill of Indictment drawn up against Monmouth, James' magistrates accused Monmouth of unlawful acts including touching for the King's Evil. James himself frequently touched large crowds of sufferers, over 4,400 in 1685 alone, but he made some alterations in the ceremony and personnel involved.[145] The Catholic king restored the Latin prayers and the Sign of the Cross, and turned to the Catholic clergy to assist him in the healing rite.

Similarly, although King James continued the appointments of the men who were in place as aulic doctors when he ascended the throne in 1685, changes were made in the royal household. Physicians were ranked numerically after 1685 and given graduated salaries; three serjeant-surgeons were reduced to one with a salary fixed at just under £370; and two apothecaries to the Person received salaries of £500 each.[146] While James made no new appointments through the Lord Chamberlain to any of the physicians' posts at court during his reign, he did, however, elevate James Pierce and James Moleyns in the surgical ranks, making way in 1687 for three new names on the medical roll: Thomas Hobbs, Thomas Fraser, and Francis Beaulieu. These three vacated their posts in December 1688 on the flight of James II from England.[147]

While retaining James Chase as one of his personal apothecaries and John Jones as a household druggist, King James raised James St. Amand and Charles Giffard into the ranks of royal apothecarial service. St. Amand, perhaps the best known pharmacist outside court circles, enjoyed royal largesse for the first time as apothecary to the Duke of York; in 1679 at the height of the Popish Plot discord he accompanied the duke to Brussels, the better to be out of sight. Active in the leadership of the Society of Apothecaries, St. Amand became Master in 1687, after James II commissioned him first apothecary. He was elected a Member of Parliament, sitting for St. Ives from 1685 to 1687, and represented Castle Baynard ward on the London Court of Aldermen until the Glorious Revolution. Despite his association with King James, St. Amand continued to flourish after 1688. As apothecary to Hans Sloane, one of the busiest doctors in the capital and an extravagant prescriber, St. Amand provided medicines for many wealthy patients. Continuing his leadership of his guild, St. Amand secured a contract for the Apothecaries' Society in 1702 to supply the fleet with medicines, personally commending the proposal to Queen Anne. He stood in vain for Parliament as a Tory in 1710 and thereafter concentrated on his business near Covent Garden. St. Amand died a wealthy man in 1728, leaving his son an annuity of £300 and ample bequests to the rest of his family.[148] Charles Giffard entered James's household staff at the same time that St. Amand became first apothecary to the king, but did not live long enough to enjoy the benefits of his position. He passed away in 1686, leaving a small estate to his wife and ten shillings to each of his brothers and sisters for the purchase of gold rings.

As heir presumptive and Duke of York, James Stuart used the services of Padua M.D. David Bruce, son of the principal of St. Leonard's College, St. Andrews, and nephew of royal doctor John Wedderbourne; his degree was incorporated at Oxford in 1660. Though he tended the duke and duchess in the early 1660s and enrolled in the Royal Society, he soon wearied of court life and retired to Edinburgh.[149] Another of James's physicians as duke was Samuel Haworth, the sort of empiric Charles II might have promoted. Calling himself a student of plague, Haworth, a Hertfordshire native, sold tinctures and tablets from his shop in London. The College of Physicians made him extra-licentiate in 1680, probably acknowledging his M.D. from the University of Paris or in response to royal pressure. Haworth wrote treatises on mineral baths and consumption. He kept his remedies for consumption confidential while denigrating traditional physicians, who, he said, only used narcotics on their patients. Though not divulging the ingredients in the remarkable elixirs he produced, he did advise his readers to avoid meat and "crude salads."[150]

According to Munk, Francis Bernard, physician to St. Bartholomew's Hospital, became a physician-in-ordinary to James II.[151] An apothecary by training, Bernard's medical degree was bestowed by the Archbishop of Canterbury in 1678 and incorporated by Cambridge University the same year. James II's 1687 charter given to the College of Physicians made Bernard a Fellow. A polyglot well-versed in literary history, Bernard accumulated a remarkable agglomeration of books at his house in Little Britain, including what was reputed to be the largest collection on physic in England. The library was sold at auction after Bernard's death in 1698; the auction catalogue lists hundreds of books in both classical and vernacular languages.[152]

The royal doctors had played a role helpful to the Stuart monarchs in the Restoration era, publicizing the king's healing powers, promoting a scientific agenda, and buttressing social and political hierarchy. One physician who proved particularly useful to James II was the faithful Robert Brady, who certified the legitimacy of the "wondrous son" born to James II and his queen, Mary of Modena, in June 1688. After years of miscarriages, stillbirths, and dead toddlers, the royal couple begot a child who lived, James Francis Edward, conjuring up to James's opponents unacceptable visions of Catholic Stuarts persisting into the foreseeable future. Even James's grown daughters by his first marriage, brought up Protestant by order of Charles II, jealously challenged the idea that the baby was really born to the queen. Princess Mary, since 1677 wife of the Dutch Stadtholder (and her first cousin), William of Orange, and Princess Anne, married in 1683 to Prince George of Denmark but living in England, were already corresponding about the dangers their "Papist" father posed to the Protestant faith even before the birth.[153] Despite the presence of sixty witnesses, including the Queen Dowager, several doctors, two midwives, the Mistresses Labadie and Wilkes, and a nurse, Pelegrine Turini, James' enemies intimated that the pregnancy had been feigned and the delivery a feat of legerdemain. Historian Edward Gregg identifies Anne as "the major perpetrator of the rumor of [the queen's] suppositious pregnancy."[154]

At a public meeting called by King James in October, Dr. Brady gave a deposition testifying to the authentic birth of the Prince of Wales.[155] He was echoed by the Countess of Sunderland and apothecary St. Amand, in attendance on the queen before and shortly after the baby's delivery. Questioned repetitiously for over a decade about the verity of the Prince's nativity, St. Amand avouched that he took a sample of the blood from the umbilicus and saw the afterbirth. He told the Privy Council on the eve of the arrival of the Prince of Orange in London that he had attended the baby every day until the King and Queen fled to France. The royal family was accompanied by William Waldegrave, a Roman Catholic physician who became a member of the exiled court and first doctor to the Prince of Wales.[156] Accoucheur Hugh Chamberlen, who had actually missed out on the birth, wrote an account intended for Sophia, Electress of Hanover, discrediting the theory that the newborn might have been surreptitiously brought into the queen's bed in a warming pan. Chamberlen pointed out that one of the midwives, Judith Wilkes, was an intractable antipapist and swore to him that the Prince was no impostor.[157]

Nevertheless, the rumors persisted, fortified in 1696 by the publication of a tract claiming to identify the baby's true mother, based on clandestine letters exchanged in 1688 by the queen's other midwife, Mrs. Labadie, and her father, and deciphered by an Oxford don. According to the pamphlet, which was dedicated to Anne's young son, the Duke of Gloucester, Mrs. Labadie must have told her father about a plot to smuggle in an infant and pass him off as a prince; her father responded that it was a hazardous undertaking, but that a successor was needed by any means.[158] As late as 1703, when James II was dead and his son was being called a pretender, St. Amand responded again to questions posed to him, this time by Queen Anne's deputies obsessed with disproving the royal birth. The apothecary boasted that he had helped the newborn child survive a large dosage of mithridate administered by Queen Mary's midwives by giving the baby a spoonful of syrup of peach blossom. He attested that six months later on his advice to Dr. Waldegrave, then the queen's physician, a drop of laudanum saved the infant's life and enabled him to suckle with a wet nurse.[159]

In the end, the birth of Prince James could not still the voices raised against his father, whose unpopular rule provoked a bipartisan group of seven statesmen to invite the king's son-in-law, William of Orange, to land an army in England. James II and his family left the country, paving the way for replacement by William III and Mary II as co-sovereigns. William and Mary ushered in an age of moderation and greater toleration; they also ushered in a cadre of new personnel at court including medical men. Supporters of James and his heirs remained active for almost sixty years after the Glorious Revolution, loyal to the repudiated king, his son, and his grandson. James II died in 1701 in exile in France, his body, minus brains, bowels, and heart, buried in the English Benedictine priory church in Paris; miracles were reported to have been performed at his sepulchre.[160] Recognized by Louis XIV as James III, "the Old Pretender" attempted an invasion of Scotland in 1708 that was stopped by James contracting measles, and participated in an open, albeit abortive, Jacobite rebellion in 1715. Charles Edward Stuart, "the Young Pretender," orchestrated the last Jacobite attempt in Britain to regain the throne for his father. After a handful of victories, "Bonnie Prince Charlie" saw his army destroyed at Culloden in 1746. During the French Revolution, vandalistic insurgents seeking lead from coffins disentombed the remains of King James II and scattered his bones in a common grave.

Notes

1. *Calendar of Treasury Books, 1660–1714*, 32 vols., (London: HMSO, 1904) 1: 195. For more on the "Merry Monarch," see Hutton, *Charles II*; Antonia Fraser, *Royal Charles* (New York: Delta, 1979); and Paul Seaward, *The Restoration, 1660–1688* (New York: St. Martin's Press, 1991).

2. Bloch mentions sermons by Archbishop of Canterbury William Sancroft, pamphlets by John Bird, and an argument in favor of the royal touch for many ailments by one of the king's surgeons, John Browne: Bloch, *Royal Touch*, 211. Robert Boyle also lauded the efficacy of touching: see Raymond Crawfurd, *The King's Evil* (Oxford: Oxford University Press, 1911).

3. John Browne quoted in Bloch, *Royal Touch*, 212. See also Richard Wiseman, *Severall Chirurgicall Treatises* (London: Flesher and Macock, 1676), a 550–page opus dedicated to Charles II that deals with, among many other things, the King's Evil, and the best contemporary account, *Charisma Basilicon* (London: Thomas Newcomb, 1684) by Browne, who enumerates 92,107 touched between 1660 and 1682.

4. A. Rupert Hall asserts that Charles "ensured the Royal Society did not cost him a penny" and did not interfere with his prerogatives. See Hall, *The Revolution in Science 1500–1750* (London: Longman, 1983), 221. Antonia Fraser is not so cynical about the king's "zealous" scientific embrace: Fraser, *Royal Charles*, 194.

5. Hall, *Revolution in Science*, 224. See also Michael Hunter, *The Royal Society and Its Fellows 1660–1700* (Chalfont St. Giles, England: British Society for the History of Science, 1982), 24.

6. Fraser, *Royal Charles*, 195.

7. Porter, *Disease, Medicine and Society in England*, 44. Medical historians use the word "empiric" to denote a person who lacks theoretical training, emphasizing practical experience or observation; contemporaries used it to mean "quack."

8. See Porter, ed., *The Popularization of Medicine 1650–1850*; and Lucinda McCray Beier, *Sufferers and Healers* (London: Routledge and Kegan Paul, 1987).

9. Archer, *Every Man His Own Doctor*. See also Roy Porter, *Health for Sale: Quackery in England 1660–1850* (Manchester: Manchester University Press, 1989). Though Charles II feared a completely self-regulating press and introduced a Licensing Act in 1662 to suppress unlicensed printing, books and pamphlets dealing with medical matters were rarely seized. I have identified nearly two hundred publishers and printers who produced medical literature during the reigns of the later Stuarts.

10. See Roger French and Andrew Wear, eds., *The Medical Revolution of the Seventeenth Century* (Cambridge: Cambridge University Press, 1989); Holmes, *Augustan England*; and Harold J. Cook, "Living in Revolutionary Times: Medical Change under William and Mary," in *Patronage and Insti-*

tutions: Science, Technology and Medicine at the European Court 1500–1750, ed. Bruce T. Morgan (Rochester, N.Y.: Boydell, 1991): 111–35.

11. For more on these disasters and their effect on public health issues, see D. R. Hainsworth and Christine Churches, *The Anglo-Dutch Naval Wars 1652–1674* (Stroud, England: Sutton, 1998) and Frank L. Fox, *A Distant Storm: The Four Days' Battle of 1666* (Rotherfield: Press of Sail Publications, 1996); for plague, see Creighton, *History of Epidemics*; Slack, *Impact of Plague*; and Gustav Milne, *The Great Fire of London* (New Barnet, England: Historical Publications, 1986).

12. In 1660 James married Anne Hyde, daughter of the Earl of Clarendon, one month before the birth of their first child, a son who died in infancy. Shortly thereafter, Anne converted to Roman Catholicism. Two daughters (out of eight births) were produced by the marriage, Mary and Anne. James converted sometime before his wife's death in 1671. In 1673 he married an Italian Roman Catholic, fifteen year-old Princess Mary Beatrice of Modena.

13. See John Hinton, *Memoires of Sir John Hinton: Physitian in Ordinary* (London: n.p., 1679); his book is actually a petition in his old age to help him meet several thousand pounds in debts.

14. Munk, *Roll* 1: 329.

15. Maurice Ashley, *Charles II* (New York: Praeger, 1971), 5.

16. Congenital syphilis would explain many of the chronic symptoms from which both Mary and Anne suffered, including watery eyes, gout, and reproductive failure. Anne Hyde broke out in sores on her face and body, so severe she avoided public appearances: see Historical Manuscripts Commission, *Manuscripts of His Grace, the Duke of Rutland* 4 vols., (London: HMSO, 1888–1905) 2: 10–11. James's salutary biographer Jock Haswell demurs from the syphilis diagnosis, as does one of Mary II's biographers, noting the robust health of several bastards: see Haswell, *James II: Soldier and Sailor* (London: Hamilton, 1972), 169; and Hester Chapman, *Mary II, Queen of England* (Westport, Conn.: Greenwood Press, 1976), 24.

17. Latham, ed., *The Shorter Pepys*, 426–27 (September 19, 1664).

18. Hutton, *Charles II*, 56, 73, 77, 119. Hutton says that Charles dismissed "Fraser" in the spring of 1659, but, if so, that marked only a temporary rift between them.

19. Latham, ed., *The Shorter Pepys*, 426–27. The diarist bluntly said that Fraizer, whom he did not much like, could help the ladies at court "slip their calves" and cure great men of "their claps."

20. Dr. Timothy Clarke (Clerke) and James Pierce, the king's surgeon, were also in attendance; Martin, "Prince Rupert and the Surgeons," 41. This James Moleyns was the grandson of the famed lithotomist (d.1639) and son of Edward (d. 1663).

21. Munk, *Roll* 1: 232, 432.

22. For more on the plot and the virulent anti-Catholicism that gave it credence, see John P. Kenyon, *The Popish Plot* (New York: Penguin, 1974). Pinpointing the precise origins of the Whigs and Tories as parties is a historical parlor game; see J. R. Jones, *The First Whigs*, rev. ed. (London: Oxford University Press, 1970); Keith G. Feiling, *A History of the Tory Party 1640–1714* (Oxford: Clarendon Press, 1924); John Miller, *Popery and Politics in England 1660–88* (Cambridge: Cambridge University Press, 1973); and Tim Harris, *Politics under the Later Stuarts: Party Conflict in a Divided Society, 1660–1715* (London: Longman, 1993).

23. *William Denton, The Burnt Child Dreads the Fire* (London: J. Magnes, 1675), 4.

24. Others, including one royal apothecary, had favored remedies for scrofula; Nicolas LeFevre advised an application of "human afterbirth and oil of grim." For LeFebvre's recipes see SL MSS 631, folios 200–223b, British Library.

25. K. Thomas, *Religion and the Decline of Magic*, 240–41; Bloch, *Royal Touch*, 216.

26. For more on the case, see John Dickinson Carr, *The Murder of Sir Edmund Godfrey* (New York: International Polygontics, 1989).

27. He could do nothing to help Queen Catherine's infertility. Though he urged her in 1663 to visit Tunbridge Wells and Bath to promote her fecundity, she suffered two subsequent miscarriages; Jack Dewhurst, *Royal Confinements*, 11.

28. For more on Wakeman's legal tribulations, see *The Tryals of George Wakeman* (London: H. Hills, 1679) and Francis S. Ronalds, "Sir William Scroggs and Sir George Wakeman," in *The Attempted Whig Revolution of 1678–1681* (Urbana: University of Illinois Press, 1937), 27–51.

29. Kenyon, *Popish Plot*, 214. Munk does not include Wakeman in his roll, but the *DNB* credits him with studying at St. Omer, Pavia, and Paris, where "he possibly graduated in medicine."

30. Harold Cook lists Bate as a First Physician, but he died long before Fraizer, also designated by Cook as First Physician; Cook, *Decline of the Old Medical Regime*, 282. Sainty and Bucholz's research does not indicate a change in Bate's or Fraizer's status; Sainty and Bucholz, *Officials of the Household*, 46.

31. Bate to Mr. Edward, SL MSS 123, f. 2b, British Library.

32. Munk, *Roll*, 1: 228; Anthony A. Wood, *Athenae Oxonienses* 5 vols., (London: Rivington, 1813–20) 3: 827–31. See George Bate, *Elenchus Motuum Nuperorum in Anglia*. Clarendon was the Duke of York's father-in-law.

33. See William Salmon, *Pharmacopoeia Bateana*, trans. by James Shipton (London: S. Smith, 1694). Evelyn narrated the recovery of one Privy Councillor beset by apoplexy in the Gallery at Whitehall: "Several famous doctors [applied] hot fire-pans and spirit of amber to his head, but nothing was found so effectual as cupping on the shoulders." De Beer, *Diary of John Evelyn*, 4: 77.

34. Latham, ed., *The Shorter Pepys*, 50 (May 24, 1660).

35. Egerton Manuscripts (Eg MSS) 2551, f. 24, British Library. The date is described as "the twelfth year of our reign," in reference to the moment when Charles II is said to have become king in the eyes of God.

36. Clippingdale, Medical Court Roll, 1: 104. LRCS.

37. "John Baber," *Notes and Queries*, 12th series, 12 (1922): 516.

38. See John Baber, *A Poem upon the Coronation* (London: R. Everingham, 1685); and *To the King, upon the Queen's Being Deliver'd of a Son* (London: Mary Thompson, 1688); *To that Most Lamentable and Most Incorrigible Scribbler Bavius* (London: "Printed for the Coffee-Houses," 1688); and *To the Poet Bavius* (London: printed for the author, 1688), attributed by Donald Wing to Aphra Behn. Another work, Robert Wild's *The Grateful Non-Conformist* (London: n.p., 1665), is dedicated to Baber.

39. *Calendar of Treasury Books*, 6: 232. Also listed are Scarburgh, Greaves, Coxe, A. Fraizer, Talbor, Dickinson, and Ferdinando Mendes.

40. Wyman, "Samuel Barrow, M.D. Physician to Charles II and Admirer of John Milton," 339; Clippingdale, Medical Court Roll, 1: 89b; for Barrow's history see Eg. MSS 2618, f. 128, British Library.

41. Whitaker is not listed in Munk (*Roll*), but he may have obtained a degree from Oxford around 1625.

42. Tobias Whitaker, *The Tree of Human Life* (London: n.p., 1638), 24. The work was enlarged and republished in 1654.

43. Clippingdale, Medical Court Roll, 1: 126, LRCS.

44. Robert Latham and William Matthews, eds., *The Diary of Samuel Pepys*, 10 vols. (Berkeley: University of California Press, 1971): 4: 132, 441.

45. Annals of the College of Physicians, vol. 4, fos. 82b, 93b, LRCP.

46. Matthews, *Royal Apothecaries*, 115.

47. Munk, 1: *Roll*, 471; Norma Perry, "Anglo-Jewry, the Law, Religious Conviction, and Self-Interest (1655–1753)," *Journal of European Studies* 14 (1984): 14–16. For more on Queen Catherine, see Gray, *The King's Wife*.

48. SL 4046, f. 132, British Library. The letter may have been written for Mendes by someone else, as the complimentary close and signature are in another, weaker hand than the body of the letter.

49. Munk, *Roll* 1: 332. Mendes' *Stadium Apollinare sive progymnasmata medica* was published in 1668. For Prujean's career, see Munk, *Roll*, 187; Prujean's Latin recipes can be found in SL MSS 2984, f.3, British Library.

50. Munk, 1: *Roll* 252; Dobson and Walker, *Barbers and Barber-Surgeons*, 125; Latham, ed., *The Shorter Pepys*, 261 (Feb. 27, 1663).

51. SL MSS 565, folios 1–20, British Library.

52. Royal College of Physicians, *Mutual Admiration: An Exhibition Catalogue*, (London: RCP, 1989), 4.

53. Scarburgh lists eleven doctors (Dickinson, Edward Browne, Brady, Short, Farrell, Witherley, Millington, Lower, Barwick, LeFevre, and himself), but omits Edmund King. The Society of Antiquaries possesses Scarburgh's manuscript, but it is reproduced in its entirety in Raymond Crawfurd, *The Last Days of Charles II* (Oxford: Clarendon Press, 1909) and recapitulated in Treue, *Doctor at Court*, 24–29. Antonia Fraser nicely sums up all differing accounts of Charles' death: Fraser, *Royal Charles*, 443–57.

54. Charles's first barber was Thomas Lisle; Young, *Annals*, 19.

55. Fraser, *Royal Charles*, 446.

56. Crawfurd and Treue diagnose Charles with chronic granular kidney inflammation, a form of Bright's Disease, the final phase ushered in by uremic convulsions. Crawfurd, *Last Days*, 19, 49; Treue, *Doctor at Court*, 25.

57. *Calendar of State Papers, Domestic Series, of the Reign of Charles II*, 28 vols., (London: Longman, Green, Longman, and Roberts, 1960–1939) 9 (1668–69): 315; Munk, 1: *Roll*, 297. Responding to criticism after 1660 that too few doctors were licensed, and again acknowledging the prerogative of bishops to license practitioners, the College granted extra-licenses, but they were little more than the right to use College buildings and attend lectures. Clark, *History of the Royal College of Physicians* 1: 316–17.

58. Clippingdale, Medical Court Roll, 1: 111, LRCS. Rattansi identifies Williams as a Helmontian. Rattansi, "Helmontian-Galenist Controversy," 11.

59. Rattansi, "Helmontian-Galenist Controversy", 22–23. According to the *DNB*, another Caroline royal physician labeled Helmontian was Thomas Shirley, grandson of the adventurer. For the refounding of the Society of Chemical Physicians, see Henry Thomas, "The Society of Chymical Physitians," in *Science, Medicine, and History* ed. E. A. Underwood (London: Oxford University Press, 1953), 56–71.

60. Munk, *Roll* 1: 394.

61. SL MSS 1586, British Library.

62. De Beer, *Diary of John Evelyn*, 4: 290.

63. Munk *Roll* 1: 448; Jesse, *Memoirs of the Court* 2: 355.

64. Munk, *Roll* 1: 394.

65. William N. Blomberg, *An Account of the Life of Edmund Dickinson*, M.D. (London: R. Montague, 1737), 63.

66. For more on this intellectual squabble between the "virtuosi" and the "wits," see Joseph M. Levine, *The Battle of the Books* (Ithaca, N.Y.: Cornell University Press, 1991); and Levine's *Dr. Woodward's Shield: History, Science, and Satire in Augustan England* (Ithaca, N.Y.: Cornell University Press, 1991).

67. Munk, *Roll* 1: 504. See, for instance, *Vomits in Fevers* (London: n.p., 1700), a twenty-four-page tract in which Chamberlen exhorts physicians to use strong medicines, especially emetics, as long as febrile symptoms persist.

68. Spencer, *History of British Midwifery*, xvi. The forceps were secreted under the floor of a closet at Woodham Mortimer Hall in Essex; found in 1813, four pairs were preserved at the Royal Society of Medicine until a World War II bomb destroyed the museum's exhibits: "Huguenot Surgeon," 70.

69. Annals of the College of Physicians, vol. 5, folios 82b-83a, LRCP. Hugh Chamberlen's brother, Paul, was a quack who invented the anodyne necklace for children's teeth and women in labor.

70. William Ramesey, *The Gentleman's Companion* (London: Rowland Reynolds, 1672), 24. For Ramesey's other publications, see *Vox stellarum* (1651); *Lux veritatus* (1652); *Astrologia Restaurata* (1653); and *De venenis or a Discourse on Poysons* (1663). Ramesey's father was a gentleman of James I's bed chamber. Ramesey himself suffered much during the Civil War, and was created M.D. at Cambridge by royal mandate in 1668; Munk, *Roll* 1: 303.

71. Clippingdale, Medical Court Roll, 1: 69, 87. The *DNB* describes Llewellyn and Denton as a sworn physicians to Charles II after the Restoration; Colladon, knighted in 1664, was physician to Queen Catherine.

72. See Peter Barwick, *Life of Dr. John Barwick* (London: J. Bettenham, 1724); Munk, *Roll* 1: 352. Barwick's letters to Hans Sloane review the efficacy of Jesuits' powder; SL MSS 4036, folios 57–61, British Library.

73. Clippingdale includes ten of the appointments found by Sainty and Bucholz among the Lord Chamberlain's warrants, but excludes Bate, Barrow, Hinton, and Whitaker, all of whom had aulic commissions, from the post-1660 list. Sainty and Bucholz (*Officials of the Royal Household*), in turn, omit Samuel Barrow, Edward Greaves, Robert Talbor, Daniel Coxe, and Ferdinando Mendes, all identified in the *Calendar of Treasury Books* 6: 232. On Clippingdale's alphabetical list are John Arnold, Baber, John Betts, Brady, Edward Browne, Thomas Burnet, Chamberlen, Clarke, Daniel Coxe, John Damascene, Richard Edward, Dickinson, C. Farrer (a misreading for Christian Harrell, whose name, Munk asserts [*Roll* 1: 452], is always misspelled), John Floyer, both Fraizers, Harrell, James Hyde, Dr. Inard, King, Martin Lister, Richard Lower, Thomas Millington, Walter Needham, Francis Prujean, Quartermaine, William Ramesey (Ramsay), Scarburgh, Thomas Shirley, Thomas Short, Theodore de Vaux, Wakeman, Waldron, Edward Warner (physician to the Regiment of Guards), Thomas Willis, John Windebank, and Witherley. Some doctors, like Gideon Harvey, claimed to be Caroline appointees; Harvey calls himself "physician-in-ordinary to His Majesty" on the frontispiece of his anti-College of Physicians book, *The Conclave of Physicians*.

74. Quoted in Munk, *Roll* 1: 372. See Browne's *Journal of a Visit to Paris 1664* (London: John Murray, 1923), written when Browne was twenty-two, which recounts his encounters at an impressionable age with great figures in medicine.

75. Moore, *History of the Study of Medicine*, 73.

76. SL MSS 1895, British Library. In this "Medical Daybook," Browne not only includes recipes and methods for making ingredients like edible pearl and coral, but lists the twenty-four physicians and surgeons with whom he conferred in 1673.

77. Lady Murray quoted in Craig, *History of the Royal College of Physicians of Edinburgh*, 53; Clippingdale, Medical Court Roll, 1: 94, 101, LRCS.

78. SL MSS 123, f. 13, British Library.

79. 6194 MSS, f. 240, British Library.

80. Daniel Coxe, *Discourses (about) Physick and Physicians* (London: n.p., 1669), 13; Jonathan Goddard, *A Discourse Setting Forth the Unhappy Condition of the Practice of Physick in London* (London: John Martyn, 1670), 19. See also Frank H. Ellis, "The Background of the London Dispensary," *Journal of the History of Medicine* 20 (1965): 197–212.

81. Kenneth Dewhurst, ed., *Thomas Willis's Oxford Lectures* (Oxford: Sandford Publications, 1980).

82. Garrison, *Introduction to the History of Medicine*, 262; Munk, *Roll* 1: 338. See also Add. MSS 4224, folios 112–127, British Library, for a short, contemporary paean of praise to Willis on his death in 1675, and Hansruedi Isler, *Thomas Willis, 1621–1675: Doctor and Scientist* (New York: Hafner, 1968).

83. See Thomas Willis, *The Remaining Medical Works*, trans. S. Pordage (London: T. Dring, 1681).

84. Quoted in Munk, *Roll* 1: 379. Moreover, by denying that catarrhal defluxions came from the brain, Lower further undercut the humoral theory: see *De catarrhis*, trans. Richard Hunter and Ida Macalpine (London: Dawsons, 1963).

85. Richard Lower, *Dr. Lower's Receipts* (London: John Nutt, 1700).

86. Annals of the College of Physicians, vol. 5, folios 80a-81a, 126a, LRCP; Cook, *Decline of the Old Medical Regime*, 208–9.

87. Morison's *curriculum vitae*, probably compiled by Dr. Archibald Pitcairne, can be found in SL MSS 3198, folios 17–29, British Library. Pitcairne was a widely respected Scottish physician, formerly Professor of Medicine at Leiden, and the arch-enemy of Sir Robert Sibbald.

88. S. H. Vines and G. Claridge Druce, *An Account of the Morisonian Herbarium* (Oxford:

Clarendon Press, 1914), lii. The authors assert that Morison's work did not meet with general approval or achieve scholarly acceptance.

89. Ibid., xxiv. According to the authors, Morison's Scottish burr was unintelligible to a visiting Moroccan ambassador.

90. Annals of the College of Physicians, vol. 4, f. 108a, LRCP.

91. Matthews, *Royal Apothecaries*, 114.

92. Clippingdale names "Joshua LeFebvre" as Charles's apothecary, but this College of Physicians member (licentiate in 1684, Fellow by James II's charter in 1687) was Nicolas's son. He attended Charles II in his last illness. Munk, *Roll* 1: 454.

93. Rattansi, "The Helmontian-Galenist Controversy," 11 n. Daniel Foote of Cambridge, who owned some of the Sloane Manuscripts, prepared an index to the text: SL 631, folios 200–23b, British Library.

94. Matthews, *Royal Apothecaries*, 112.

95. LeFevre, *Discourse upon Sir Walter Rawleigh's Great Cordial*, passim. LeFevre advised that the cordial should be used as a base in many different beverages.

96. An anonymous Frenchman, quoted in "Tabor's (or Talbor's) Cure of the Ague," *Journal of the Royal College of Physicians of London* 21/1 (1987): 66.

97. Rudolph E. Siegel and F.N.L. Poynter, "Robert Talbor, Charles II, and Cinchona," *Medical History* 6 (1962): 83. The annuity was granted by a patent issued under the Privy Seal in August 1678. Sainty and Bucholz do not list Talbor's appointment.

98. Reports of the amount of the subsidy vary: Jaime Jaramillo- Arango puts it at £2,000: see "A Critical Review of the Basic Facts in the History of Cinchona," *Journal of the Linnaeus Society* 53/351 (March 1949): 301. One writer (unfortunately uncredited) has suggested that Talbor may have been involved in political activity on Charles's behalf at the French court: "Tabor's (or Talbor's) Cure," 66. See also Laurence Brockliss, "The Literary Image of the *Médecins du Roi* in the Literature of the Grand Siècle," in *Medicine at the Courts of Europe 1500–1838*, ed. Vivian Nutton (London: Routledge, 1990), 130–32.

99. Talbor, in Nicolas de Blegny, *The English Remedy or Talbor's Wonderful Secret* (London: J. Wallis, 1682). The subtitle states that "the secret was sold by the author to the Most Christian King, and since his death ordered by His Majesty to be published in French for the benefit of his subjects." Of course, Talbor had published *Pyretologia*, touting Jesuits' bark, a decade earlier!

100. De Beer, *Diary of John Evelyn*, 4: 325, 333. He related that "the cortex [was] mingled with a little chalk, which qualified the ebullition." Not everyone recognized the efficacy of Jesuits' bark; Gideon Harvey denied that "chinchina" powder cured anything: Harvey, *Conclave*, 141.

101. Matthews, "Italian Charlatans," 2; Maple, *Magic, Medicine and Quackery*, 114.

102. Matthews, *Royal Apothecaries*, 137–38; C.J.S. Thompson, in his *Quacks of Old London*, calls Tilborg a Stuart medical phony. Despite Tilborg's ignominy, William III renewed his license.

103. Archer, *Every Man His Own Doctor*, 137. Appropriate foods for those with dry, hot bodies included turkey, goose liver, and salmon; he suggested figs for women right before their terms and for everyone he advised river water over rain water (too thin) or well water (too thick).

104. Mercury was also used as a vomitory for fever in a preparation called "mercury of life," consisting of mercury sublimate and antimony: de Beer, *Diary of John Evelyn*, 3: 220.

105. John Archer, *Secrets Disclosed of Consumptions* (London: The Author, 1684), 3.

106. Clippingdale, Medical Court Roll, 1: 118, LRCS.

107. Young, *Annals*, 215.

108. Munk, *Roll* 1: 388. A grateful John Knight bestowed a number of heraldic manuscripts on the college.

109. SL MSS 206a, f. 21, British Library. Evelyn mentions this use for millipedes: de Beer, *Diary of John Evelyn* 4: 290.

110. See E. M. Calvert and R.T.C. Calvert, *Serjeant Surgeon John Knight* (London: Heinemann, 1939).

111. Garrison, *Introduction to the History of Medicine*, 276. See also L. M. Zimmerman and I. Veith, *Great Ideas in the History of Surgery* (Baltimore: William and Wilkins, 1961).

112. Quoted in Louis Bakay, "Richard Wiseman, a Royalist Surgeon of the English Civil War," *Surgical Neurology* 27 (1987): 415.

113. T. Longmore, *Richard Wiseman* (London: Longmans, Green and Co., 1891), 95–96. Pyle and Painter probably felt Wiseman breathing down their necks. During the Civil War Wiseman assisted Pyle in service to the Prince of Wales while on the Isle of Jersey, and in 1665 Wiseman garnered an extraordinary serjeant- surgeoncy, waiting in the wings for his elders to retire. Power, "Serjeant Surgeons of England," 83–84.

114. See P. W., *Elegy for Richard Wiseman* (London: n.p., 1676), an apprentice's lament. The union of the Barber-Surgeons started to unravel and in 1684 Charles II was petitioned by the surgeons to set them free from their ignorant colleagues; nothing was done, however, and the confederation persisted until 1745.

115. Latham, ed., *The Shorter Pepys*, 735; Young, *Annals*, 372.

116. Add. MSS 38854, f. 73, British Library; Clippingdale, Medical Court Roll, 1: 119, LRCS.

117. Latham, ed., *The Shorter Pepys*, 386, 932.

118. The verdict of James St. Amand, repeated in Matthews, *Royal Apothecaries*, 121.

119. John Browne, *Preternatural Tumours* (London: R. S., 1678), 76, 120, 379.

120. John Browne, *Adenochoiradelogia: Treatise on the King's Evil* (London: T. Newcombe, 1684), 188. Part three of this tripartitie treatise is *Adenographia,* on the royal gift of healing.

121. For the controversy surrounding Browne, see K. F. Russell, "John Browne, 1642–1702," *Bulletin of the History of Medicine* 33/5 (1959): 393–414, 503–22. Browne remained active in the Barber-Surgeons' Company throughout his career. See Young, *Annals*, 4, 95, 406, 429, 497.

122. Thomas R. Forbes, "The Case of the Casual Chirurgeon," *Yale Journal of Biology and Medicine* 51 (1978): 583–88. Forbes concludes that Browne was guilty of malpractice, though the record of the outcome of the case is lost. Besides the royal surgeons already identified, Clippingdale classifies these men as Caroline surgeons: Laurence Arbillear (a French surgeon from Besançon), Michael Andrews (until his death in 1661), Alexander Beucher (granted surgeon-in-ordinary board wages for 1663, "not withstanding the suspension"), Florent Fourcade (referred to 1672 and 1675 as surgeon-in-ordinary), Charles Peter, John Troutbeck (principal surgeon-in-ordinary in 1666), Charles Turland (bone setter-in-ordinary in 1664), and John Watson (granted his petition to be surgeon-in-ordinary in 1660): Clippingdale, Medical Court Roll, 1: 36, 112, 116b, 118, 126, LRCS.

123. In her 1665 petition, Anne asked for reversion of office of controller of customs in Devonshire for herself and her two sisters, but no record of the grant has been found: Matthews, *Royal Apothecaries*, 103.

124. Ibid., 104–6. Matthews notes that in 1669, to compensate Chase somewhat for his losses, he was granted two-thirds of the prize goods (to the value of £1,500) that he had discovered to have been embezzled at Plymouth.

125. Ibid., 115–16. Another example of a Lambeth doctor is the charlatan Thomas Saffold, originally a weaver, who sold nostrums from his shop near Blackfriars, taught astrology, and kept a boarding-house for his patients. In 1688 Saffold personally reported "eight treasonable and seditious libolls" against James II to the Secretary of State at Windsor: Add. MSS 41805, f. 38, British Library.

126. Matthews, *Royal Apothecaries*, 116. Jones is similarly referred to in *Calendar of Treasury Papers, 1556–1728*, 6 vols., (London: Longmans, Green, Reader, and Dyer, 1868–89) 1 (1556–1696): 134, 203.

127. Matthews, *Royal Apothecaries*, 141–42.

128. Ibid., 107.

129. Ibid., 102–3, 129.

130. William Munk incorrectly gives Leiden as Sibbald's medical alma mater, but later historians have found that Sibbald and other aspiring physicians matriculated at Angers, which had lower fees and academic standards. Munk, *Roll* 1: 439; E. A. Underwood, *Boerhaave's Men at Leyden and After* (Edinburgh: Edinburgh University Press, 1977), 89–90; and Charles D. O'Malley, ed., *History of Medical Education* (Los Angeles: University of California Press, 1970).

131. See Roger L. Emerson, "Sir Robert Sibbald, Kt., the Royal Society of Scotland, and the Origins of the Scottish Enlightenment," *Annals of Science* 45 (1988): 41–72.

132. Craig, *History of the Royal College of Physicians of Edinburgh*, 139–42. Sibbald founded the Edinburgh Botanical Garden with Balfour in 1670. Balfour also helped in the formation of the Royal College of Physicians of Edinburgh: Clippingdale, Medical Court Roll, 1: 124, LRCS.

133. See *The Memoirs of Robert Sibbald*, ed. Francis Paget Hett (London: H. Milford, 1832), a history of the Royal College of Physicians in Edinburgh, begun but not finished by its president.

134. See *Autobiography of Sir Robert Sibbald* (Edinburgh: n.p., 1833).

135. Curiously, Roger Emerson omits any reference to Sibbald's religious swings in his meticulous account of the doctor's role among the virtuosi of the Scottish Enlightenment.

136. Emerson, "Sir Robert Sibbald," appendix III, 70. Emerson notes that Sibbald's professional rival, Archibald Pitcairne, was pointedly omitted from the proposed membership.

137. SL MSS 4036, f. 237, British Library.

138. Clippingdale, Medical Roll Call, 1: 124, LRCS.

139. SL MSS 4077, f. 15, British Library. Clippingdale erroneously calls Stevenson "Archibald," and credits him with being Charles's first physician in Scotland in 1681. Clippingdale, Medical Court Roll, 1: 124, LRCS.

140. Andrew Balfour, *Letters Write (sic) to a Friend* (Edinburgh: n.p., 1700), passim. He recommended seeing Covent Garden while in London, and travelling to Italy in the autumn. Balfour also praised the work of Charles II's botanist, Robert Morison, whose gardens in London and Blois Balfour admired.

141. Clippingdale, Medical Court Roll, 1: 124, LRCS.

142. See John Durkan, "The French Connection in the Sixteenth and Early Seventeenth Centuries," in *Scotland and Europe, 1200–1850*, ed. T. C. Smout (Edinburgh: John Donald, 1984). Burnet's son, also Thomas, got his M.D. from Leiden.

143. Clippingdale, Medical Court Roll, 1: 124, LRCS.

144. James II is enjoying a renaissance of sorts as revisionists appreciate his gifts and bemoan the Whig interpretation of history. See this progression from the unsympathetic to the enthusiastic in F. C. Turner, *James II* (London: Eyre and Spottiswoode, 1948); Maurice Ashley, *James II* (Minneapolis: University of Minnesota Press, 1977); John Miller, *James II* (Hove, England: Wayland, 1978); J. R. Jones, *The Revolution of 1688 in England* (New York: Norton, 1973); and Michael Mullett, *James II and the English Revolution* (New York: Routledge, 1994).

145. James in exile after the Glorious Revolution continued to touch in France and Italy, and belief in the healing ritual was cultivated by Jacobites in England: Bloch, *Royal Touch*, 221.

146. Sainty and Bucholz, *Officials of the Household*, 45–49.

147. Hobbs is the only one of the three listed in Young's *Annals*, as Master of the Company in 1687 and a licentiate of the College of Physicians in 1684. It is likely that he came from a long line of surgeons. Young, *Annals*, 10, 18; Munk, *Roll* 1: 433. For their withdrawals from office, see Sainty and Bucholz, *Officials of the Household*, 122, 107, and 71 respectively.

148. Matthews, *Royal Apothecaries*, 118, 121.

149. Munk, *Roll* 1: 297.

150. Samuel Haworth, *Method of Curing Consumptions* (London: Samuel Smith, 1683), 14.

151. Munk, *Roll* 1: 449.

152. *Catalogue of the Library of Dr. Francis Bernard* (London: n. p., 1698).

153. See Benjamin Bathurst, ed., *Letters of Two Queens* (London: R. Holden, 1925). James acknowledged four bastard children by his mistress Arabella Churchill and one by Catharine Sedley.

154. Edward Gregg, *Queen Anne* (London: Routledge and Kegan Paul, 1980), 53; J. Dewhurst, *Royal Confinements*, 21. The delighted father paid the midwives 500 guineas each for his son's safe delivery, but his royal generosity only added grist to the scandalmongers' mills, as did the news that the Pope had consented to be one of the prince's godfathers: Ashley, *James II*, 228–29.

155. Munk, *Roll* 1: 418. Brady became a Fellow of the College of Physicians in 1680.

156. Munk, *Roll* 1: 335. Waldegrave had encouraged Mary to visit Bath spa in 1687, for which she was grateful. King James and his queen produced another child, Princess Louisa Mary, born in June 1692 and died of smallpox in August 1712.

157. SL MSS 4107, f. 150, British Library. W. F. Bynum calls Mrs. Wilkes a Roman Catholic,

but he derives his information from an unscholarly secondary source: W. F. Bynum, "Medicine at the English Court, 1688–1837," in *Medicine at the Courts of Europe*, 265, 285. During the five labors that Mary of Modena endured before Prince James was born, Elizabeth Cellier, a celebrated midwife, tended to her and suggested that the queen take therapeutic baths. In June 1687 Mrs. Cellier proposed a midwives' college, a proposal King James reviewed with sympathy: Antonia Fraser, *The Weaker Vessel* (New York: Vintage, 1985), 454–62.

158. William Fuller, *A Brief Discovery of the True Mother of the Pretended Prince of Wales* (London: n. p., 1696). Fuller said the real mother was Mary Grey and that Dr. Wallis, a Professor of Geometry at Oxford, decoded the letters.

159. Matthews, *Royal Apothecaries*, 119–20. It was Waldegrave, however, who was knighted for his service to the crown.

160. Besides Waldegrave, James's doctor in France was Guy Fagon, first physician to Louis XIV; Clippingdale, Medical Court Roll, 1: 131, LRCS.

Chapter 7

The "Glorious Revolution" and the Medical Household of the Dual Monarchs (1688–1702)

In a virtually bloodless coup in November 1688, William of Orange, the foremost Protestant in Europe, seized the English throne for himself and his wife from James II, his uncle and father-in-law. Opponents of the increasingly autocratic Catholic king found in the Dutch prince the consummate alternative, while William procured the men and material needed to reinforce his extended military campaign against France and at the same time prevented a possible Anglo-French alliance. It was a perfect match. Moreover, William himself, Stadtholder of the United Provinces, had Stuart blood in his veins, his mother being the sister of Charles II and James II; William's wife had an even stronger claim as the elder daughter of the king, but by continental standards the entitlements of females meant little. Together, the royal pair was an irresistible force, crafting for the nation a "Glorious Revolution," as the calibration in government came to be called by its advocates. In return for control of the army and navy, the Dutch prince reluctantly accepted a Declaration of Rights, a keystone of the constitutional resolution and a vindication of the rule of law protecting citizens from arbitrary actions by the state. The Declaration also fixed the succession on Mary's children, if any, next on her sister Anne and Anne's heirs, and lastly on any children William might have by a later marriage. The Prince of Orange's acceptance of these arrangements made possible the coronation of the Dual Monarchs, William III and Mary II.[1]

The Revolution of 1688 maintained several traditions in Britain and altered others, as King William reformed his government and found new sources of funding for his wars, which included a belated showdown between his forces and those of James II in Ireland. In general the medical establishment welcomed the innovative sovereigns, but William's reforms soon affected its professional traditions. The consequence of the military in British life directly altered the dynamics among doctors, surgeons, and apothecaries. The Royal College of Physicians was diplomatically silent upon the arrival of William and Mary, probably because the institution had received a new and favorable charter from James II in 1687, supportive of the regulatory activities of the College. Giving the Fellows more authority over surgeons and apothecaries than their previous constitutional document had given them, the new charter enabled a doubling of the membership in the College from forty to eighty and a significant increase in its number of licentiates and honorary Fellows.[2] However, since the Revolution of 1688 bestowed more domestic authority on Parliament while William was assigned international responsibilities, the legislature controlled the fate of institutions like the College of Physicians. Rival medical corporations like the Society of Apothecaries could appeal directly to Parliament for new legal privileges, bypassing the crown altogether. As long as Parliament provided the king with sufficient funds for war, he conceded to it the details of national politics including medical management.

At the same time, William and Mary's reign ushered in medical metamorphoses in institutions and personnel, in no small part because of the regime's emphasis on revamped military medicine.[3] To fulfill the medical needs of an active army and navy, the king at first turned to the College of Physicians, which promised to help select medicines and even paid for some drugs while William's forces were in Ireland during 1690 and 1691. William had no experience with such a body, as there was no comparable institution in the Netherlands, but if the Fellows could assist him in creating a better medical service for the army and navy, he could tolerate their corporate authority. Before long, however, rancor developed between the Fellows and the Lords of the Admiralty over who should choose doctors to tend the sick and wounded. Their quarrel extended to medical supply questions as the armed forces contacted suppliers themselves rather than wasting time with an intermediary like the College or burdening an expedition with complex College-recommended medicines that were of no use when simple and efficient cures were called for. By the mid 1690s, the Society of Apothecaries and the Barber Surgeons' Company were contributing the medicines and tools for surgeons' chests and for military hospitals. Inadvertently, the military establishment had "further legitimized an increasingly respectable medical empiricism," while King William himself favored experimental trials of new medicines for the sick and wounded, some bordering on quackery, if they brought about recovery.[4] He did not care about ineffective physicians who claimed to be superior on the basis of hypothetical learning alone, but only about those trained practitioners, often battle-tested surgeons, who could deliver immediate cures for wounds and diseases.

The two monarchs kept courts in the Netherlands, Scotland, and in England, where they maintained two official households, each with a medical staff. Initially naming four king's physicians, two queen's doctors, and a household physician, the efficient William eliminated the household position in 1690 during a reduction in the royal staff. Though he employed many doctors, surgeons, and apothecaries, some out of political gratitude, William's medical corps was never as large as that of Charles II. Clearly, William of Orange had as pragmatic a view of medicine as he did of politics. Accordingly, he eschewed magic and miracles, and so as king, William refused to touch for the King's Evil. Educated in the tenets of Calvinism, he saw only superstition in the healing rite, not a role for himself as the first physician of the nation. His deferential Stuart queen, Anglican by upbringing and conscious of the popularity of touching when performed by her uncle and father, did not perform the ceremony either. In abandoning the royal ritual, which may have seemed ludicrous to the practical Dutchman, the new monarchs doubtless contributed to a lessened sense of awe and allegiance on the part of their subjects, a topic of much discussion after the revolution.[5] Besides his failure to recognize the potency of the people's belief in sacred royal powers, William may have been directed away from touching contagious, scrofulous subjects by his own fragile health.

The Prince of Orange had been a sickly child, beset with asthma that left him gaunt, hollow-chested, and prone to debilitating coughs. His father had succumbed to smallpox before he was born, but the death of his mother from the same disease ten years later so physically and emotionally devastated the boy that his guardians feared for his life. Even after his recovery, he required a harness to support his back. The prince's frailty was exacerbated by the demands of his office, requiring travel for diplomatic and military purposes even while he was still an adolescent.[6] At seventeen, William had such a badly infected and swollen throat that some thought he would die, but the real threat came in 1675 when he himself contracted smallpox, hovering between life and death for a fortnight. As an adult William was described by Bishop Gilbert Burnet, who knew him well, as "always asthmatical [with] a constant dry cough, his body thin and weak," with the look of a hunchback.[7]

His health deteriorated after his arrival in England. The polluted London air exacerbated William's respiratory condition, the city smog penetrating into his weak lungs and blackened rain chilling him to the bone. He coughed constantly, bringing up great quantities of phlegm, and collapsing, exhausted with the effort. As soon as Mary came to England, the two repaired to Hampton Court, which needed significant restoration, and though some courtiers complained that living there distanced the king from the capital, William knew it benefited his health. The king and queen purchased Kensington House a few months later, hiring Christopher Wren to supervise the reconstruction of the Jacobean house and grounds. Hoping to emulate the tranquility of the formal Dutch gardens beloved by the royal couple, William and Mary both spent considerable time on flora and fountains. However, the sovereigns' attempt to improve the uncongenial environment of their new kingdom did not rid William of his maladies. In early 1690 another serious bout of bronchitis and fever depressed the king as he prepared to battle the Jacobite forces in Ireland. After the Irish war, as he returned to England, William was involved in a coach accident, wrenching his shoulder. Though usually healthy enough on his continental campaigns, the king endured colds and headaches in the summer of 1694, and back in England for the winter he caught a chill, taking quinine, apples, and milk for his ailment. By 1700 he was, at the age of forty-nine, a careworn old man, plagued by colds, constipation, and swollen legs. Even sojourns at his cherished palace at Het Loo near the Zuider Zee and the wholesome air of Holland no longer offered any respite from his many aches and pains.

As for Mary, poor eyesight was a perennial problem, but far more lamentable was her inability to produce a child, a torment compounded by her awareness of William's extramarital affairs. She miscarried twice early in her marriage, the first time when she was seventeen, despite the presence of an illustrious continental doctor, Jacob Senaer, and thereafter she complained of rheumatism and chills. She had a serious bout of fever in 1680, probably malarial, and even after her return to England in 1689 she suffered from nervous depression, insomnia, fatigue, agonizing headaches, and other undiagnosed ailments, frequently dosing herself or submitting to phlebotomy as a remedy for her pains.[8] After a dozen years in Holland, she described herself as a "perfect stranger in my own country." No doubt her illnesses after the Glorious Revolution were partially provoked by the tribulation of seeing her husband and father at war with one another. In anguish over the prospect of William and James in personal combat with one another, Mary wrote to the Electress Sophia, her Hanoverian cousin, that "I have every reason to be in distress for a husband, but I am a daughter as well, and I do not know what wishes I ought to make for a father." Mary became bitterly estranged from her sister Anne, the heiress presumptive, over Anne's household revenues, and she came to "look on this disagreement as punishment on us for the irregularity by us committed on the revolution."[9] By 1694, at thirty-two, the queen was worn out from the rigors of her responsibilities, submitting to a regimen of asses' milk, the fashionable tonic of the day for weak constitutions, recommended by her physician, James Welwood. Welwood knew of the salubrious effects of asses' milk from various manuals, like the *Pharmacopoeia Londinensis*. Under *assinus* is recorded:

> The milk is alexipharmick [a poison antidote, which] nourishes and cleanses; it helps in consumptions, diseases of the stomach and lungs, impostumes and exulcations of the reins [kidneys], stone in the bladder and gout; it loosens the belly, provokes urine and the terms. Outwardly it is costinetick [cosmetic], softens the gums, and eases arthritic pains; give inwardly from half a pint to a pint.[10]

Naturally, any change in regime produces some fluctuation in personnel, none more than change by revolution, and a revolution involving foreign participants at that. Charles Scarburgh and Thomas Witherley, both loyal to the previous administration, lost their posts as royal physicians, although Scarburgh petitioned successfully to keep the lodgings assigned to him by Charles II in Scotland Yard for life; the new government also dismissed Edmund Dickinson, so he gave up the practice of medicine entirely.[11] New medical men accompanied William up the steps of power, including many who received aulic appointments. At the same time, William and Mary were sufficiently canny to include in their households some veteran members of the London medical establishment and suitable holdovers from earlier reigns, confirming the sovereigns' hope for peace within the medical profession. By supporting the men they did, however, the co-sovereigns demonstrated that they favored the resourceful healer over the paternalistic consultant. In their choice of royal doctors, the king and queen emphasized commercial and clinical medicine rather than the scholarly management of the College of Physicians.[12]

A Scotsman, John Hutton, became the principal physician to William and Mary in February 1689 by virtue of his loyalty to the House of Orange. Though from a lowly background as a herd-boy to a minister in Dumfriesshire, Hutton had the good fortune to receive an education, including medical studies at Padua, financed by his employer. He practiced for a while among the important English-speaking community in Holland, where he caught the attention of the future queen of England when he ministered to injuries she incurred falling from her horse. Hutton subsequently treated Mary's diminishing vision, though with little success. He rose to become Physician-General to William's forces in the Netherlands and was also involved in the prince's spy network before 1688.

Hutton developed the codes and ciphers used in the planned invasion of England. William's key agent in London, James Johnston, provided The Hague with intelligence and assessments of the political situation in the form of ordinary letters. Missives resembling routine business correspondence were in fact messages that revealed secret information when soaked in a solution prepared by Dr. Hutton.[13] Given Hutton's remarkable role in the revolution of 1688, it is not surprising that William installed Hutton in a special apartment in Whitehall in preparation for Mary's arrival from Holland. Hutton then went with William to Ireland and was present at the Battle of the Boyne, where William was slightly wounded in the leg, and at the siege of Limerick. He traveled to Flanders when the king made a visit there in 1691 and was a leader in the formation of a commission to inspect all drugs and medicines supplied to the British army and its hospitals. Dr. Hutton spearheaded the effort to improve the military medical system in William's domains.

Hutton's medical degree (not conferred until 1690) was from Padua, but he soon accumulated the requisite national credentials, becoming a Fellow of the Royal College of Physicians in 1690 and of the Royal Society in 1697. Like other continentally trained doctors, Hutton had his degree incorporated at an English university, in his case Oxford, in 1695. Besides giving his medical expertise to the reform-minded administration, he advised the king's council on German affairs. Given his long association with the king and varied positions of responsibility, Hutton was the most influential medical adviser of the Williamite regime. After the king's death, he returned to Scotland, but served as a Member of Parliament for Dumfries in 1710, and he seems to have preferred political writing to medical or scientific activities. However, Hutton's assiduous fidelity to William did not mean prompt payment from the crown for services rendered. As late as September 1717, five years after his death, Hutton's heirs were still trying to collect £950 in back salary.[14]

Another physician who accompanied the Stadtholder to England in 1688 was Pierre Silvestre (Peter Silvester), a Huguenot with an M.D. from Montpellier, whose career in France had been ruined by Louis XIV's revocation of the Edict of Nantes. Silvestre escaped to Amsterdam, attracted the attention of Prince William, and became his physician in Holland. Like Hutton, he was with William at the Boyne. Described in the College of Physicians' Annals as a French Protestant "refugee from Orange," Silvestre was admitted as a licentiate in 1693. The College returned half his of fees when he pleaded poverty, though Richard Blackmore, a royal doctor himself four years later, opposed the reimbursement. At no time did the Fellows, those for him or those against him, assert that Silvestre was a royal doctor, a usual accolade upon introduction to the College.[15] Silvestre soon developed a large London practice and joined the Royal Society. Serving as both physician and adviser on the arts, Silvestre accepted the patronage of Ralph, Duke of Montagu, Caroline ambassador to France and master of the wardrobe under William. Silvestre's eclectic interests and erudition brought him admission to the most brilliant circles. After William's death, the naturalized physician still served on numerous boards and commissions, such as those for the naval sick and aged and, appropriately, "poor French proselytes."[16] He died in 1718.

Among the Stuart medical holdovers employed by William and Mary was Charles Fraizer, son of Alexander Fraizer and himself the doctor of Charles II and James II from 1677. Fraizer had all the right connections to the prerevolutionary professional establishment, including education at Westminster School and Trinity College, Cambridge. His M.D. from Cambridge was obtained by royal mandate in 1678 and he joined the College of Physicians in 1684. Though his father was a resolute Royalist and ally of the Stuart kings, Alexander Fraizer demonstrated his allegiance to the Dual Monarchs by going with William on his early military maneuvers in Ireland. William therefore confirmed Fraizer in royal employment as second physician. Fraizer stayed at his post until he fell ill in late 1697; his sister picked up his pay, £300, because he was indisposed. He expired early the following year.[17]

Not much has been recorded about Dr. William Stokeham. His warrant as Physician to the Person is dated July 2, 1689, making him the third appointee of the Dual Monarchs.[18] Born in Nottinghamshire, he obtained his arts degrees at Queen's College, Cambridge, but relocated to Padua for an M.D. in 1671. An honorary Fellow of the College of Physicians in 1680, he attained full Fellowship status in 1687 and participated fully in the College's struggle against empirics. Stokeham appears to have headed a committee that petitioned Parliament in 1690 for permission to sue unlicensed frauds in order to reassert the Fellows' authority. He did not, however, support the establishment of a Physicians' Dispensary, a major issue for the College, and he played a key role among the group of Fellows who opposed what they perceived as authoritarian actions by the institution's leadership. In 1697 Stokeham and others beseeched the official "visitors" of the College to investigate by-laws violations committed by the Dispensarians, but confusion over the visitors' legal control blunted the inquiry.[19] Stokeham quit his post as a royal doctor in 1693, and was replaced by Walter Harris. Historian Harold Cook speculates that politics may have motivated Stokeham's resignation, since the timing of his departure coincided with the Tories losing control of William and Mary's Council; Stokeham's inflexible Anglicanism may also have been a factor.[20] William Stokeham died in 1698, his medical eminence acknowledged in a magnificent funeral.

Christian Harrell was the Dutch-born son of Adam Harel, apothecary from the University of Vienna and in service to Charles II in 1654 at Aix-la-Chapelle. The younger Harrell, who had a doctorate from Leiden, went on to serve the household of Charles II from 1670 as "operator" and then "professor in chemistry," for which he was to receive £150 plus an additional £40 as apothecary; other emoluments included bouche and an allowance for laboratory fuel. Harrell, too, often went unpaid, and by 1677 more than £1,100 was due to him. Eight years later he obtained a certificate acknowledging that at the time of Charles II's death the tab had risen to more than £2,600, including a bill of £109 for acting as royal mistress Nell Gwyn's doctor during her last illness. Harrell even had to borrow £800 from the royal treasury in 1685 to pay for his lodgings near St. James' palace. Harrell was paid £1,918 by the Exchequer later that year, an amount that did not cover everything due him in arrears.[21]

Undaunted, Harrell, who was married to the daughter of the Dutch court physician, accepted appointments as fourth physician-in-ordinary to William and Mary in May 1689 and as queen's apothecary, also in 1689. Although he was an honorary Fellow of the Royal College of Physicians after 1687 and a prominent participant in its conflict with the Apothecaries' Society over the establishment of a philanthropic dispensary run by doctors, no evidence of Harrell's medical degree exists. He wrote of Mary's fatal battle with smallpox in late December 1694, describing the frighteningly rapid and inexorable worsening of her condition. At first, feeling slightly out of sorts, she dosed herself with Venice treacle, a powerful diaphoretic often recommended for fever by London society doctor Richard Lower. On December 21, however, when she developed a severe headache and nausea, and became flushed "like St. Anthony's fire," her physicians were called in. They administered carduus possets, blistered her shoulders, and bled her vigorously. After three days, the doctors acknowledged that she had smallpox, the disease that had killed William's father and mother. Since he himself had survived a bout of smallpox, the king could help nurse his wife. As variolous pustules and livid petechiae covered her body, her physicians bled her again and applied plasters to her feet. Unable to sleep but resigned to her fate, she passed away three days after Christmas.[22] Mary's death had great import, not only for William, who was shattered by her passing, but for the nation as well. Since Mary had died childless, her sister Anne or Anne's offspring would one day rule Britain. Dr. Harrell's final task for Mary was as her embalmer. He charged and received £200 for creating a perfumed lining for the queen's coffin, washing the body in scent, and stuffing it with spices.[23] After Mary's death, Harrell became nonessential at court, but in 1702 King William awarded Harrell a pension of £200 per year.

Neither John Radcliffe's treatment of James II's nosebleeds nor his outspoken disapproval of the 1688 coup undermined his professional endorsement by the new king and queen. Born in Yorkshire and educated at Oxford, Radcliffe moved to London in 1684 and settled in Covent Garden. An avowed Tory and Jacobite, Radcliffe was physician to the Princess Anne from 1686, and had taken over the lucrative London practices of former Roman Catholic Richard Lower and lifelong Catholic Thomas Short. Unlike his erudite comrades in medicine, Radcliffe studied the works of Thomas Willis and little more; he ridiculed knowledge gained only from a library. Radcliffe was one of the new Fellows admitted by the 1687 College of Physicians charter; indeed, obtaining the affiliation of this illustrious practitioner was one of the reasons the College wished to enlarge its membership.[24]

When King William's asthmatic coughing grew intolerable in 1689, Radcliffe's prescription gave him so much relief that, notwithstanding the doctor's Tory politics, William offered Radcliffe an official position at £200, a higher rate of pay than any other doctor at court. The irascible Radcliffe refused the appointment, preferring to treat William and Mary at his convenience; he made as much as 600 guineas a year by such an arrangement.[25] Radcliffe probably did not need the extra income, as he astutely invested in various overseas voyages, such as his partnership in the outfitting of the *Lyon*, which returned from the South Seas in 1693. His suit in Chancery Court against the ship's manager over the division of the profits of the cargo reveals the doctor's attention to business details.[26] Dr. Radcliffe became a governor of St. Bartholomew's Hospital in 1690 and appears to have been deeply concerned about the well-being of poor patients treated there. His bedside manner was often brusque, however, when it came to treating the royals. Radcliffe reportedly declared to William, when summoned to examine his periodically swollen ankles, that "I would not have your majesty's two legs for your three kingdoms."[27]

Regardless of Radcliffe's lack of finesse, William called on him in 1694 to attend the dying Mary. Bishop Gilbert Burnet, director of the Williamite propaganda chorus and one of the king's most influential advisers, unfairly castigated Radcliffe for Mary's demise. Radcliffe correctly diagnosed the queen's disease as smallpox two days before her regular doctors concurred.[28] Because of his fame in the healing arts and despite his politics, in 1699 William asked once again for Radcliffe's opinion on his own health. The doctor reportedly told the king that he drank too much: "your juices are all vitiated, your whole mass of blood corrupted, and the nutriment for the most part turned to water; I'll engage to make you live three or four years longer, but beyond that time no physic can protect your Majesty's existence."[29] Finally tired of Radcliffe's rudeness, William never allowed the doctor in his presence again. An acute observer of symptoms and an effective campaigner in the constant war against disease, Radcliffe was habitually at odds with his medical colleagues. Nevertheless, he was the first London physician to use the gold-headed cane, bestowed on the city's outstanding physician by the Royal College of Physicians, in which he was a Fellow from 1687.

Of less stature in the medical community than Radcliffe, but adamantly Williamite in his politics and accomplished as a polemicist, Scotsman James Welwood served William and Mary in a different way. Welwood's medical credentials were certainly adequate, since he had obtained an M.D. degree from Reims in 1684. Before returning to Scotland later that year, he had spent some time at The Hague, getting to know key figures in Prince William's circle. By the spring of 1689 he was in London, anonymously penning an influential, erudite journal of political opinion, *Mercurius Reformatus*. Moreover, Dr. Welwood made astute references in a January 1690 issue of *Mercurius Reformatus* to the health of soldiers fighting in Ireland and the possible threat of pestilence to them. Welwood's pro-revolutionary, anti-French commentary coupled with his medical knowledge drew the attention of Bishop Gilbert Burnet, who in turn promoted the doctor at court. Welwood's first aulic appointment in England as physician extraordinary in March 1690 was prompted as much by his early enthusiasm for the House of Orange as by his medical prowess; a month later he became Physician to the Person. Disturbed by derogatory published remarks about her grandfather, Queen Mary asked Welwood to write an authorized history of the reign of Charles I.[30] Welwood's book evolved into a Whiggish summary of the seventeenth century, and became a source used by influential historians like Thomas Babington Macaulay and G. M. Trevelyan.

Because of his steadfast dedication to the medical reforms the king had in mind, the government in early 1691 appointed Welwood Superintendent of the Surgeons of the Fleet and Principal Physician for the Sick and Wounded at various Thames forts, assignments he undertook with his usual seriousness and dedication to duty.[31] In spring 1691, Welwood became a member of the Commission for the Sick, Wounded, and Prisoners of War, and through it, he came to appreciate the particular needs of military medicine, especially its reliance on the standardization and regularization of diagnosis and treatment. The Commission for the Sick and Wounded had been the recipient of some reproof, but during Welwood's tenure it became a vehicle through which improvement of military medicine was achieved and a key expression of the government's understanding that future recruitment depended on the conscientious care given its past and present soldiers and sailors. A crusader for humane treatment for both home forces and foreign captives, Welwood secured provisions for military hospitals, located people's lost relatives among prisoners of war, and helped defuse explosive social conditions in London caused by the detention of hundreds of Irish soldiers at the Savoy chapel and at the Marshalsea jail. No commissioner matched Dr. Welwood's energetic devotion to the king's objectives in medical advancement; he became a Williamite emblem of virtue and dedication to duty.

Welwood was warmly welcomed into Fellowship by the Royal College of Physicians in 1690, and in particular by its effusive President, Walter Charlton, who referred to Welwood in his salutation as "regis et reginae communis medicus."[32] All these honors, however, could not protect Welwood from censure by his and the king's political opponents. In November 1691 the House of Commons severely reprimanded Welwood for criticism in his newspaper of Parliament's reduced military appropriations for William's wars, forcing the physician to grovel in penitence. Shortly after, Welwood ceased publication of *Mercurius Reformatus*, but he continued to write political tracts, sometimes designed by the government to parry the thrust of Jacobite literature. After the queen's death, however, Welwood spent more time compiling innocuous almanacs and translating classical works. His only medical publication was an introduction to a case study of the presumably miraculous cure of a crippled girl.[33] Welwood accepted several College of Physicians' offices in his later years and enjoyed the life of a gentleman-scholar during the reigns of Queen Anne and King George I. In the final year of his life, 1727, the aged doctor acted as a go-between in the acrimonious separation of the mistress of the Prince of Wales, Mrs. Henrietta Howard, from her obstreperous, extortionate husband. Covering all corners in the royal triangle probably killed him.[34]

Sir Thomas Millington served as physician-in-ordinary to William and Mary from April 1691, moving up into the second rank in 1701 and later he held the same post under Queen Anne, though his own infirmity limited his endeavors in his final years.[35] Born in Berkshire, Millington earned an M.D. in 1659 from Oxford and in 1675 became Sedeleian Professor of Natural Philosophy there, a post he held until his death, though in later years he was represented by a deputy. Another inaugural Fellow of the Royal Society, widely respected and admired, the wealthy Millington was knighted by Charles II in 1679. Like Dr. Fraizer, Millington forged a good connection to the medical establishment for the co-sovereigns, as he was particularly active in the College of Physicians. In 1686 he was the treasurer and head of a committee negotiating with Sir Christopher Wren to remodel some rooms at the College, careful that their plans would not lead to architectural disaster.[36] Despite his successes with the crown and with his colleagues, Millington found himself embroiled in two major public imbroglios, both sullying his medical reputation in London.

First, he and John Radcliffe quarreled openly over Millington's diagnosis and the treatments he prescribed for Queen Mary at the time of her fatal smallpox attack and for King William as his health deteriorated later in the reign. Millington, quickly recognizing variola, had ordered that the queen be bled, but Radcliffe, diagnosing measles, thought bleeding should have begun earlier or been deferred until the pox actually erupted.[37] They differed, too, on what to do about the king's painful conditions towards the end of his reign, carrying their disquieting arguments into the sickroom. Radcliffe judged that William had dropsy, and prescribed asses' milk and purging; Millington demurred from that diagnosis and treatment, advising garlic instead. Radcliffe countered that garlic would damage the king's already weak lungs, and Millington retaliated that William's lungs were "the soundest part about him."[38] Millington compounded his contradiction of Radcliffe by pleading that Dr. Hutton, the first physician, be called in for consultation, a direct challenge to Radcliffe's authority.

More publicly, Radcliffe explicitly confuted Millington's position in the famous Dispensary controversy. Millington served as President of the College of Physicians from 1696 to 1704, the most critical years for the institution. Although Millington tried to curry favor with the court, encouraging Samuel Garth to deliver an extravagant panegyric of William III in the 1697 Harveian oration, he could not camouflage the ugly dispute between the Fellows and the London apothecaries over treatments and dominion. Simmering for decades, the doctor-druggist hostility exploded in 1698 with the launching of the first free outpatient clinic in the city in buildings adjacent to the College of Physicians in Warwick Lane.[39] The Dispensary essentially consisted of two rooms where charity patients received medicines financed by £10 contributions from fifty-three of the Fellows. However, an equal number of the College's physicians refused to contribute, and some dissidents, led by Radcliffe and Richard Blackmore, another royal doctor, renounced the Dispensary and boycotted meetings. So-called "society physicians" like Radcliffe ridiculed the Dispensary subscribers as inferior and undistinguished, threatening the beleaguered College from within. Perhaps as a counterthrust, the "Dispensary physicians" among the Fellows designated yet another physician to William and Mary, Christian Harrell, to hire resident assistants for the Dispensary, stock its laboratory, and outfit it with furnaces and stills pleasing to both Galenic and chemical doctors. Harrell likewise supervised the storage of preparations in an abutting coach-house. Poor patients came in droves to the Dispensary, necessitating the opening of branch clinics in Westminster and Cornhill.

But, in spite of this apparent success, internal divisions within the College widened and attacks on the Dispensary from apothecaries and elsewhere persisted. Wits and poets took up the cudgel, creating a public relations nightmare for Dr. Millington. Samuel Garth, respected College Fellow, prominent Whig poet, and later physician-in-ordinary to George I, lampooned the apothecaries' opposition to outpatient rooms and their own filthy establishments in *The Dispensary*, a six-canto poem which went through three editions in a few months. Moreover, the poem poked fun at certain College physicians, like William Gibbons, who contested the Dispensary. Millington and others accused the Apothecaries' Society of setting up a party within the College, but there was hardly unanimity among the schismatics themselves. Radcliffe impugned the ability of fellow "society doctor" Gibbons, calling him a "nurse," and railing over his use of "slops" to treat patients.[40]

Nonetheless, in the midst of this disorder, Millington determined to test the Fellows' coercive powers and regulatory authority. The College censors first charged one of their own, Johannes Groenvelt, a cohort of the schismatic anti-Dispensarians, with malpractice, exposing the College to further public ridicule and political risk. Then in 1700, after a complaint was made against

William Rose, an apothecary in St. Nicholas Lane, the Fellows prosecuted Rose in the Court of King's Bench for improperly practicing physic. When the verdict went against Rose, he petitioned the Privy Council, asking for a writ of error from the House of Lords, which had established in 1695 that the members of the Society of Apothecaries had equal rights with other professionals in London. After intense lobbying by both the College and the Society, the House of Lords in 1704 reversed the verdict against Rose and denied the regulatory authority of the College in London. The government ruled that medical privileges grounded in practical, empirical experience had nullified the dominion of an educated, judgmental elite; the *Rose* case acknowledged what had already happened in the medical marketplace: apothecaries were giving advice to the sick.[41] Stunned by the collapse of his organization's juridical power and the diminution of the doctors' collective moral weight, his own health ravaged by the ordeal, Millington died following a bladder operation later in the same year.[42]

Even before the Restoration of the Stuarts, the unpredictable Walter Charlton had been a physician to Charles II in exile, and with the return of the monarchy, Charlton was retained as a medical consultant, became a member of the Royal Society, and, at long last, a Fellow of the College of Physicians in 1676.[43] The delay in his approval by the Fellows, due to his sudden shifts from Galenist to Helmontian to mechanical philosophy, did not ultimately impede his activities within the College. He gave the Harveian oration in 1680, 1702 and 1706, and the Cutlerian lectures in 1683; he took on the post of Harveian librarian (at £20 per annum), too. During his public addresses, Charlton enthusiastically advocated iatromechanical principles, a system based on the belief that the blood was composed of particles in corpuscular agitation in a body made up of mechanical tubes, engines, and implements.

Charlton's mutable medical views did not hinder his acceptability as a leader of the Fellows anymore than they had limited his enterprise, for he served as President of the College from 1689 to 1691 during political and professional times nearly as turbulent for the College as those of the Civil War and Interregnum.[44] While President, the licensing of mountebanks was Charlton's responsibility, an ironic task given his own prior status as a blackballed physician, but by then Charlton had metamorphosed once again, mellowed by his rise in his colleagues' esteem. He now opined that the only authentic cures by irregular medical practitioners were due to the use of mercury and antimony.[45] Charlton had become something of a moderate on philosophical and jurisdictional matters, but more importantly, the College Fellowship now encompassed a majority of members interested in the new science and chemical medicine. King William made Charlton Physician to the Person in November 1691, even though the long-lived Charlton was criticized for spending too little time at his patients' bedsides and being "too much given to romances." Two years later, forgetting Charlton's cumulative effort as former President of the College, the Fellows remarked on his absences from meetings; Charlton rejoined that he had been busy serving His Majesty in wartime.[46]

He was not, however, too busy to write. A voluminous essayist on various themes before and after the Restoration, Charlton's post-Helmontian publications include a curious piece on Stonehenge in answer to architect Inigo Jones, who had argued that the monument was a Roman temple. Charlton identified Stonehenge as Danish, "because it looks Danish."[47] In the Sloane Manuscripts is a thirteen-page undated folio of Charlton's, written in English, on the differences between man's brain and that of animals, perhaps the basis for one of his lectures.[48] The catalogue of the British Library lists dozens of works by Charlton, many in Latin, written during a forty-year-span; he authored treatises on *Epicurus's Morals* (1656), *The Lives of the Ancient Philosophers* (1668), *A Natural History of the Passions* (1669), and *Enquiries into Human Nature* (1680). Walter Charlton left London during the reign of Queen Anne when his practice shriveled, and he died at eighty-eight in 1707.

Walter Harris, third physician-in-ordinary to William on the resignation of Dr. Stokeham, had an established practice in London and a learned reputation when tapped for aulic duties. Nothing is known of his parentage, but he was born in Gloucestershire in 1647. A scholar at Winchester College, he became a Fellow of New College, Oxford, in 1666. Harris received his arts degree in 1670, but, following his conversion to Roman Catholicism around 1673, he studied medicine in France and obtained a medical degree from the University of Bourges in 1675. Moving to London in 1676, Harris turned his attention to translating French medical manuals into English. He first translated Nicolas Blegny's book about curing venereal diseases with mercury; this was followed by a rendering of Nicolas Lemery's popular *Cours de Chymie*, which contained descriptions of various chemical medicines used by continental physicians with suggestions for their easy preparation.

However, Harris's Catholicism remained an impediment to his medical career, and amidst the turmoil of the Popish Plot he renounced the Catholic Church and published *Farewell to Popery* in 1679.[49] This pamphlet is in the form of a letter to Dr. John Nicholas, Vice-Chancellor of Oxford University and a warden of New College, justifying his return to the Church of England. Political correctness could definitely boost a medical career in Stuart England and keep one professionally unmolested. Consequently, Harris's M.D. was incorporated by Cambridge in 1680; Fellowship in the College of Physicians came in 1682, along with invitations to deliver Harveian orations on four occasions and Lumleian lectures during his later career. A protégé of the great Thomas Sydenham, whom he praised profusely in his Lumleian lectures, Harris often asked Sydenham for guidance in his continuing medical education. Sydenham purportedly suggested he read *Don Quixote* and learn how knowledge comes through observation.

In 1683 Harris published his best-known work, *Pharmacologia Anti-Empirica, or a Rational Discourse of Remedies both Chymical and Galenical*, on the six great medications: mercury, antimony, vitriol, iron, quinine bark, and opium. The book included discussion of superstitious cures such as broth in which gold has been boiled, amulets, and charms. In his chapter on gout, Harris emphasized the prevention of acute attacks, rejected a rigid diet in management of the ailment, and remarked on the higher incidence of gout among men of intellect. He also justified the concentration by a physician on a single disease. Harris hoped to vindicate "natural remedies" in the book, which additionally lambasted "diverse empiricks and mountebanks." Calling for a judicious and methodological administration of medicine buttressed by interventionist authorities, Harris ridiculed Paracelsus as an impetuous chemist who wrote like a "heathen" and never said his prayers.[50]

In 1689 Harris authored his most noteworthy contribution to medicine, a treatise in Latin on acute diseases in infants, *De Morbis Acutis Infantum*, first translated into English in 1693 by William Cockburn. Reprinted multiple times, the work became the standard pediatric monograph for a century and was translated into French and German. Harris addressed the difficulties of diagnosing and treating young patients; he estimated the effect of heredity on disease in children and the importance of correct diet in infancy. Harris was particularly concerned about the noxious effects of childhood acidosis, attributing the etiology of various digestive troubles to intestinal acid. He recommended first neutralizing the acidity with powdered oyster shell, followed by a rhubarb purge to rid the body of abnormal elements. Harris also advised parents to administer beer and wine to children in order to make their obstreperous offspring more docile.[51]

Walter Harris provided some medical services to Charles II in 1683, but was out of favor with Catholic James II. After the revolution, the Archbishop of Canterbury, John Tillotson, promoted Harris to King William as much for his renunciation of Roman Catholicism as for his talent as a physician. Harris moved from the post of queen's physician to physician to the king in 1693.[52] He attended Mary during her fatal bout with smallpox in 1694, contributing to the diagnostic dissension at her bedside. Harris disagreed with the advice that Dr. Richard Lower had given the indisposed queen to take Venice treacle, an opiated sudorific and popular panacea since Roman times, and reported that he had warned her not to provoke a permanent fever with an intensely hot medicine. Following the queen's death, Harris accompanied King William to Holland, where he was much impressed by Dutch gardens. In 1699 he wrote *A Description of the King's Royal Palace and Gardens at Loo*; it included Harris's observations about diseases in the Netherlands.[53]

Applauded by the College of Physicians for his well-timed broadside against quacks, Harris supported the Dispensary and was active during his later years in the College's governance and intellectual enterprises. He brought his medical addresses into print in the 1720s. His 1707 oration, about the queen's decease, was published in 1720 as *De morbis aliquot gravioribus observationes*. Two of his lectures appeared in print: *De Peste Dissertatio* in 1721 and *Dissertationes Medicae et Chirurgicae habitae in amphitheatro collegii regalis medicorum Londiniensium* in 1725. Harris penned a religious tract, *The Works of God*, in

1727. He died in 1732 at age eighty-five, having encountered in his life most of the religious, political, and medical turmoil of the era.

In February 1697, King William named Richard Blackmore Physician to the Person.[54] A prominent Whig and poet manqué, Blackmore was born in Wiltshire and educated at St. Edward's College, Oxford. He worked for a time as a schoolmaster, then traveled to the continent for medical study, receiving his M.D. from Padua. Returning to England before the Glorious Revolution, Blackmore became a Fellow of the College of Physicians in 1687, and a decade later at the height of the Dispensary discord, to which he was an outspoken contributor, King William named him physician-in-ordinary. The monarch may have elevated Blackmore to royal service as much out of appreciation for an epic poem the doctor had penned as for his medical aptitude. In 1695 Blackmore had written *Prince Arthur*, a popular Whiggish paean to the Prince of Orange as the legendary British champion. When a conspiracy to assassinate William was uncovered that year, the king determined to use the incident as propaganda against his adversaries. John Somers, a leading Whig lawyer and then William's Keeper of the Great Seal, chose Blackmore to write a book about the plot and supplied him with documents.

Blackmore got rather carried away by his assignment and ended up blaming the French for the intrigue; Somers had to revise Blackmore's draft. Ultimately, the government decided that since it was entering into delicate peace negotiations with France, the time was not right for a contentious book, even with Somers' alterations. Blackmore finally brought *A True and Impartial History of the Conspiracy against the Person and Government of William III* to publication in 1723 when the populace had cooled off considerably.[55] In 1697 however, at the behest of the Crown, Blackmore was able to augment his poetic saga and rename it *King Arthur*. The king repaid Blackmore for this splendid literary analogy with an aulic appointment. Despite his denunciation of the College's Dispensary, Blackmore became a censor and elector of the College in 1716.

The career of Thomas Lawrence (Laurence) demonstrates the possibilities for upward mobility within the medical profession. The son of a London apothecary, Lawrence matriculated at Merton College, Oxford, ultimately receiving a master of arts degree from St. Alban's School in 1655 and an M.D. from Padua before 1664 when he became an honorary Fellow of the Royal College of Physicians.[56] In attendance to Charles II though not with an official appointment, Lawrence was given responsibility for the British garrison at Tangier, a possession that came in Catherine of Braganza's dowry.[57] He had returned to London by 1685, when he participated in the post-mortem on the king's body, then held the post of Physician-General under James II. After the Glorious Revolution, William gave Lawrence's job to Hutton, but moved Lawrence to Ireland in a similar capacity. Lawrence additionally served as physician to the hospital in Flanders, the office with which he is identified in the 1698 warrant for his new allowance as third physician-in-ordinary to William III, the final regular appointment of the reign.[58] Thomas Lawrence continued in medical service to Queen Anne, as her first physician and as Physician-General to the army.

With two households to maintain, William and Mary wanted additional doctors available for their needs. Besides Welwood's short-lived stint as an extra physician, Guy Babanks and William Briggs received these appointments. Records show that a warrant of authorization for Babanks as an Extra Physician to the Person was issued in April 1694. As he is not listed among the College Fellowship, Babanks was doubtless another continental import, perhaps a Huguenot, whom King William summoned to England for aulic duties. William Briggs, extra physician-in-ordinary to William from 1696 to 1701, was the son of Norwich Member of Parliament Augustine Briggs. After obtaining a medical degree in 1677 from Corpus Christi College, Cambridge, Briggs's specialization in eye disease brought him to the attention of the Royal Society and led to his appointment as physician to St. Thomas's Hospital in 1681.[59] Like many other London physicians of the time, Briggs was interested in the efficacy for fever of Jesuits' Bark, especially as it influenced his specialization. One Simon Blenckerne wrote Briggs in October 1681 about his use of the drug on four patients who reported dizziness and temporary blindness after a second dosage.[60] Like other royal doctors, Briggs had trouble getting his pay on time even with the king's promise that it was forthcoming; he was not paid at all during 1698.[61] Fortunately, Briggs had the postrevolutionary patronage of the wealthy, if unprincipled, Duke of Montagu to support his work on the retina and the optic nerve, particularly after he lost his post at St. Thomas's due to the machinations of a rival oculist.[62]

The sole Physician to the Household appointed during the Dual Monarchy was Thomas Goodman, whose warrant dated from March 1690 and whose tenure stretched until William's death. Though his life is not described in Munk's compendium of the College Fellows, Goodman was probably a longtime resident of London. In 1739 his extensive library was sold at auction in the capital by Fletcher Giles; the catalogue of its contents ran to 260 pages.[63]

According to Clippingdale, William and Mary used the talents of several other doctors during their reign, some seasoned on previous household staffs, some new to the Lord Chamberlain's department. However, a number of the people listed, like George Howe and Theodore Colladon, were merely signatories to royal autopsy reports and not regular appointees. Howe was better known as an anti-Dispensarian, "Querpo" in Garth's poem; Colladon, a Mayerne on his mother's side, was physician in Queen Anne's reign to the Royal Hospital at Chelsea.[64] Other names, like Richard Morton, cannot be validated as those of physicians to the Dual Monarchs. Morton, William's physician during an English visit in 1670, maintained his close connections with the House of Orange. King James had purged Morton's name and the names of three others from the list of Fellows enumerated in the College of Physicians' 1687 charter, but it was restored on the recommendation of the College members and Morton became a College officer. The *DNB* calls Morton a physician-in-ordinary to

William III, but the entry may refer to his 1670 responsibilities; Morton does not appear to have obtained an aulic appointment when the Dutch prince became king of England.[65] William retained Thomas Burnet, brother of Bishop Burnet and friend of Dr. James Welwood, as physician-in-ordinary in Scotland and added Thomas Dalrymple, son of Lord Stair, Secretary of State for Scotland, to the staff there in 1691.

William and Mary appointed and employed equally renowned surgeons for service to the court, but in this category the monarchs indisputably favored familiar doctors from Holland over their English counterparts and drew upon those with impeccable political credentials. All of the Jacobean surgeons in the three discrete categories of aulic service vacated their offices on the "abdication" of their sovereign, acceding to a polite fiction that bolstered William and Mary's claims to the throne and their right to organize their own household.[66] The new king and queen brought several medical men with them to England at the time of the Glorious Revolution including two foreign surgeons, a Dutchman, William van Loon, and Stephen (Etienne) Ronjat, a Protestant refugee from France.[67] The Barber-Surgeons objected to this importation of competitors and ruled that no foreigner could become Master of the Company, though the monarch's serjeant-surgeon traditionally occupied this post. Later rescinded, the rule epitomizes the xenophobia that took hold in England after 1688.[68] Van Loon, who had been the Prince of Orange's Surgeon- General to the army and navy of the United Provinces, was someone King William could trust with renovating the military medical services. Van Loon's warrant is dated March 1689, confirming that the previous holder of the office under King James, the Catholic James Pierce, lost his post with the revolution. At the instigation of the new monarchs, van Loon immediately moved to gather together a group of skilled surgeons for the armed forces by conscripting the past masters of the Barber-Surgeons' Company into military service, perhaps another reason for the guild's objection to immigrants in the livery.[69]

Stephen Ronjat, who had been Surgeon to the Person for a few years, succeeded van Loon as serjeant-surgeon in November 1701 when the Dutchman died. David Elder briefly filled the post of Surgeon to the Person after March 1689, appointed on the same day that Charles Peter became surgeon to the household; Ronjat followed Elder up the surgical ladder, receiving the precise salary of £317 15s. per annum by warrant of the king.[70] The new and larger armed forces under King William depended on medical practitioners who could offer more effective treatment for the sick and wounded, practitioners who themselves had learned the trade on the battlefield. Ronjat based his surgical philosophy on rugged medical experience rather than effete Latin learning; he was exactly the sort of man the king wanted on the job. Charles Peter may have been one of those medical professionals who, William and Mary hoped, would bridge the gap between officeholders at court and occupational leaders in the community. He had been surgeon to Charles II and served under him in the Dutch wars; he had also tended James II. Besides his duties to the household, Charles Peter was surgeon to the Horse Guard. However, Peter was discharged in 1693 and Thomas Gardiner assumed his duties, staying in that office until 1707.[71] Gardiner was well-established within the London community and a leader in the Barber-Surgeons' Company; he was licensed by the College of Physicians, a distinction not often awarded to surgeons.[72] He must have had a particularly impressive scholarly reputation among his colleagues, as he was chosen to deliver the prestigious Linacre lectures at St. John's College, Cambridge. William II employed two barbers, William Germaine and Richard Longbottom, each at a salary of £170, and retained Hugh Brown as his Scottish surgeon-apothecary.[73]

The top-ranking member of the pharmaceutical staff was Abraham Rottermondt, Apothecary to the Person during the whole of William's reign. Like his English counterparts, Rottermondt, a native of the Netherlands, came from a family of court druggists and he himself had served the House of Orange in The Hague. Rottermondt journeyed extensively with the king, including missions to Ireland and Flanders, receiving "riding expenses" on each occasion. Highly regarded by William and Mary, he shared a coach with the household physician when the monarchs moved from one residence to another; in 1692 the king gave Rottermondt precedence over other attending apothecaries. Besides their responsibilities to the royal persons, Rottermondt and Dr. Hutton were charged with examining drugs and medicaments supplied to the military; further, Rottermondt kept the herb garden at Hampton Court. In fact, Rottermondt was kept so busy that his salary was raised in 1692 from £127, when not in residence, to £500 including bills for materials.[74] At the king's death in 1702, the Dutch apothecary prepared the perfumed crimson and white taffeta for the royal coffin.[75] Though named by Queen Anne as apothecary at her accession, Rottermondt retired to his native Holland later in 1702, still owed £446 by the government.

The other Apothecary to the Person under William and Mary was James Chase, longtime aulic servant to several monarchs and third generation member of a family of apothecaries to the Stuarts. Chase's grandfather, Stephen Chase, served Charles I and II; his father, John, worked for Charles II. Even though John Chase's salary and supply money often arrived late, he secured a reversion of his post for his son.[76] James Chase, second apothecary to James II from 1685 to the Glorious Revolution, lost his commission upon the arrival of William of Orange. However, as James Chase headed the Society of Apothecaries as Master in 1688–1689, his professional status was doubtless obvious to the new monarchs as they searched for competent medical men during their first months in England. Accordingly, Chase recaptured his appointment in May 1690; he continued as a royal apothecary into the reign of George I. Chase could not have been too surprised at delays in payments for his services similar to those that had plagued his father; even the bouche no longer existed. The warrant for Rottermondt's and Chase's allowance specifies that each was to receive £52 for lodging out of court, but in 1692 James Chase was forced to rent a room in Whitehall for which he still sought reimbursement after Queen Anne's death.[77] In 1701 he became Member of Parliament for Marlow, Buckinghamshire, and was reelected intermittently until 1710, a rather unusual situation for a royal servant; he died in 1721, aged seventy-two.

Providing posterity with the only surviving record of a royal apothecary's professional work, James Chase chronicled the pharmaceutical needs of William and Mary's court in a fascinating five hundred-page daybook. Affording a glimpse of health care among the Stuart elite and covering over two years, the journal lists what mixtures Chase prepared and for whom during the period April 1691 to May 1693. Many of the prescriptions are for the king and queen, but Chase made medicines for courtiers and administrators, too. Chase did not include the names of the physicians who prescribed the medicines, perhaps an indication that oral instructions were given to him. The more common concoctions he prepared were purgatives, vomitories, laudanum for pain, and amalgamations to ward off everything from melancholy to intestinal worms. Chase lists thirty-five categories of frequently used medications including eleven different waters and the patients for whom they were prepared. He used such remarkable ingredients as the slime of earthworms, raspings of ivory, bruised millipedes, half an ounce of human skull, and the urine of a healthy man; saffron, tea, and cinnamon are among the less startling ingredients that he employed. While the task of venesection sometimes fell to apothecaries, Chase did not perform that operation himself, probably enlisting another apothecary from his workshop. He supplied perfumed potpourri, colognes, and soaps to the court; the king's periwig-maker had Chase's powders delivered directly to his shop in Leicester Fields.[78]

Although King William, in the interests of economy, tried to reduce the size of his medical staff, he found himself with too many apothecaries to the household after a grant of reversion for John Jones' son was misplaced. The senior Jones, apothecary to the Stuarts for thirty years, petitioned that his apprentice son, William, receive that post upon his own retirement or death. Ample precedent existed for such a request, and the wealthy royal servant, who owned stock in the Royal African Company, loaned the Exchequer nearly £2,400 due to him in back salary to cement the arrangement. Consequently, William Jones asserted his right to the court apothecary's post when his father died in 1693. But another claimant, John Soames, had already drawn wages as the new court mixer of potions. William Jones brought suit in Exchequer Court, claiming his right to the job and producing evidence of the 1677 grant of reversion. The government recognized his right, dismissed Soames, and awarded Jones the post by patent in 1697. He held the job throughout the reigns of William and Anne, whom he accompanied on progresses.[79]

Irregulars on the royal medical roll after the revolution included the controversial oculist-in-ordinary, Thomas Woolhouse. From childhood on, Queen Mary, like her sister Anne, suffered from sore, watery eyes, possibly a symptom of congenital syphilis. Treatment for defluxion, as it was called, included bleeding, and Mary had leeches set behind her ears to relieve ocular inflammation.[80] Woolhouse proposed iridectomy, but the queen instead restricted her reading and card playing so that her eyesight might have a chance to improve. She prudently resisted the solicitation of a one-eyed "oculist extraordinary" from Wapping, Roger Grant, who repeatedly tried to get appointed to court without success.[81] While an "operator for the teeth" did not become part of the royal household staff until 1727, dental problems often required special expertise. Dr. Radcliffe, that acute observer of symptoms, recommended two grains of opium for sore teeth, and for bleeding teeth a preparation of gum arabic and dragonwort.[82]

Besides responsibilities as physician to the king-stadtholder, Govert Bidloo, who received an M.D. from Franaker in 1682 and pursued a career as professor of anatomy and surgery at The Hague and Leiden, acted as royal dentist for William III. He was called to England to tend the king's loose teeth in 1695 and 1699; those teeth caused William misery while in Holland at Let Hoo in 1697. Bidloo blamed most dental problems on scurvy, and advised the king to use a mouthwash made of tincture of myrrh and "fair water."[83] William's legs were acting up again and Bidloo was shocked at their condition: the left leg swollen above the ankle and the right foot up to the heel. The Dutch physician prescribed rubbing the king's legs with flannel covered with a powder of crabs' eyes, flour, and cumin seed, together with hot poultices; William later complained that the poultices kept him awake and he discontinued their use.[84] Bidloo inquired after the king's general well-being and William sheepishly admitted that he hunted hard in order to violently exercise his lungs. He confessed to Bidloo that he was eating and drinking more than he had as a younger man, notwithstanding the warnings of his palace doctors back in England.

Bidloo was a fascinating if prickly character. The offspring of Mennonite parents, Bidloo was apprenticed to a surgeon in 1670. After his university studies, he became a specialist in military medicine, in 1688 a professor of anatomy at the Hague and in 1694 professor of medicine at Leiden, but despite his professional successes the Amsterdam resident wrote indignant plays, poems, and occasional broadsides directed at esteemed Dutch judges. Bidloo was imprisoned for defamation, but the Stadtholder interceded and he was freed. He was himself the injured party in what has become a famous case of plagiarism in medical literature.[85] In 1685 after nine years of work, Bidloo produced an anatomical atlas in Latin and Dutch to be published by a Dutch company, created by three investors for the sole purpose of distributing the most beautiful medical book ever published. One hundred five anatomical drawings by Gerard de Lairesse were based on autopsies performed by Bidloo. Critics, including Bidloo's own teachers at Leiden, charged that the engravings were aesthetically pleasing but their accompanying explanations were useless, and that Bidloo's anatomical knowledge was incomplete, particularly regarding the muscles. The atlas, despite of the hopes of its sponsors, did not sell well.

Nevertheless, in 1698 William Cowper, a London surgeon and member of the Royal Society, issued a version of Bidloo's atlas, with the original illustrations and an improved text, under his own name. Furious, Bidloo turned to the Royal Society in protest, demanding that it expel the well-respected Cowper, but in the end the Society gave no judgment.[86] Cowper claimed that his London publisher had signed an agreement with Bidloo's company for use of the engravings and for translation of the text; no international copyrights existed at that time. Cowper actually issued a pamphlet, "Eurcharistia," replying to Bidloo's complaints made to the Royal Society, but while Cowper feigned an apology in the tract, he actually further insulted Bidloo's work.[87] In spite of the controversy, Bidloo became William III's supervisor of all physicians, surgeons, and apothecaries in Holland, and he managed all Dutch civilian and military hospitals. In 1692, the king extended Bidloo's oversight to the British army. By 1701 old disagreements were forgiven sufficiently for Bidloo himself to become a member of the Royal Society. He presented to the members his findings that the nerves are not hollow, nor do they contain fluid, but consist of fibers.[88]

Cowper's association with King William III centered around two autopsies. The first was that of little William, Duke of Gloucester, son of Princess Anne, heiress apparent after Mary's death; Cowper was among the surgeons who signed the post-mortem report in 1700. The analysis of the surgical dissection was sent to William in Holland since Gloucester had been Anne's only living child and his death generated great concern for the succession. William had not worried about Anne's loyalty to the revolution as long as Gloucester lived, but with his death the king feared that Anne might contact her father in France and establish some sort of accord with her half-brother. As for Cowper, his career had blossomed after 1691, when he was awarded membership in the Barber-Surgeons' Company. The surgeon-scientist authored two important anatomy books and the first English-language text on general physiology for surgeons.[89] In 1694 Cowper presented a paper to the Royal Society denying the hemostatic effects of a styptic powder invented by a surgeon named John Colbatch.[90] Cowper suggested such medications be tested in experimental cases before being made available to the public. Two years later he reviewed for the Royal Society the process of digestion and "chyfilication," further enhancing his reputation as a thorough and ingenious scientist. The fellows of the Royal Society responded later that year by electing to membership Cowper and the queen's surgeon, Charles Bernard, the first two surgeons chosen for the prestigious association.[91] Cowper continued to publish on a variety of subjects: the eponymous glands of the urethra, canine and feline capillaries, and pulmonary arteriovenous shunts. Some scholars rate his 1705 paper on arteriosclerosis as "a landmark in the history of surgery."[92]

Cowper was also a signatory to William's own autopsy, performed at Kensington Palace two years later; he was part of a medical team led by Dr. Millington, whose report was delivered to the Privy Council. Everyone had noticed a significant decline in King William's vitality as the new century commenced, and in the summer of 1701 during an inspection of his Dutch armies, eyewitnesses at The Hague thought he looked like a dead man. He could barely walk; gout made his left hand useless and riding difficult. In the autumn he caught a raging cold after hunting in a downpour. His doctors tried everything possible to reduce his discomfort, and William was able to once again make the voyage to England, bringing his favorite Dutch physician, Govert Bidloo, along with him. By February 1702, the king's health rebounded from the usual rigors of winter, but when he was out riding in Richmond Park, his horse stumbled on a molehill. William was thrown and broke his collarbone. Serjeant-surgeon Ronjat set the fracture at Hampton Court, but the king insisted on returning to Kensington. On the bumpy coach ride the bone was jolted out of place again and Dr. Bidloo had to reset it. Although the king seemed in reasonable health in the week afterward, the break did not mend properly; the king gradually weakened, grew feverish, and experienced great pain. His physicians dosed him with herbal decoctions, Raleigh's cordial, and cinchona. Bidloo remained by his side, feeding the king by hand and holding him upright, but, despite the doctor's devotion, William III died on March 8, 1702, just six months after the death of the outcast James II in France.

Like Cowper, Ronjat was a signatory to William's autopsy report to Queen Anne, a summary making it unambiguous that the king was already seriously ill before his disastrous riding accident: he was asthmatical, dropsical, and scorbutic. The post-mortem examination revealed the king's emaciated condition, pulmonary pleurisy, and curiously little blood.[93] In an open letter in French to Bidloo, published the following year as *Lettre Écrite de Londres à un Médecin*, "premier chirurgien" Ronjat squabbled with the physician about who could claim credit for the late monarch's health care in Holland and about the reasons for his death. Ronjat objected to Bidloo's boastful journal and supposed singular insight by listing all the medical men at the autopsy: physicians-in-ordinary Millington, Hutton, Blackmore, and Lawrence, plus "Professeur" Bidloo, Doctors Harrell, Theodore Colladon, Edward Hannes, George Howe, surgeons Charles Bernard, and himself.[94] With his patron dead and medical foreigners in Britain in disrepute under a new, very English sovereign, Ronjat retired to Switzerland.

By the end of the Williamite era in British politics, the people and Parliament were openly disenchanted with the Dutch ruler and his policies. William had found spoken English hard to follow and admitted few Englishmen into his confidence. Ironically, though he despised politicians, as a foreigner he had to depend on them, thereby devaluing his regime. Even Bishop Burnet, William's great propagandist, criticized the king for taking "little pains to gain the affections of the nation."[95] Throughout his life, William's heart lay in the Netherlands. He would not abjure his position there as Stadtholder, and he chose Dutch favorites as his primary advisers in England. For some years foreigners persisted as commanders of English troops in the field, and William kept Dutch guards around him in England. Many Englishmen were envious of the Dutch and French Protestant émigrés who had come with the Prince of Orange to England, later obtaining lands and high offices from him. Dutch-style geometric gardens, evergreen shrubbery, and neat red-brick houses, so popular in 1688 with Englishmen, assumed political meanings in the late 1690s and attracted criticism; Tories even denounced topiary because it was associated with Dutchmen. Of course, some English indignation stemmed from nativist cultural arrogance, but much of it signaled partisan animosity. Everyone knew that complaints about aliens were really thinly disguised assaults on the government and the king himself. Daniel Defoe noted that "the word Foreigner was the shibboleth of a party, who made it popular, that they might better affront that great foreigner, that had made them all denizens. I mean King William."[96]

In 1701 Parliament passed an Act of Settlement forbidding an English monarch of foreign birth from taking the country into "any warr for the defence of any dominions and territories which do not belong to the crown of England," and from leaving the kingdom; the same legislation disqualified any alien from a governmental or Parliamentary position. So when Queen Anne delivered her first speech to Parliament in March 1702, a surge of loyalty greeted the new monarch as her countrymen rejoiced to have an Englishwoman on the throne again. Mindful of her bifurcated political heritage, she wore double mourning clothes: black for her father, James II, and purple for her brother-in-law and cousin, William III. Her immediate predecessor had not believed that women were capable of a political or governing role but, though Anne did not attempt to imitate William's style of rule, she would not be taken for granted. Queen Anne's strong preferences, for causes as well as for persons, had considerable political relevance throughout her kingdoms. Her inclinations lent a distinctive focus to royal medicine during the reign of the last Stuart sovereign, returning to some established healing traditions while complementing the changes begun under William and Mary.

Notes

1. For more on the lives of the joint sovereigns, see Henri and Barbara van der Zee, *William and Mary* (New York: Knopf, 1973; John Miller, *William and Mary* (London: Weidenfeld and Nicolson, 1974); and Tony Claydon, *William III and the Godly Revolution* (Cambridge: Cambridge University Press, 1996.

2. Annals of the College of Physicians, vol. 5, f. 52b, LRCP. For the Fellows' reaction to William, see the College exhibition catalogue, *Mutual Admiration*, 1.

3. See Harold J. Cook, "Practical Medicine and the British Armed Forces after the 'Glorious Revolution,' " *Medical History* 34 (1990): 1–26; Simon Schaffer, "The Glorious Revolution and Medicine in Britain and the Netherlands," *Notes and Records of the Royal Society of London* 43 (1989): 167–90.

4. Cook, "Practical Medicine," 14, 16. King William gave charlatan Cornelius Tilborg, Charles II's former surgeon, a license to sell a poison antidote despite the Fellows' frantic objections: Matthews, *Royal Apothecaries*, 137.

5. For more on the allegiance controversy, see Mark Goldie, "The Revolution of 1689 and the Structure of Political Argument," *Bulletin of Research in the Humanities* 83 (1980): 473–564.

6. While the Prince of Orange was in England in 1670, Richard Morton, a Suffolk-born chaplain in Worcestershire, was his Physician to the Person, accompanying William to Oxford. Upon the prince's nomination, Oxford awarded Morton an M. D.

7. Gilbert Burnet, *History of His Own Time*, 2nd ed., 6 vols. (Oxford: Oxford University Press, 1833) 4: 562.

8. Chapman, *Mary II*, 231.

9. Richard Doebner, ed., *Memoirs of Mary, Queen of England* (London: David Nutt, 1886), 7, 45, 78–79.

10. William Salmon, *Pharmacopoeia Londinensis or New London Dispensatory*, 5th ed. (London: J. Dawk, 1696), 198–99.

11. *Calendar of State Papers, Domestic Series, for the Reign of William and Mary*, 5 vols., (London: Eyre and Spottiswoode, 1895–1906) 1: 237, 317.

12. Cook, "Living in Revolutionary Times," 120.

13. John Carswell, *The Descent on England* (New York: John Day, 1969), 131.

14. Munk, *Roll* 1: 481. Cook tallies over £3,000 in salary and riding charges earned by Hutton from 1690 to 1702: Cook, "Living in Revolutionary Times," 125.

15. Annals of the College of Physicians, 6: 72–73, LRCP; Munk, *Roll* 1: 502, LRCS. There is no record of payment to Silvestre other than his Dutch pension.

16. Vigne, "Mayerne and His Successors," 224–25.

17. Cook, "Living in Revolutionary Times," 126.

18. Sainty and Bucholz, *Officials of the Household*, 46. Cook calls him Stockholm, but gets the reign correct; Munk dates his service from 1680, as physician-in-ordinary to Charles II. Cook, *Decline of the Old Medical Regime*, 283; Munk, *Roll* 1: 447.

19. Annals of the College of Physicians, vol. 5, fos. 103a, 104b, 105b-107a; vol. 7: 93–97, LRCP. Starting with volume 6, page numbers rather than folio citations are used.

20. Cook, "Living in Revolutionary Times," 126.

21. Munk, *Roll* 1: 452. Munk says the bill was paid by a banker named Child in 1688.

22. See Norman Moore's introduction to *Album Amicorum of Adam Harel* (London: n.p., 1914) and W.F. Bynum, "Medicine at the English Court, 1688–1837," 268–69. Christian Harrell was Adam's son.

23. See *Calendar of Treasury Books*, 1693–96: 1078; or Add. MSS 5751, folios 50, 90, British Library. His June 1695 receipt of payment from Edward Nicholas is recorded in Add. MSS 5751A, f. 50, British Library.

24. Royal College of Physicians, *Mutual Admiration*, 5.

25. Campbell R. Hone, *The Life of Dr. John Radcliffe* (London: Faber and Faber, 1950), 55–56.

26. *Calendar of Treasury Papers, 1691* 1: 335.

27. Narcissus Luttrell, *A Brief Historical Relation of State Affairs, 1678–1714*, 6 vols. (Oxford: Oxford University Press, 1857) 4: 310; Hone, *Life of Radcliffe*, 51.

28. Kenneth Dewhurst, "The Death of Queen Mary II: A Mistaken Diagnosis by Dr. Radcliffe," *Oxford Medical School Gazette* 14 (1962): 104–6. Bishop Burnet repeated the tale that Radcliffe was negligent in treating Mary, when actually Walter Harris was in charge of her care. See also Royal College of Physicians, *Mutual Admiration*, 5; Munk, *Roll* 1: 455.

29. Quoted in William MacMichael, *The Gold-Headed Cane* (London: Longmans, 1884), 55.

30. It became something more in Welwood's enthusiastic hands: see *Memoirs of the Most Material Transactions in England* (London: T. Goodwin, 1700). The history was dedicated to William III, a widower by the time of its publication.

31. Historical Manuscripts Commission, 12th Report, App. VII (London: HMSO, 1890) 17/2: f. 313; *Calendar of State Papers, Domestic, William and Mary*, 1694–95: 178–79; *Calendar of State Papers, Domestic, William III*, 1695: 256.

32. Munk, *Roll* 1: 483.

33. *A True Relation of the Wonderful Cure of* M. *Maillard to which is added a letter from Dr. Welwood upon that subject* (London: R. Baldwin, 1694).

34. For more on Welwood's life and times, see Elizabeth Lane Furdell, *James Welwood: Physician to the Glorious Revolution* (Conshohocken, Penn.: Combined Publishing, 1998).

35. Cook dates Millington's appointment from 1701, but Sainty and Bucholz found the earlier one. Cook, "Living in Revolutionary Times," 126; Sainty and Bucholz, *Officials of the Household*, 142.

36. See the letter from Wren to Millington in SL MSS 3984, f. 245, British Library.

37. E. M. Thompson, ed. *Correspondence of the Family of Hatton*, 2 vols. (New York: Johnson Reprints, 1965), 2: 209; Bynum, "Medicine at the English Court," 275.

38. James Vernon, Under Secretary of State, quoted in van der Zee, *William and Mary*, 419.

39. See Frank H. Ellis, "The Background of the London Dispensary," *Journal of the History of Medicine* 20 (1965): 197–212.

40. Samuel Garth, *The Dispensary, A Poem* (London: John Nutt, 1699). For more on Garth see Richard I. Cook, *Sir Samuel Garth* (Boston: Twayne, 1980) and John F. Sena, *The Best-Natured Man* (New York: AMS Press, 1986); for Gibbons, see Munk, *Roll* 1: 490. An Oxford graduate in medicine, Gibbons is recognized by social historians for introducing mahogany furniture to London.

41. Wall, *The London Apothecaries*, 6; Howard Bayles, "The Rose Case," *Chemist and Druggist* 132 (1940): 473; Harold J. Cook, "The Rose Case Reconsidered: Physicians, Apothecaries, and the Law in Augustan England," *Journal of the History of Medicine and Allied Sciences* 45 (1990): 554. For the Groenvelt case, see Harold J. Cook, *Trials of an Ordinary Doctor* (Baltimore: Johns Hopkins Press, University 1994). Dr. Gibbons, by the way, testified at the behest of Dr. Groenvelt.

42. Munk, *Roll* 1: 363.

43. Munk says Charlton was retained as Charles II's physician after the Restoration, but Sainty and Bucholz cite November 1692, during the reign of William and Mary, as the date of the warrant commissioning Charlton. Munk, *Roll* 1: 390; Sainty and Bucholz, *Officials of the Household*, 46.

44. For a brief description of Charlton's presidency see Cook, *Decline of the Old Medical Regime*, 220–22.

45. Matthews, *Royal Apothecaries*, 143–44.

46. Munk, *Roll* 1: 390, LRCS; Annals of the College of Physicians, 6: 76–78, LRCP. Harold Cook errs in calling Charlton a physician extraordinary and in defining the extra physicians, like William Briggs, as not on a regular salary or enjoying tenure in office. See Cook, "Living in Revolutionary Times," 132; Sainty and Bucholz, *Officials of the Household*, 46, 77, 84.

47. Walter Charlton, *Dissertation on the Vindication of the Antiquity of Stonehenge* (London: J. Brown, 1730), 6; reprinted in Inigo Jones, *The Most Notable Antiquity of Great Britain* (Farnborough, Surrey: Gregg, 1971).

48. SL MSS 698, fos. 74–87, British Library.

49. Walter Harris, *Farewell to Popery* (London: Walter Kettilby, 1679).

50. Walter Harris, *Pharmacologia Anti-Empirica, or a Rational Discourse of Remedies both Chymical and Galencial* (London: Richard Chiswell, 1683).

51. Walter Harris, *De Morbis Acutis Infantum* (London: Samuel Smith, 1689); Samuel X. Radbill, "Pediatrics," in *Medicine in Seventeenth-Century England*, ed. Allen G. Debus (Berkeley: University of California Press, 1974), 251.

52. Munk, *Roll* 1: 423, LRCS.

53. Walter Harris, *A Description of the King's Royal Palace and Gardens at Loo* (London: R. Roberts, 1699).

54. For Blackmore's life see Harry M. Solomon, *Sir Richard Blackmore* (Boston: Twayne, 1980).

55. Richard Blackmore, *A True and Impartial History of the Conspiracy against the Person and Government of King William III. Of Glorious Memory, in the Year 1695* (London: J. Knapton, 1723).

56. Munk, *Roll* 1: 347, LRCS. Lawrence's grandson, also Thomas (1711–83), was a College member and friend of Samuel Johnson.

57. See James Henry Lawrence, "History of the Antient Family of Lawrence," *Gentleman's Magazine* 85/2 (1815): 12–17.

58. Add. MSS 5763, f. 60, British Library; Lawrence received £250 per annum. Sainty and Bucholz found an appointment for a Lawrence as Physician to the Person in 1692 but without any additional identifying information: Sainty and Bucholz, *Officials of the Household*, 132.

59. Briggs published *Ophthalmo-graphia* in 1686.

60. SL MSS 123, f. 7, British Library. Sloane 123 is a collection of letters to Briggs and fellow physician Edward Hulse. Folio 1 to Briggs asks for consultation on what to do about a young

woman in Peterborough so despondent over her mother's death that she had regular 6 P.M. fits and about a case of a laudanum-induced cough.

61. See *Memorial to Dr. William Briggs* (London: n.p., 1702).

62. Munk, *Roll* 1: 424, LRCS. Jonathan Swift referred to Montagu, who shifted his political allegiance with remarkable ease, as "arrant a knave as any in his time."

63. *Catalogue of the Entire Library of Thomas Goodman, Physician* (London: n.p., 1739).

64. Clippingdale listed the following physicians in service to William and Mary: Govert Bidloo, Richard Blackmore, William Briggs, Theodore Colladon, Edward Hannes, Christian Harrell, Walter Harris, George Howe, John Hutton, John Inglis, Thomas Lawrence, Thomas Millington, Richard Morton, John Radcliffe, Peter Silvester, Charles Scarburgh, and James Welwood. He omitted William Stokeham, Walter Charlton, Guy Babanks, and Thomas Goodman.

65. Munk, *Roll* 1: 398, LRCS.

66. Proponents of the legal invention that James's escape equated to abnegation of the throne often buttressed their de jure argument with de facto reinforcements: Goldie, "Revolution of 1689," 488.

67. No biographical information on either van Loon or Ronjat is available in the usual medical compilations—the *DNB*, Young, Munk, or Dobson and Walker. See instead G. A. Lindeboom, *Dutch Medical Biography* (Amsterdam: Ridopi, 1984) and Royal College of Physicians, *Mutual Admiration*. A July 1694 request for hospital linens in Dutch from van Loon is in Add. MSS 38699, f. 3, British Library, and a pass for van Loon to travel to Holland in April 1690 can be found in *Calendar of State Papers, Domestic Series, William and Mary*, 1: 539.

68. Young, *Annals*, 197.

69. Cook, "Practical Medicine," 4.

70. See Add. MSS 5763, f. 55, British Library. The keeper of the gondola, by comparison, received £50 and the royal ratkiller £48. Ibid., folios 57, 60.

71. Young's *Annals* list Thomas Hobbs as the serjeant-surgeon until 1697, but he vacated his office in December 1688. Furthermore, Young's index calls Thomas Gardiner Hobbs's successor, but Gardiner was surgeon to the household from 1693. See Sainty and Bucholz, *Officials of the Household*, 48–49, 107, 122, 152; Young, *Annals*, 18; and Cook, "Living in Revolutionary Times," 130–31.

72. Munk, *Roll* 1: 433, LRCS; Young, *Annals*, 10, 18.

73. Add. MSS 5763, f. 28, British Library.

74. Add. MSS 5763, folios 43–45, British Library.

75. Matthews, *The Royal Apothecaries*, 133.

76. Chase's salary is set in the same warrant as Rottermondt's. Add. MSS 5763, fos. 43–45, British Library.

77. Matthews, *Royal Apothecaries*, 138. For Chase's appointment see *Calendar of Treasury Books*, 1689–92: 609.

78. Matthews, "Day Book of the Court Apothecary", 161–73.

79. *Calendar of Treasury Papers*, 1691–93: 134, 344; 1694–95: 991, 1022.

80. Matthews, *Royal Apothecaries*, 137.

81. See Leslie G. Matthews, "Licensed Mountebanks in Britain," *Journal of the History of Medicine* 19 (1964): 30–45.

82. Dobson, "The Royal Dentists," 286. Radcliffe agreed that diet affected dentition, and his bequest to St. Bartholomew's Hospital was aimed at raising the nutritional standards of the indigent sick. See Norman Moore, *History of St. Bartholomew's Hospital*, 2 vols. (London: C. A. Pearson, 1918), 2: 356.

83. Dobson, "The Royal Dentists", 285; C. Gysel, "Dental Aspects of Bidloo's 'Anatomy,' " *Medical Hygiene* 44 (1986): 2212–13.

84. Add. MSS 5724, British Library; Hone, *Life of Radcliffe*, 58.

85. See K. B. Roberts, "Bidloo, Cowper and Plagiarism of Anatomical Illustrations," *Canadian Social History of Medicine Newsletter*, September 1970, 7–10.

86. Some scholars have argued that the controversy over the borrowed illustrations has ob-

scured the prescience of Cowper's scientific text. See Robert F. Buckman, Jr., and J. William Futrell, "William Cowper," *Surgery* 99 (1986): 587–88.

87. G. A. Lindeboom, "Cowper's Brutale 'Plagiaat' van Bidloo's Anatomische Atlas," *Nederlands Tijdschrift voor Geneeskunde* 126/41 (1982): 1878–82. I wish to thank Mrs. Letty Jolly of Neptune Beach, Florida, for her translation of this article from the Dutch.

88. Bidloo's nephew, Nicolas, was physician-in-ordinary to Tsar Peter the Great from 1702. Nicolas Bidloo is recognized as the founder of the first hospital and the first botanical garden in Russia. Like his uncle, he wrote and staged plays. Lindeboom, *Dutch Medical Biography*, 135.

89. *Myotomia Reformata* appeared in 1694, *Anatomy of Humane Bodies* in 1698, and *Glandularium Quarundam* in 1702. Publication of the text on anatomy embroiled Cowper in a nasty dispute with Dutch surgeon Govert Bidloo, whose engraved anatomical illustrations in an earlier publication Cowper had expropriated for his own. The plagiarism charges Bidloo leveled at Cowper have obscured the scientific content of the text.

90. For more on Colbatch and medical entrepreneurialism, see Harold J. Cook, "Sir John Colbatch and Augustan Medicine," *Annals of Science* 47 (1990): 475–505.

91. For a discussion of Cowper's anticipation of John Hunter, see Buckman and Futrell, "William Cowper," 582–90.

92. Ibid., 589.

93. Add. MSS 5724, British Library; Royal College of Physicians, *Mutual Admiration*, 11. The lifeless king was found to be wearing Mary's gold ring and a lock of her hair on a black ribbon around his neck.

94. Stephen Ronjat, *Lettre Écrite de Londres à un Médicin* (London: n.p., 1703), 26–28. Hans Sloane and Edward Browne may have been observers at the autopsy; Hannes asked them to go with him to the "dissection" at 8 A.M. March 10. See SL MSS 4059, folios 117–119, British Library. The diary that irritated Ronjat is Govert Bidloo, *Verbaal van de Laatste Ziekte en het Overlijden van Willem III* (Leiden: n.p., 1703).

95. Quoted in John Miller, *William and Mary*, 120.

96. Quoted in Daniel Statt, *Foreigners and Englishmen* (Newark: University of Delaware Press, 1995), 115. See also Gary S. DeKrey, "Political Radicalism in London after the Glorious Revolution," *Journal of Modern History* 55 (1983): 613.

Chapter 8

The Medical Personnel in Queen Anne's Court (1702–14)

Until 1694, no one expected Anne Stuart, Protestant younger daughter of James II by his first wife, to become queen of England.[1] Her birth to the Duke and Duchess of York during the plague year of 1665 went unrecorded even by the fastidious diarist Samuel Pepys. Her mother died in 1671, then her father wed a teenage girl in 1673 only seven years older than Anne. Deprived of her mother's affection and unhappy with her Catholic stepmother, at age eight Anne established a great friendship with a thirteen-year-old attendant in the service of Mary of Modena—Sarah Jennings, later Sarah Churchill, Duchess of Marlborough; their friendship lasted almost to the end of Anne's life. After an unpleasant, failed meeting in 1681 with potential spouse Prince George of Hanover, Lady Anne accompanied her father to Scotland during the exclusion crisis that threatened his succession. While she was in the northern kingdom, the Danish envoy proposed to Charles II that Anne marry Prince George of Denmark, a Lutheran and the thirty-year-old second son of Frederick III. No one had any serious objections and since Protestant princes of any denomination were hard to come by, the engagement was announced. John Evelyn described George, as blonde, heavy, and reticent, but known for his valiant combat rescue of his brother, the Danish King Christian V.[2] Following the nuptials in 1683, Sarah became Anne's lady of the bedchamber and persuaded her to keep a low profile during James's unpopular reign. Though Prince George escorted King James to Salisbury when William of Orange invaded, he soon deserted James and Anne fled to Nottingham for safety. Throughout the revolution, Anne was strongly influenced by the Churchills, who advised the princess to support the triumphant claims of her brother-in-law to be co-monarch with her sister, Mary. As a consequence of that support, the title would settle on Anne and her offspring if Mary's line failed.

Anne and her sister had always been close, but after Mary's coronation an estrangement, magnified by Sarah Churchill and her husband, took place over Anne's apartments, allowance, and rights to James II's private estate. After Mary's death, King William reconciled with Anne and treated her with every courtesy, mindful that her court could become a magnet for any plots to depose him. In 1701, being childless, Anne acquiesced to the Act of Settlement, which named Sophia, Electress of Hanover, and her progeny in line for the crown on the grounds of their descent from James I. On March 8, 1702, Anne, last of the

Stuart sovereigns, acceded to the throne. She was only thirty-seven, yet so infirm from various physical ailments that she had to be carried to her coronation.

The following month, the College of Physicians sent Queen Anne a letter congratulating her on her accession and reminding her of the Fellows' prerogatives as caretakers of the English medical establishment. Despite this advice, Anne's government sided straightaway with the medical challengers on two significant occasions. First, when the College tried to contract with the crown in 1702 to supply medicines again to the armed forces, a contract it had lost during the previous decade to the apothecaries, Anne's government accepted the Society of Apothecaries' proposals, shutting the physicians out. Under administrative mandate, the Apothecaries' organization furnished drugs to the army and navy, the East India Company, and the crown colonies. Clearly, in the judgment of the government, apothecaries had overcome any vestiges of the "tradesman" stigma to be acknowledged as legitimate medical competitors with a respected knowledge of physic.[3] Second, after William Rose, the apothecary whom the College sued for malpractice, decided to appeal his conviction in King's Bench, he petitioned the Privy Council for a writ of error. Anne's government in November 1703 furnished Rose with his writ, filed the following February in the House of Lords, the highest appellate tribunal in England. The law lords decided the *Rose* case in favor of the apothecary and rebuked the arbitrary harshness of the medical monopolists in the College. Like William and Mary before her, Queen Anne had dealt the elite medical establishment a severe blow, at the same time officially recognizing the alternative medical corps of surgeons and apothecaries. The psychological effect on the Fellows in the College of Physicians was devastating. In 1711 some complaints were still being brought against apothecaries, but by 1714 the amount of business in general conducted by the Fellows was minimal and the record of the minutes was sparse.[4]

However, the association of Queen Anne with medicine is not simply her relationship with the College of Physicians. Most students of British history have some awareness of the fragile health of Anne, who in a relentless quest for a Stuart heir conceived eighteen children, only one of whom survived beyond the first few years.[5] During a fifteen-year period before ascending the throne, when she was between the ages of nineteen and thirty-five, Anne endured eleven miscarriages out of seventeen pregnancies. In addition to her tragic fecundity, she experienced lifelong discomfort from sore, myopic eyes, dangerous obesity, and, from middle age onward, enervating gout.[6] Because of her precarious physical condition and her persistent hopes for a child, the queen placed great importance on having adequate medical care for herself and her household. As a sovereign, she sought the best cures, some of which were hers to dispense through God's gift to her subjects, and as a noblewoman, she practiced the civilized feminine art of nurture. In doing so, she consciously pursued wellness for herself and the nation.

Queen Anne revived the monarch's claim to be the nation's first healer by resuming the ancient practice of touching subjects for the King's Evil. Given her devotion to the monarchy and the Anglican church as twin pillars of English life, some of Anne's more orthodox subjects, urged on by a bevy of scrofula sufferers, easily persuaded the queen to reinstate the miraculous tradition of the rite. She began to touch again shortly after her accession, hanging coins around the necks of the afflicted, but she used a simplified ceremony and shorter liturgy. As part of his duties, Thomas Gardiner, surgeon to Anne's household, screened applicants for the queen's touch at Bath in October 1702.[7] The queen introduced a protective magnet into the ritual, placed between her curing fingers and the sick person's affected parts, but she still distributed gold pieces. In April 1706 she wrote to Sarah, asking her to order 200 pieces of healing gold, for she intended to touch the sick at the Banqueting House before hot weather arrived.[8] Anne's touching engendered patriotic enthusiasm, particularly among the Tories, who applauded the rebirth of regal protocol. Jonathan Swift, Tory propagandist and Anne's speechwriter, lauded the efficacy of the royal hand and denounced the excesses of skepticism in the souls of those who denied the truth of the matter. A popular card game played in Anne's reign and sold in London bookshops depicted her on the nine of hearts touching her sick subjects.[9] Queen Anne continued the touching ritual throughout her reign, performing the ceremony for the last time on April 27, 1714. Anne's finale, actually a coda, signals the permanent end of the royal observance; no English sovereign from that day onward has touched the sick or distributed medical amulets. In reality, of course, the political revolutions of the seventeenth century in England had simultaneously toppled two imperial governments and the people's faith in the supernatural character of royalty.

Though an unlikely medical renegade, like most gentlewomen of her era without professional credentials, Queen Anne freely advised friends and relatives to drink asses' milk, treacle water, and elixirs.[10] She asked about the efficacy of certain prescriptions for the illnesses of her friends, and felt that the Duchess of Somerset's "gravel" might be eased by authentic Tipping's water, not the counterfeit liquor excoriated in *Post Boy* advertisements.[11] Regardless of class distinctions, English women were expected to provide for the well-being of their families with effective home remedies. For instance, Lady Grace Mildmay, who married into an aristocratic Puritan Northamptonshire family, had been educated at home in "phisicke and surgerie," and often read William Turner's popular herbal. Lady Mildmay kept a journal from 1570 to 1617 which tells of a variety of medical activities; the recurrence of these activities attests to their centrality in her life. She regarded healing as part of her religious duty: "It is good sometimes to be alone and meditate, but it is also good to call on one's neighbours to comfort their souls and bodies."[12] One celebrated patrician practitioner was Elizabeth Grey, Countess of Kent, the originator of "Kent's powder," a much-favored mixture of steel filings, ground pearl, and sugared spices for a condition known as the green sickness; it was similar to a recommendation made by famed London physician Richard Mead.[13] The Countess's "rare and selects secrets in physick and churgery" were collected and published as *A Choice Manual*, selling for one shilling and going through seventeen editions, a clear indication of its popularity.

Given the scarcity of qualified M.D.s in England, some physicians inadvertently contributed to their own decline by providing helpful hints to "petticoat doctresses."[14] George Hartman wrote *The Family Physitian* to be "useful for families and serviceable for country people."[15] Dozens of similar titles appeared in Stuart Britain, some written by women, a tacit acknowledgment of the importance of the amateur caregiver to the nation's health. Most wives' pharmaceutics remained unpublished, treasured legacies for their daughters to use in their households, but Lady Margaret Hoby's diary of her record of attendance at births, sicknesses, and recoveries was printed, as were the notes of Scotswoman Lady Grisell Baillie.[16] London stationers distributed several editions of Hannah Woolley's ambitious recipe book, *The Accomplish'd Ladies Delight in Preserving, Physick, Beautifying and Cookery*. This fashion for amateur pharmaceutics disclosed a lack of confidence in traditionally trained doctors. Long before the Augustan Age, so-called for the literati's fascination with the Rome of the Emperor Augustus, criticism of physicians had become widespread. Some of that criticism was self-serving, emanating from competitors in the medical marketplace, but much was honest observation from the patient's perspective and could be read in the biting ridicule of Joseph Addison and Richard Steele in *The Tatler* and *The Spectator*.[17]

Anne's health demanded more than faith in her own healing powers; it needed "physic," too. Dogged all her life by physical problems, Princess Anne had been a delicate toddler whose incessantly watering eyes caused alarm at the age of three. Anne was sent into the care of her grandmother, Henrietta Maria, to consult an eye specialist outside Paris. She never outgrew this secretory condition, which, coupled with severe myopia, caused her to prefer small rooms and niches even as queen, possibly creating an unsocial court life and damaging court culture.[18] Between the ages of four and six, while she was in France, Anne lost her grandmother, her aunt Henriette-Anne, and her mother, creating a sense of insecurity that she "never successfully overcame."[19] Bereavement plagued the princess's world; within months of her mother's death, Anne's four year-old brother Edgar and infant sister Katherine died. When rumors that poison might have killed her aunt frightened James, he ordered Anne home from France and declared that she was cured of her eye ailments.

A few days before her sister's wedding to the Prince of Orange in November 1677, Anne contracted smallpox, and she was too ill to attend the ceremony. Her governess, Lady Frances Villiers, caught the disease and died just as Anne was recovering; her infant half-brother, Charles, also died. The tally of Anne's seventeen miscarriages and unsuccessful pregnancies began with a daughter, stillborn in May 1684. Two daughters, Mary, born in 1685, and Anne Sophia, born in 1686, survived the rigors of delivery only to die from smallpox within days of each other in February 1687; Princess Anne thought the foul air of London had adversely affected her girls and took up residence temporarily at Hampton Court, but King James ordered her back to Whitehall.[20] After three miscarriages, one of which she attributed to dancing the rigadoon, Anne delivered a son, William Henry, in July 1689; the baby was named after the king, the boy's godfather, who promised him a separate residence and made him Duke of Gloucester. Premature babies born to Princess Anne died in 1690 and 1692, followed by eight more miscarriages from 1693 to 1700, including an unusual double miscarriage in September 1696 following a "convulsion fit."[21] Each pregnancy caused her more anguish and required a longer recovery period, making her an invalid before she was thirty. Even in the seventeenth century, so many pregnancies with so few live births was exceptional. Despite her continued efforts to conceive again, there were no more pregnancies after 1700. A pelvic infection may have cut short her fertility far before the usual seventeenth-century age for menopause.[22]

What was wrong with Princess Anne that only three of her babies lived to be baptized and none lived to survive her? A number of explanations, none of them satisfactory, have been offered over the years. Contemporaries of Anne and her consort might have pointed out that their marital union violated the common belief that prolific marriages were those between opposites; the Princess and George were too alike in their reticent, stolid ways. Augustan Age physicians differed over whether or not maternal impressions could affect the unborn child.[23] Since Anne's doctors thought that pregnancy was a condition somewhere between sickness and health, their advice focused mainly on the mother's digestive problems. The diet and purges prescribed for constipation and febrile illnesses probably killed a large number of seventeenth-century babies. Midwives still recommended that amulets like the "eagle stone" (iron oxides) be worn during pregnancy to prevent miscarriage and held during delivery near the "privy parts" to draw out the child and the "after burthen." Elizabeth Cellier, a proponent of midwife regulation, reported in her royal petition of 1687 that in the previous twenty years six thousand women had died in childbirth and more than five thousand infants of less than a month old had been buried; two-thirds of those deaths she attributed to lack of midwifery skill.[24] Of course, royalty did not rely on "wise women" for their deliveries; Anne had the best *accoucheurs*.

More modern condemnation of the treatment visited on Anne has focused on her physicians' clinging to Galen's outdated theories on pregnancy. Despite the triumph of practical medicine over ancient principles, Augustan doctors still believed that the fetus was nurtured by menstrual blood in the womb, which later was diverted into milk. They thought that corrupt menstrual blood or a bad womb could cause scabby, measly babies.[25] Although one critic of Anne's obstetrical treatment has suggested that today a caesarean section would be performed on a patient with a possible pelvic abnormality, the first caesarean section from which the mother recovered did not take place in England until 1773, when Charles White demanded that surgical cleanliness pertain also to obstetrics.[26] Amazing as it seems, observing the patient's symptoms did not become *de rigeur* until the publication in 1707 of Sir John Floyer's *The Physician's Pulse Watch*, which encouraged physicians to examine their charges more closely.[27]

However, more than the treatment Princess Anne received must have been involved in the deaths of her children, and, despite Cellier's claims, there had been a marked improvement during the seventeenth century in the ratio of fetal deaths to christenings from six times to what it is in modern industrialized countries to less than double; Anne's register of failed pregnancies far exceeds the norm.[28] Twentieth-century historians provide an array of ideas explaining Anne's litany of loss. Rhesus incompatibility or some other blood-group antigens might be the culprit, some have submitted; by a second pregnancy, sufficient antibodies develop in the mother's bloodstream to cause hemolytic disease in the fetus and subsequent stillbirths.[29] But Gloucester, who lived the longest, was Anne's sixth child, and most of her pregnancies ended in miscarriage. James Kemble has concluded that Anne had a deformed pelvis and Hester Chapman postulates that a "dropsical" infection developed during her first pregnancy caused the miscarriages and premature deliveries, several of which, she states, were of hydrocephalic babies. R. Scott Stevenson insists that Anne's consort had syphilis, perhaps carried in his Danish line, producing hydrocephalus in young Gloucester.[30] Of course, Anne's sister was also cursed with miscarriages and beset with sore eyes for which the Danes cannot be blamed.

Jack Dewhurst rejects these explanations and the labeling of Anne's failed pregnancies as miscarriages, asserting instead that in seven of eleven of the purported miscarriages the fetus was carried to viability and was born dead some time later. Dewhurst postulates intra-uterine growth retardation due to placental insufficiency as a likely cause of Anne's reproductive tragedy. Often associated with raised blood pressure in the mother, if the placenta is poorly formed or if some of its blood vessels become thrombosed, the fetus may die before the end of the pregnancy or be born very small and sickly.[31] Another diagnosis has been porphyria, a hereditary metabolic disorder that can be traced back to Mary, Queen of Scots, and was observed in the characteristic purple urine of James I by his royal physician, Dr. Mayerne. The malady manifested itself most famously in the madness of George III, a collateral relative much further removed from the early Stuarts than Queen Anne.[32] Finally, Queen Anne's lifelong medical problems, reproductive and otherwise, have often been ascribed by others to her father. The verdict has persisted that James II infected both of his wives and eleven of his fifteen legitimate children with venereal disease. Syphilis, the "great imitator," has many faces and mimics the features of other diseases including gout, psoriasis, gastric distress, and sore eyes, so while it may be easy to dismiss the diagnosis of congenital syphilis as the product of Whig propagandists, there could be merit to the syphilis hypothesis.[33] However, despite persuasive arguments by historians and biographers seeking to understand Anne's reproductive tribulation and the consequent end of the Stuart dynasty, no single explanation is without flaw or dependence on tenuous conjecture.

The symptoms of what Anne's physicians called chronic gout commenced in 1698, a most unusual malady for a thirty-three-year old woman. She characterized herself in a letter to Sarah that year as "a perfect cripple" with gout in her knee and foot. By her coronation, she wrote, "she was so lame that she could hardly walk the length of a room, and that with two sticks."[34] Physicians thought females escaped the torture of gout because they did not drink excessive amounts of wine and ale, and because their menstrual discharges gave them some immunity. Of course, Anne was a monarch, like her predecessor Elizabeth I with "the heart and stomach of a king."[35] Men, stout and indolent like Queen Anne, developed gout, observers opined, therefore she suffered because of her unwomanly intemperance. Anne grew fat as she aged, due to an excessive fondness for eating and a violent antipathy for exercise. She was gluttonous, even in grief; card playing and hunting from a specially designed cart were her only forms of recreation. For her use at Windsor, carpenters built a chair with pulleys to hoist her from floor to floor and a machine to lift her from her coach. Doctors attributed gout to indigestion due to overeating that became manifest in interior putrefaction, which traveled all over the body in hideous attacks; some believed gout was caused by vitiated lymph discharged from the brain through the nerves in the extremities.[36] Besides the monstrous swelling, gout produced grotesque postures and flatulent contortions, and crampy "gout in the stomach" that could move to the head, a condition for which Queen Anne was treated frequently.[37]

Anne often received therapy for what was thought to be erysipelas, an acute inflammation of the skin that can strike other parts of the body. For this malady she called upon the prescriptions of former surgeon Daniel Turner, a licentiate of the College of Physicians. The inventor of Turner's cerate, an oil, wax, and calamine mixture, he wrote extensively on skin diseases, advocating the treatment of shingles by applying blood from the tail of a black cat. Turner's prescriptions for Anne's complexion must have had little effect, for in her later years the queen appeared in public slathered in cosmetics.[38] Presumably she did not avail herself of another of Turner's specialties, the treatment of syphilis and gleets, an infected urethral discharge usually due to gonorrhea.[39]

Queen Anne sampled whatever remedies might be proffered for her eye troubles, even seeking out the services of quacks. William Read, an itinerant tailor who advertised that he could cure wens, harelips, and cataracts, became Anne's oculist-in-ordinary. Inventor of styptic water to be used in place of cauterization, he claimed cancer removal as another of his specialties, but in his book, *A Short But Exact Account of All the Diseases Incident to the Eyes*, Read combined conventional Galenic treatment with his own recipes for eye health. In the book, he corrected the errors of other oculists, especially those whose remedies "heat the brain" and therefore dull the sight; he recommended drinking beer in the morning, to help those with "dry brains," plus the usual bleeding and cupping. Read described the use of a "couch needle" to remove coagulated, viscous humors and prescribed an eyewash of sulphur, turpentine, vivum, and honey of roses. He became very wealthy through advertisements in *The Tatler* and, according to Swift, was able to afford lavish parties where good punch was served in golden vessels.[40] Queen Anne likewise consulted Roger Grant, the quack oculist of Wapping whose advertising tenacity her sister had weathered. When Gloucester developed badly swollen eyes, Anne consulted former royal apothecary James St. Amand and personally called on Dr. Luke Rugeley, an aged physician in Bloomsbury who claimed to have a secret liquid for curing sore eyes.[41]

Since Anne often complained of ague, she spent much of her time confined to a hot, airless room, dosed with an herbal concoction of hart's tongue, colt's foot, and comfrey, or with pills made from tar and elecampane. By Anne's era, however, Jesuits' bark had become the standard ague treatment, regarded by most doctors as safe and effective for periodic fevers. Taken over prolonged periods of time and in significant doses, however, the bark may produce cinchonism, a systemic poisoning. Symptoms include ringing in the ears, dizziness, blurring of vision or blindness, rashes, and a decrease in blood pressure. In addition, and most important for Anne, quinine induces uterine contractions and can cause spontaneous miscarriage in pregnant patients.[42] Robert Talbor, the man most closely associated with the post-Restoration popularity of cinchona, had been aware of the potentially deleterious side effects of the bark. In his book, *The English Remedy*, he catalogued convulsions, seizures, and constipation as possible results if the drug was administered by someone unfamiliar with pharmaceutics.[43]

Nevertheless, Talbor's directions for dosages to be given to gravid patients recommended stronger than usual concentrations of cinchona powder in a lemon syrup, four to six drachms twice daily. Ironically, the remedy was not to be used by women "during their courses," the one time during their monthly cycles when there was no danger of inducing miscarriage.[44] Cautionary notes are now routinely included in over-the-counter quinine remedies for nocturnal leg cramps. Consumers today are advised not to ingest such products if pregnant or of child-bearing capacity. Such warnings were not available, of course, to those seventeenth- and eighteenth-century women who routinely took massive doses of Jesuits' bark. Surely an important question to be asked by future researchers concerns the correlation between the taking of cinchona by pregnant women and miscarriage. Queen Anne herself may offer the startling example of the age: the wealthy, frequently pregnant patient whose recurrent bouts of ague were treated with huge doses of the bark. Modern demographers have noted the higher incidence of miscarriage among the wealthier classes of early modern England, but even seventeenth-century observers agreed that poor women had fewer problems in childbirth.[45] Some of the many miscarriages endured by aristocratic women may have been attributable to the ingestion of quinine. Although a number of physical problems could be the cause of Queen Anne's reproductive woes, indiscriminate use of quinine cannot be ruled out; nor should the vertigo of her young son, the Duke of Gloucester, be attributed solely to arrested hydrocephalus or rickets. He, too, received massive doses of Jesuits' Bark.[46]

As princess and heiress presumptive, Anne was attended by such eminent doctors as Richard Lower, John Radcliffe, and the venerable Charles Scarburgh; they shared many professional associations, but often disagreed on diagnoses or treatment. After his daughter's first unsuccessful pregnancy, King James appointed the eminent if curmudgeonly Radcliffe to attend Anne along with Scarburgh and Lower; the last-mentioned was said to be the princess' favorite physician until his death in 1691. Consulted often on Anne's gravid condition, Lower provided a decisive opinion that she ought to take the waters at Bath during her pregnancy in 1688. Scarburgh disagreed with the treatment, but Anne opted to follow Lower's advice, thereby enabling her to be conveniently absent from birth in London of her Catholic stepbrother.[47] At about the same time that the trio began ministering to Anne, Scarburgh also accepted an appointment as physician to Prince George, an assignment he carried out until his death at the age of eighty-eight in 1694.[48]

No physician epitomized the quarrelsome and fractious nature of Stuart medicine more than Dr. Radcliffe. His outspoken disapproval of the Glorious Revolution did as much eventually to undermine his credibility with Anne as his intemperate categorization of her as a hypochondriac. When Anne's ailments were described to him as gout in the stomach that became gout all over, Radcliffe sarcastically added "excepting the joints."[49] The foremost physician of his day, Radcliffe also ministered to other members of the royal household. In 1691 Radcliffe saved Gloucester, then two years old, from a serious illness; the boy's family was so grateful that the doctor was given 1,000 guineas. Princess Anne recommended him to her friends, once telling Sarah Churchill that since Radcliffe was going out of town for a while, they had better get whatever medicines they needed from him before he left.[50] In addition to his care for the royals, Radcliffe had a lucrative London practice, bolstered by support from the apothecaries for whose status he showed respect by writing his prescriptions in English, thereby giving them standing as attendants with knowledge denied the public. His Fellows at the College went so far as to expel him for not using Latin directions, but they readmitted him upon payment of a forty shilling fine.[51] Radcliffe disdained the philosophical study associated with erudite members of his profession, and boasted about the more practical contents of his library: herbs, vials, and a skeleton.[52] Radcliffe's bedside manner also left something to be desired. His habit of speaking his mind even to royalty outraged his patients and made them indignant; William III never forgave Radcliffe for his intemperate remarks, but he did continue to use the doctor's prescriptions.

Like many physicians of the Augustan age, Radcliffe conducted his business in one of London's many coffee houses or taverns. His consultations were held at the Bull's Head Tavern and he advertised his remedies in broadsides and pamphlets. His recipe for cough syrup calls for conserve of roses, gilly flowers, Venice treacle, and flower of brimstone, washed down by the ubiquitous asses' milk. He prescribed purges and "restorative" cordials for his patients, including one consisting of ox flesh, marrow, and prune broth.[53] Radcliffe, a lifelong bachelor, grew wealthy with his medical success, acquiring estates in the north of England and mansions in and around London; paintings by Rubens and Rembrandt hung in his house in Bloomsbury Square.

Radcliffe, something of a specialist in children's diseases, was assigned regular responsibility for taking care of little Gloucester, whose delicate health was problematic from the start.[54] Not all physicians recommended wet-nursing. Some, like Henry Newcome in *The Compleat Mother* (1695), deplored the custom and urged women, especially "those of rank and quality," to nurse their own babies. However, most aristocratic women handed over their newborns to suckle at the breast of another. Choosing the right wet-nurse, whose milk and morals could help or hinder the baby's development, fell to Gloucester's father, who held interviews for the job. Critics carped that he had chosen poorly. The boy's head grew too big, a sign of hydrocephalus, and after his third birthday fluid had to be drawn from time to time. Gloucester's legs were rickety, and as he developed through childhood, he had difficulty climbing stairs; his locomotion was never stable and if he fell, he could not get up. Prince George could not understand his son's physical weakness and wanted to beat the boy during these episodes of debility. When Gloucester was ill with ague, Radcliffe prescribed quinine, which made him vomit violently. When he caught whooping cough, the doctor ordered his head shaved, blistered, and dressed.[55]

On his eleventh birthday, Gloucester became overheated and fatigued from dancing; he was bled, still the standard practice for such indulgence. Dr. Radcliffe, who had been dismissed by Anne as the duke's regular physician for his rudeness the year before, was appalled to learn that the child had been bled, and when called to see the boy diagnosed scarlet fever. Often at war with his medical brethren, Radcliffe was one of a few Stuart era physicians who opposed wholesale bleeding, preferring the shaving of heads and blistering for treatment of fevers.[56] His fear that Gloucester was doomed proved true; six days later, the boy "died hard, shouting and chattering." Autopsied, Gloucester's body, "turned green and yellow," revealed that a "malignant fever" killed him.[57] His corpse was ferried by royal barge to the House of Lords and on to burial in Westminster Abbey. His mother was described as dry-eyed and stunned; some said that she believed her bereavement was sent as a visible punishment from heaven for her cruelty to her father.

Despite the prominence of the royal physicians who tended Gloucester and the household, they had their critics, as evidenced by a pamphlet published in February 1702 accusing Anne's doctors of deliberate malpractice. The broadside, entitled "Some Few Queries about the Preparations of Making Way for a Prince of Wales in the Year 1687," charged those who had attended Princess

Anne with destroying her babies and those of Queen Mary II through the medicines prescribed. The anonymous author accused Catholics of being at the heart of this murderous conspiracy, offering as evidence the successful pregnancy of Lady Powys, who followed the same regimen as Anne for eight days, but stopped it and had a healthy son.[58] Anne herself unfairly blamed Radcliffe for Gloucester's death, and refused to patronize him in any capacity after 1700, though the doctor's reputation sustained him in London. Sidney Godolphin, Anne's Lord Treasurer and a prominent Whig, tried to persuade her after her accession to reinstate Radcliffe as a royal doctor despite his politics, but the queen rejected the idea.[59]

After Gloucester's death, Anne referred to herself, using an informal pseudonym employed in correspondence with her friend Sarah Churchill, as "your poor, unfortunate Morley."[60] The death of Gloucester meant that when Anne became queen, she did so knowing that her successor was likely to be the head of the House of Hanover, and since the Electress Sophia was over seventy, the crown would probably pass to Prince George, the cousin who had spurned her as a wife. A theme of Anne's twelve-year reign would be keeping him and his relations out of England and out of the political spotlight as long as possible; according to one governmental official, this was "common enough amongst princes when their subjects begin to make more than ordinary court to their successors and when people begin to adore the rising sun."[61] The queen used the scandalous marital relations of George and his wife, as well as his Low Church sympathies, to keep him and his entourage at a distance regardless of the liaison efforts by King William's physician, Dr. Hutton, and the Whig party to bring the Hanoverians over to England. Despite Anne's loathing for her German relative, she was determined to avoid a Catholic heir and reminded her subjects that their cherished freedoms would be lost in the arbitrary "designs of a Papist pretender."[62]

Notwithstanding the greatness of Britain's power, its monarch suffered intensely during her time in office. While in England in 1706–7 negotiating a Treaty of Union with Scotland, one of the great accomplishments of Queen Anne's reign, Sir John Clerk met with the sovereign and had an opportunity to observe her on a number of occasions. He remarked on how pathetic she looked: her face red and spotty, her dress negligent, surrounded with "plaisters, cataplasms and rags," her foot tied up with "pultis and nasty bandages." She appeared, he felt, "as the meanest of her subjects," and he pitied her for her solitary life and frequent illnesses.[63] Clearly, Queen Anne needed a great deal of medical attention. Four physicians-in-ordinary at a time served her and her court; they were ranked by number and given graduated salaries of £400, £300, £250, and £200 per annum. From 1689 extra physicians to the Person were also appointed by royal warrant, usually one at a time, at a salary of £200. Queen Anne ignored the reduction in medical personnel ordered by her predecessor in May 1690.[64] Although two physicians to the household usually attended the later Stuarts, the office was inexplicably left vacant during all of

Anne's reign. After 1685 one serjeant-surgeon received a fixed salary of nearly £400 per annum; Queen Anne also left the office of Surgeon to the Person vacant, but used two royal apothecaries. Remuneration varied during her reign between £320 and £372 to cover an apothecary's salary and all supplies, down considerably from the £500 paid to both the apothecaries to William and Mary.

Sir Thomas Millington, greatly respected physician to William and Mary, was reappointed by Queen Anne in 1702; he stayed on until his death two years later. Likewise, she retained Thomas Lawrence in his post, which he held along with physician-generalship to the army until he died in 1714. Her Majesty's first new medical appointment went to Edward Hannes, named Physician to the Person in July 1702. Hannes had attended Gloucester during the boy's terminal illness and headed the team performing his post-mortem. His published account of the dissection of Gloucester's body provoked an unpleasant anonymous satire, *Doctor Hannes Dissected* (London: 1700), but two years later Hannes functioned on King William's autopsy team. An arch-enemy of Radcliffe, who called him the son of a basket-maker, Hannes incurred the disapproval of the Royal College of Physicians by ignoring mandatory meetings of the Fellows and by employing disreputable practices, like stopping carriages in the street, to get more patients.[65] Nevertheless, he continued to practice with impunity and was knighted in 1705 at Windsor. Ill health removed Hannes from the medical spotlight after 1709.[66]

On the same day that Hannes was named an aulic doctor, Martin Lister became one, too. A man of many interests, Lister enjoyed Stuart favor throughout his career. He studied at St. John's College, Cambridge, before the Restoration, becoming a Fellow there by royal mandate in 1660. After receiving a master of arts degree, Lister practiced medicine in York without an M.D. for twenty years. A medical degree was essential to acceptance in the capital, so before moving to London, Lister obtained one from Oxford in 1683 upon the recommendation of the Chancellor; Fellowship in the Royal College of Physicians followed in 1687.[67] Lister's important studies in geology and natural history earned him membership in the Royal Society, which has preserved his work on shells and spiders. In 1698 and 1699, Lister attended William Bentinck, Earl of Portland, on a mission from William III to the court of France, and thereafter counted Portland as a patron.[68] Anne knew Lister by reputation, as he had earlier publicized the salubrious effects on gouty patients of mineral waters, such as the queen had experienced at Bath.[69] Not everyone found him a figure deserving of unstinting respect. After Lister published a book about the "soups and sauces of the ancients," William King responded with *The Art of Cookery* (1709), a satirical take on Horace's *Art of Poetry*, skewed to ridicule Lister.

The Scotsman David Hamilton had a large practice and a fine reputation as an *accoucheur* when Queen Anne, past needing those services, appointed him third physician-in-ordinary in 1703. Hamilton, who received an M.D. from Reims, also published in the area of psychological medicine, but is perhaps best remembered for the diary chronicling his years at court. His moderate Whiggery made him useful for political errands, like acting as liaison between Anne and Sarah Churchill during the final acrimonious days of their disintegrating friendship. He became the chief negotiator in the ousting of the Duchess from her various court offices, speaking with the queen on fifty-five occasions in 1710 about the situation, and concluding that anxiety was wearing down the monarch. The deaths of Gloucester in 1700 and Prince George eight years later, coupled with her estrangement from Sarah, devitalized Queen Anne, and although he marveled at how her personal piety had maintained her, he thought that she needed a true friend upon whom she could rely "for strength of mind." Dr. Hamilton worried that all the political disquiet around Anne might cause a "translation" of her gout, and he often interceded with courtiers not to tease or take advantage of Her Majesty.[70]

Perhaps because of his genuine devotion to Queen Anne and personal service to her, Hamilton chafed under the title "third physician-in-ordinary," and was relieved to move up to the number two slot when Martin Lister died in 1712. He feared that John Shadwell, who was a partisan of the Hanoverians, the dynasty waiting in the wings to succeed the last Stuart, might outrank him in a new household, despite Shadwell's being only fourth in line under Anne. Rather than bear the indignity of an aulic demotion, Hamilton recorded that he would prefer instead to be the sole doctor to another member of the royal family and when the German entourage arrived in England, he accordingly solicited such a position.[71]

His prescriptions for Anne's various ailments included recommending that she take millipedes powder in fresh butter internally for her gout, scurvy, and eye trouble. Hamilton viewed "that little insect called millipedes" as "the next esteemed specific," useful also for "curing any sore throat." For dropsy Hamilton suggested drinking iron filings brewed in boiling water.[72] In Hamilton's opinion, the queen's gout had been particularly exacerbated when she was agitated during her menstrual period, and, confirming his earlier prognosis, cited stress as a specific cause of her deadly seizure in 1714, noting that in addition to her feverish condition, Anne suffered from headache and nosebleeds.[73] Years later, Hamilton published a dissertation on miliary fever, a disease that took its name from "pustles or vesicles in some sort, resembling the form of gromwel seeds." The disorder targeted those with decrepit constitutions, he wrote, those with too spare a diet, with blood too thin, and too weak-minded, especially women and effeminate men. After Queen Anne's death, Hamilton, while minimizing his prowess as a man-midwife, received the appointment he desired as physician to Caroline, Princess of Wales. He speculated in securities, and apparently lost £80,000 in the 1720 South Sea Bubble.[74]

John Arbuthnot, perhaps better known for creating John Bull in his political writing, prescribed for Prince George when Anne's consort became ill at Epsom. The queen later remembered his skill, and in 1705 appointed him an extra physician assigned to the prince, who suffered from asthma.[75] Alas,

Arbuthnot's medical talent did not save George from death by dropsy in the autumn of 1708. For all his faults, Queen Anne loved her husband and had persuaded Parliament to agree to settle £100,000 on him annually in case she predeceased him. During Prince George's final months, she nursed him in a small house at Windsor near the park entrance, and she took him to Bath in late August. He developed a violent cold and cough, which irritated his asthma and kept him sleepless. The queen was so distraught that she even consented to call in Dr. Radcliffe, who, as usual, said he had been consulted too late. Prince George died a few days later, aged fifty-five. The lack of concern for Prince George evident in the heartless behavior of the Duchess of Marlborough, from whom Anne was already somewhat estranged, and in the actions of other prominent Whigs upset the queen. Even as her consort lay dying there were demands that he step down at the Admiralty; three months after his death, when she was plainly disconsolate with grief, members of Parliament exhorted her to marry again.[76]

Despite the calamity of the prince's demise, Arbuthnot moved up in rank to Physician to the Person on the retirement of Hannes in 1709. A Scot holding a medical degree from St. Andrews, Arbuthnot taught mathematics after moving to London and wrote a paper on the male-female birth ratio that appeared in the *Philosophical Transactions* of the Royal Society, to which he had been elected a Fellow in 1704.[77] Friendly with Jonathan Swift, Arbuthnot dabbled in Tory politics, authoring several popular tracts aimed at the Whigs. He also helped found the famous Scriblerus Club, became a Fellow of the Royal College of Physicians and a physician to Chelsea Hospital. Arbuthnot, whom Swift called "the Queen's favorite," remained as Anne's physician, taking lodgings at St. James's.[78] Toward the end of his career, he penned the seriously scientific *Concerning the Nature of Ailments* (1731) and the *Essay Concerning the Effects of Air on Human Bodies* (1733), the latter prompted, he wrote, by curiosity about weather and disease. In these works, Arbuthnot catalogued the necessity of chewing well, the perils of nightly dew, and the evil effects of liquor and coffee. Highly praised and admired by his contemporaries, Arbuthnot is remembered for his medical skill, political satire, and literary criticism.[79]

Queen Anne appointed Sir John Shadwell, son of William III's poet laureate, to Arbuthnot's vacated position as a physician extraordinary in 1709. Shadwell next succeeded Lister in 1712 as Physician to the Person. Born in London, he was educated at All Souls, Oxford, and received his M.D. in 1701 following his attendance on Charles Montagu, Earl of Manchester, Anne's envoy to the court of Louis XIV from 1699 to 1701. Shadwell enjoyed an illustrious medical career and was a Fellow of the Royal Society. His letters to his friend and patron, Charles Talbot, Duke of Shrewsbury, recount the queen's last year, one in which Shadwell agreed with Hamilton that Queen Anne was subject to unbearable tensions brought on by bickering servants. At Christmas in 1713, the queen suffered from fever and a painful infection in the inner portion of her right thigh. Shadwell argued that Her Majesty grappled not with gout but with "a violent inflammatory fever from a translation of the gout." He prognosticated the danger of an "imposthumation" in the queen's leg and along with Dr. Lawrence recommended bleeding.[80] Dr. Arbuthnot overruled this diagnosis and said that an ague was at the root of the queen's fever, administering several doses of Jesuits' bark. Although Anne recovered from her winter illness and by spring addressed Parliament, her physicians prescribed snake root to fortify her for the long afternoon's activities. Once again, Shadwell demurred, instead calling for traditional cupping and bleeding to prevent "too great a load of ill-humors from falling upon the leg." Though the queen consumed a large meal of a whole chicken the following day, Shadwell remained worried about her health. He believed that the pressures of political life exacerbated her symptoms and, when in July 1714, the queen complained of lost appetite, lack of sleep, and low spirits, Shadwell feared the worst. As Anne's condition deteriorated and she slipped into unconsciousness, Shadwell speculated that the "gouty humor [was] translating itself upon the brain." After Queen Anne's death, having ingratiated himself with the House of Hanover, Shadwell continued his service to the crown in the households of George I, who knighted him in 1715, and George II.[81]

The name of Hans Sloane is familiar to those who know the Chelsea district in London, for its streets and square commemorate his celebrity as president of the Royal College of Physicians and the Royal Society from 1727–41, succeeding Sir Isaac Newton. Born in Ireland where his father was head of a colony of Scots settled in Ulster by James I, Sloane studied on the continent and procured his medical degree at Orange in southern France. He moved to London in 1684. At the suggestion of Peter Barwick, he went to the Caribbean in 1687 as physician to the Duke of Albemarle, then Governor of Jamaica. His gathering of eight hundred samples of flora and fauna, obtained over the next two years, and his drawings of the things he could not bring home, provided the basis for the British Museum collection.[82] He considered himself a natural historian and wrote on life, death, and disease in the West Indies: in his *Discourse on the State of Health in Jamaica,* Sloane remarked on the absence of certain illnesses and the ease with which Caribbean women gave birth, though he did believe that the natives bathed too much. After his return from Jamaica, Sloane helped to establish an informal botany club at the Temple Coffee-House, which met to encourage the exchange of botanical information and to identify exotic species; club members probably went on botanizing expeditions in the nearby countryside.[83] Later, Sloane was honored by membership in the French, Spanish, and Russian Academies of Sciences and he corresponded with academicians who conveyed to him news of discoveries being made throughout continental Europe while he, in turn, supplied them with the *Philosophical Transactions* of the Royal Society.[84] His library of over forty-two thousand books and countless manuscripts was kept together by a Parliamentary purchase of £20,000 after he offered his collection to the nation.[85]

Due to an early illness, Sloane throughout his life believed in sobriety and moderation, which endeared him to Queen Anne, who made him Extra Physician to the Person in February 1712. As well as fulfilling his aulic duties, Sloane served as physician to Christ's Hospital. Along with his apothecary, James St. Amand, Sloane often discussed health matters with the queen, especially her persistent eye problems. In a pamphlet that he wrote later, *An Account of an Efficacious Medicine for Distempers of the Eyes*, Sloane mentioned investigating the cures of Anne's oculist, Luke Rugeley, whose papers, along with Dr. Mayerne's, Sloane had acquired. Both Rugeley and Dr. Stokeham, physician to William III, recommended a concoction that supposedly produced many cures; Sloane reported that it called for a variety of powdered ingredients—tutty (zinc oxide), lapis, hematite (bloodstone), aloes, and pearls—blended together in a mortar with viper's grease to make a liniment. Sloane preferred spring water for eye-baths, and admonished sufferers not to apply coverings lest they make their eyes too warm.

Sloane was not without his own critics, particularly for his use of mercury to treat syphilis. One of those critics was Daniel Turner, the physician Queen Anne had consulted about her skin problems. Turner, originally a member of the Barber-Surgeons, had been granted permission to leave that Company and joined the Royal College of Physicians in 1711. Turner asked that Sloane meet with him to examine a close relative who was losing his sight, perhaps as a result of the "French pox," but later he had cause to disparage Sloane's apparent use of quicksilver for the man's symptoms. Turner conducted a post-mortem that produced half a pound of mercury from the patient's intestines. Turner expounded on the dangers of mercury for use in venereal diseases in published medical notes that refuted practices like Sloane's. Dr. John Woodward, another who publicly belittled Sloane, may have done so out of jealousy; he was a rival for influence at the Royal Society.[86]

Sloane's career did not end with the last of the Stuarts. He enjoyed even more prestige and prosperity in the years after Anne, being influential with George I's ministers and busy in his profession. His house must have been a sort of lending library, as Sloane frequently received letters from colleagues requesting the loan of certain books on subjects as diverse as the geography of Fifeshire and curious plants.[87] As medical adviser to the House of Hanover, Sloane supported inoculations for the military, and even performed such procedures on members of the royal family. A Whig and a philanthropist, he worked as Physician-General to the army, wed the daughter of a wealthy London alderman, and lived to see his children married into the Cadogan and Stanley families. He died in 1753 at the age of ninety-two.

In addition to the royal doctors on regular appointment, other physicians treated the queen and her court. During Anne's final year of life, these medical consultants included such established practitioners as Richard Mead, Samuel Garth, and Richard Blackmore. Mead, Whig counterpart to Arbuthnot, was physician to St. Thomas's Hospital and vice-president of the Royal Society. A fellow of the Royal College of Physicians who held a medical degree from Padua, Mead's friendship with Radcliffe and his myriad scientific publications on poison assured his reputation.[88] He inherited Radcliffe's practice, house, and gold-headed cane, the famous emblem of superiority among the College Fellows awarded to the most prestigious London doctor until the nineteenth century.[89] Mead startled his colleagues at the Royal College of Physicians by swallowing snake venom to prove that poison needed to be introduced into the blood before it did harm. He lectured on anatomy to the Barber-Surgeons, declined the presidency of the Royal College of Physicians, citing advanced age, and later received an appointment as George II's physician-in-ordinary. He became an expert on preventing plague, and along with Arbuthnot and Hans Sloane gave advice on quarantine regulations to George I's Privy Council. He presented a cogent recommendation for dividing the city, educating searchers, and providing examinations of premises. Mead often prescribed at Batson's coffee house on the basis on his apothecary's report without actually seeing his patients, charging ten shillings instead of his usual fee of £1 for a house call. When Dr. John Woodward denounced Mead for this practice, Mead challenged his detractor to a duel and silenced him.[90] While on the Board of Governors of the London Foundling Hospital, Mead advocated a national health council for sanitary reforms and pharmaceutical dispensaries in hospitals.

Samuel Garth, the *Dispensary* poet, was a good friend of Sloane and a prominent Whig. Born in Durham in 1660 and educated at Cambridge, Garth became associated through the Kit-Kat Club with the most prominent literary and political men in London including Richard Steele, William Congreve, Sidney Godolphin, and the Duke of Marlborough. Garth was the only medical member and was probably brought into the club by his publisher, Jacob Tonson. A Fellow of the Royal College of Physicians from 1693, Garth delivered the Gulstonian lecture in 1694, an honor given to the most respected of the junior Fellows, but he was passed over shortly thereafter as Regius Professor of Physick at Cambridge in favor of Thomas Green, the choice of the Archbishop of Canterbury. Garth and John Dryden developed a close friendship, perusing and subscribing to one another's works. Dryden not only read *The Dispensary*, but recorded his admiration for the College Dispensarians.[91] When Dryden died in 1700, it was Dr. Garth who helped provide a suitable mausoleum for the former poet laureate and delivered the eulogy; some thought Garth would be Dryden's natural literary successor.

Dr. Garth was consulted during the fatal illness of Prince George and exchanged many notes with Sloane on medical matters, but he spent most of his time writing verse and translating classics like Ovid's *Metamorphoses* and Plutarch's *Life of Otho*.[92] As a staunch supporter of the war against France and its commander, the Duke of Marlborough, Garth visited the Duke's military headquarters in Holland in 1711, bringing letters from Whig partisans in England. When the doctor returned to London, the Tory campaign against the war and the Duke reached a crescendo and Queen Anne was persuaded to dismiss Marlborough from all his offices. Garth was unhappy with the Treaty of Utrecht, negotiated by the Tories in 1713, and expressed his discontent in a poem, "On Her Majesty's Statue in St. Paul's Churchyard," a reproof to those who settled for a peace too favorable to the French.[93] Following Anne's death, in appreciation for his Hanoverian enthusiasm, Garth was knighted by George I and made physician-in-ordinary to the king and Physician-General to the army, posts he held until his death in 1718.[94]

Another Whig physician who tried his hand at verse and prose, with indifferent success, was Sir Richard Blackmore, an attendant with Queen Anne at the end. A member of the Royal College of Physicians for thirty-five years, his enthusiasm for the Glorious Revolution had made him a suitable royal physician to William III, who knighted him in 1697; he held the post of Physician to the Person until the king's death. Though some of his colleagues in the profession might have demurred, Blackmore was considerably more successful as a medical practitioner than a poet, one of the most prosperous of his time. Some of his fortune probably came from speculation, as evidenced by a letter he wrote to Sloane in 1721 about "running loans by lottery."[95] Like Dr. Radcliffe, Blackmore served as governor of St. Bartholomew's hospital and made it his special task to supervise the work of the institution's apothecaries. Blackmore wrote up the report in 1702 on William's post-mortem, conducted at Kensington at the behest of Queen Anne's Privy Council. The examining doctors concluded that the king died of pneumonia after breaking his collarbone, a report that no doubt relieved the queen and her government. Blackmore composed many dull poems for public consumption as well as lengthy articles for his professional colleagues: in 1725, his service to Queen Anne long finished, he wrote a dissertation on the spleen; in 1726, he published a treatise on "Gout, Rheumatism and the King's Evil," in which he recommended surgery, not the royal touch, for easy tumors; and in 1727 he published on dropsy. Blackmore died in 1729.[96]

Although Queen Anne never needed a major operation, she experienced the usual amount of bleeding, cupping, and blistering inflicted on patients in the Augustan Age. Anne's royal surgeons included such celebrated names as Charles Bernard, Ambrose Dickens, and Thomas Gardiner. Bernard, Anne's serjeant-surgeon from 1703 to 1710, rose up through the ranks in the customary way. He apprenticed to Henry Boone in Croyden for seven years, was a member of the Barber-Surgeons' Company in 1677, and became Master in 1703. A High Churchman and a Tory, he was surgeon at St. Bartholomew's Hospital from 1686 until his death, while his older brother, Dr. Francis Bernard, who ministered to James II, wrote prescriptions for the hospital.[97] Serious about the importance of dissection to surgeons, Charles Bernard got the sheriff of London dismissed for not delivering the bodies of hanged criminals to the surgeons on time![98] When sold at auction, the Bernard family's marvelous library brought newsworthy prices and the attention of Jonathan Swift. Charles Bernard died in 1710.[99]

Ambrose Dickens was originally certified to practice as an apothecary, an indication how some of the lines in the medical profession had blurred by the

Augustan Age. He became the queen's serjeant surgeon in 1710, succeeding Bernard, whose surgical apprentice he had been and whose son-in-law he had become. He attended Anne's autopsy in 1714, and continued royal service under the first two Hanoverians during an uncommonly long tenure until his death in 1747. Master of the Barber-Surgeons' Company in 1729, he also functioned as surgeon to Westminster Hospital from 1721 and St. George's from 1733. Upon the separation of surgeons from barbers in 1745, Dickens became an assistant, comparable to a member of the board of directors of the surgeons, and a frequent examiner of license applicants.[100]

Although Queen Anne left the office of Surgeon to the Person vacant during her reign, she called upon the Gardiner family to fill the post of Surgeon to the Household. Thomas Gardiner, a holdover from William and Mary's regime, continued in that capacity under Anne. She referred to him as her chief surgeon, and it was Gardiner who screened applicants for the royal touch at Bath in 1702. Later that year he wrote a long letter to his friend Henry Watkins, in the service of the Duke of Marlborough in combat in Flanders, telling Watkins news of family, friends, and a bountiful cabbage crop.[101] In 1707 Gardiner stepped aside so that his son William could fill his shoes. William Gardiner remained as an aulic surgeon until 1716.

Queen Anne employed two Apothecaries to the Person, James Chase and Joseph Pitt. Though payments to the royal apothecaries had been delayed during earlier administrations, by Anne's reign this bureaucratic delinquency had decreased.[102] Joseph Pitt ministered to Anne's court for its first two years, receiving a salary of £115 plus £205 for medicines dispensed. He died early in 1704 and was buried in Hillingdon. Middlesex, where his carved table tomb can be found in the old churchyard of St. John the Baptist. The last Apothecary to the Person was Daniel Malthus, whose apprentice-nephew, Daniel Graham, discharged the same duties for the House of Hanover. Malthus, the son of a vicar and former apothecary to Thomas Sydenham, replaced Pitt as Apothecary to the Person in July 1704 and received the usual salary and expenses, though he made frequent demands for partitioned chests, mixing glasses, and silver vessels for Her Majesty's medicines. Malthus furnished drugs for the royal family at Windsor, Winchester, and Newmarket, and reported on the queen's health to Arbuthnot.

William Jones, second son and apprentice to John Jones, served as Apothecary to the Household during the reign of Anne, as well as at the courts of her predecessor and successor. Jones had asserted his right to the job in 1693 by virtue of a grant of reversion made to his father by Charles II in 1681. Since John Soames claimed the office, too, the younger Jones brought suit in the Exchequer Court and regained the post by patent in 1697, holding it through the reign of William III, whom he accompanied to Flanders in 1702. Jones went with Anne on her official journeys, including a progress to Newmarket in 1707, bitterly complaining about his reduction in salary since her accession. Though his salary sometimes arrived late, Jones continued to function as an aulic apothecary well into the reign of George I, and won some local fame in 1716 after treating a mail delivery boy wounded by a brick that fell off the facade of the London Post Office.[103] Patrick Hepburn was Anne's apothecary in Edinburgh from 1708 at £40 per annum. George I reappointed Hepburn, and his son succeeded him at the same salary.[104]

When Queen Anne was fatally stricken in July 1714, Abigail Hill Masham, the monarch's closest friend after the break with Sarah Churchill, sent for Dr. Radcliffe, but he refused to rush to Anne's bedside, indelicately citing a recent self-administered purgative as his excuse.[105] He doubtless thought the queen was not seriously ill, especially when he heard that she had consumed an inordinate amount of black-heart cherries. More than once Radcliffe pronounced Queen Anne, who suffered so many miscarriages, to be as healthy as anyone; she merely, like other women, often succumbed to "the vapors," apparently dyspepsia.[106] She had, of course, rallied from her Christmas malaise and returned to take up her royal duties. But this time, Anne's multiple ailments combined with enormous emotional strain brought on by political bickering among her councilors. Her spirits low and her usual voracious appetite lost, she canceled a meeting of her cabinet at Kensington scheduled for July 29, reporting herself "dispirited, flushed, and her head full." The next morning, after vomiting and twice convulsing, the queen lost consciousness; when she awoke, she could not speak. The queen revived temporarily under Dr. Arbuthnot's care, and his ministrations received praise from fellow Scriblerus member John Gay in the poem "Shepherd's Week."[107]

But Arbuthnot remained concerned about the queen's pallor, and ordered that her head be shaved and blisters applied; Dr. Sloane advised that Anne be bled, a conventional prescription for apoplexy, and she shed ten ounces.[108] According to apothecary Daniel Malthus, "cupping was used and cephalic medicines inwardly."[109] Following custom, the queen received these treatments before a large number of onlookers, to the chagrin of the patient, but this insured that no mistreatment of the monarch occurred. She weakened further, however, becoming insensible to what was happening around her, and Dr. Mead told John Evelyn that "anybody would have been in her condition, if they had the gout in their head six and thirty hours without anything done to them."[110] She died in the morning of August 1, 1714, at the age of forty-nine. Her autopsy, performed by Dr. Lawrence, revealed little in the internal organs that was remarkable. However, physicians found an ulcer they described as scorbutic. In a diary entry oddly signed as "J. Smith," the name of a moderate Whig leader in the House of Commons, Dr. Shadwell yielded to the opinions of his colleagues and attributed her death to fits of gout.[111] There was no official announcement of Queen Anne's death, but by mid-afternoon on the day of her death, George I was proclaimed King of England, Scotland, and Ireland.

After Queen Anne's death, Dr. Radcliffe, who sat in the House of Commons for Buckinghamshire, found himself the object of much opprobrium, some of it emanating from his fellow members of Parliament. One M.P., an old friend of the doctor's, demanded that he be censured for not waiting upon the queen when summoned. Radcliffe confided to Richard Mead that he had received several anonymous threats and feared an assassination attempt. Radcliffe publicly defended his refusal to attend the dying woman by admitting that, since Anne loathed him, his presence might have caused her more harm than good, but with popular feeling aroused against him, he decided it would be prudent to leave the capital for his house in Surrey.[112] Radcliffe did not survive his queen by many months, and in his will left generous grants to his alma mater, Oxford University, for medical fellowships and for construction of the Radcliffe Infirmary, the Observatory and an extension to the Bodleian Library known as the Radcliffe Camera.[113] Knowing that Radcliffe had denigrated theoretical studies for physicians, a rival London doctor found his beneficence puzzling. Samuel Garth remarked that "for Radcliffe to found a library was about as logical as if a eunuch should found a seraglio." Radcliffe, as a former governor, also bequeathed a gift to St. Bartholomew's Hospital that advantageously "altered the diet for the sick poor."[114] John Radcliffe may have been the most prosperous physician of his time, but, like the profession of medicine itself, he had both passionate admirers and vehement enemies.

Queen Anne died intestate, having refused to sign drafts of wills prepared for her. Her body remained at Kensington Palace for three weeks while preparations were made for burial. Royal apothecary Malthus, who had been at Anne's deathbed, faithfully prepared the queen's body for interment in a coffin that was almost square. After her funeral in Westminster Abbey, which George I insisted take place before his arrival in London, Malthus blended the anointing unguents for the new king's coronation, submitting a bill of £206 for oils, balsams, and perfumed spirits.[115] The first Hanoverian, who spoke no English, arrived to claim his new dominion with ninety people in his entourage including two dwarfs, two ugly mistresses, and two Turkish slaves. His ex-wife, Sophia Dorothea of Celle, did not accompany her husband to England; he had divorced her in 1694 and imprisoned her for life on the grounds that she had committed adultery with Philip von Königsmarck. His son, George, Prince of Wales, was estranged from his father and soon established a counter-court at Leicester House.

In October 1714, the College of Physicians sent King George its stock letter of congratulations and, as before with monarchs who chose to ignore the cue, a reminder of the Fellows' prerogatives.[116] The practice of foreign successors bringing physicians with them to England lingered when the new king brought George Lewis Tessier from Germany, had him naturalized, and named him physician to the household in 1715. He also brought another favorite doctor, Johann George Steigherthal, a Utrecht M.D. and the king's physician at the University of Helmstad, who immediately joined the Royal Society and became an honorary Fellow of the College of Physicians.[117] Nonetheless, the remainder of the royal medical appointees in the years after Queen Anne were not aliens, but holdovers from Anne's reign or native Britons. In part because the new rulers were foreigners and because the medical marketplace had already been thoroughly transformed by both external and internal factors, the watershed years of crown involvement in medicine and transition within the profession had already passed.

Notes

1. Biographies of the last Stuart include Gregg, *Queen Anne* and David Green, *Queen Anne* (London: Collins, 1970); see also Geoffrey Holmes, *British Politics in the Age of Anne* (London: Melbourne, 1967) and Iris Butler, *Rule of Three* (London: Hodder and Stoughton, 1967).

2. The Earl of Stanhope later wrote that "if there were in England any person duller than Her Majesty, that person was Her Majesty's consort": quoted in John Beresford, *Gossip of the Seventeenth and Eighteenth Centuries*, 2 vols. (London: R. Cobden-Sanderson, 1923), 1: 43.

3. *Calendar of Treasury Books*, 1702, 1: 334–35. The Apothecaries' Company established a physic garden in Chelsea in 1676, further expanding local knowledge of materia medica and assisting the research of leading doctors; Kew Gardens followed in 1730.

4. Annals of the College of Physicians, 7: 186; 8: 14, 22, 60–61, LRCP.

5. Henry Keepe prepared a genealogy of Prince George and Princess Anne, published in London by Nathaniel Thompson in time for their wedding in 1684, an indication of the sort of dynastic pressure Anne was under. See also Toni Bowers, *The Politics of Motherhood: British Writing and Culture, 1680–1760* (New York: Cambridge University Press, 1996).

6. For a discussion of the possible causes of Anne's ailments see Green, *Queen Anne*, appendix I.

7. Young, *Annals*, 18. Spas like Bath, known for purging and bleeding regimens as much as for their waters, were frequented by quacks. Each spa had a particular purpose: Tunbridge was for colic, and Bath for ennui. See Maple, *Magic, Medicine and Quackery*, 114.

8. Bloch, *Royal Touch*, 407 n; Beatrice C. Brown, ed., *The Letters and Diplomatic Instructions of Queen Anne* (London: Cassell, 1935), 185. For more on Anne's touching and progresses, see R. O. Bucholz, "'Nothing But Ceremony': Queen Anne and the Limitations of Royal Ritual," *Journal of British Studies* 30 (1991): 288–323.

9. James Brown, "Historical Cards," *Gentleman's Magazine* 84/1 (1814): 129. For more on these games with political import, see Elizabeth Lane Furdell, "'At the King's Arms in the Poultry': The Bookshop Emporium of Dorman Newman," *London Journal* 23 (1998): 8–9.

10. William King, ed., *Memoirs of Sarah, Duchess of Marlborough* (London: Dutton, 1930), 48; and Stubbs, "Royal Recipes," 792–94.

11. King, *Memoirs of Sarah*, 57 (*Post Boy*, January 1, 1712).

12. For excerpts from the diary and commentary, see Rachell Weigall, "An Elizabethan Gentlewoman: The Journal of Lady Mildmay," *Quarterly Review* 215 (1911): 119–36. For an overview of gentlewomen and medicine, see Lynette Hunter, "Women and Domestic Medicine," in *Women, Science and Medicine 1500–1700*, ed. Lynette Hunter and Sarah Hutton (Stroud, England: Sutton, 1997), 89–107.

13. The green sickness or chlorosis was anemia. In her *Choice Manuall of Rare and Select Secrets in Physick and Chirurgerie* (London: W[illiam] J[arvis], 1653), which went through nineteen editions, the Countess advised mixing the sifted powder with rhubarb, taking it three times daily, and walking after the morning dosage. See the excerpt relating to the powder in Charlotte F. Otten, ed., *English Women's Voices 1540–1800* (Miami: Florida International University Press, 1992), 184. At a lower social level Elizabeth Ray, the smithy's wife at Black Notley, developed a reputation for botanical competence and herbal therapies.

14. The derisive phrase, from a seventeenth-century Stafford apothecary, is quoted in Dorothy Porter and Roy Porter, *Patient's Progress: Doctors and Doctoring in Eighteenth-Century England* (Stanford, Calif.: Stanford University Press, 1989), 24–25.

15. George Hartman, *The Family Physitian* (London: R. Wellington, 1696, frontispiece.

16. See the *Diary of Lady Margaret Hoby*, ed. Dorothy Meads (London: Routledge, 1930), *The Household Book of Lady Grisell Baillie*, ed. Robert Scott-Moncrieff (Edinburgh: Scottish History Society, 1911); and Hole, *The English Housewife in the Seventeenth Century*. Lucinda McCray Beier discusses Hoby as a case study of the woman healer in *Sufferers and Healers: The Experience of Illness in Seventeenth Century England* (London: Routledge and Kegan Paul, 1987), 218–24.

17. See *The Tatler*, October 21, 1710; *The Spectator*, August 14, 1711; and Fielding Garrison, "Medicine in *The Tatler, The Spectator*, and *The Guardian*," *Bulletin of the Institute of the History of Medicine* 2 (1934): 477–503.

18. See R. O. Bucholz, *The Augustan Court: Queen Anne and the Decline of Court Culture* (Stanford, Calif.: Stanford University Press, 1993).

19. Gregg, *Queen Anne*, 8.

20. Ibid., 51–52. Anne and George lived in The Cockpit at Whitehall, present site of No. 10 Downing Street.

21. In the judgment of the attending physicians, the dead fetuses from Anne's double miscarriage were not twins. One was a son of about seven months gestation; the other was about two to three months in development and of indeterminate sex. For a litany of Anne's pregnancies, see Green, *Queen Anne*, 76, appendix 1. Gregg (*Queen Anne*, 55–56) discusses the possibility of a hysterical pregnancy in 1689, plausible even among those who have borne children and are familiar with the symptoms; see also M. B. Rosenthal and D. H. Smith, eds., *Psychosomatic Obstetrics and Gynecology* (New York: Karger, 1985).

22. W. B. Saxbe suggests that Anne developed pelvic sepsis from an infection by listeria: see Saxbe, "Listeria monocytogenes and Queen Anne," *Paediatrics* 49 (1972): 97. The general age span for the onset of menopause at the beginning of the eighteenth century was forty-two to fifty; Crawford, "Attitudes to Menstruation," 65.

23. H. Smith, "Gynecology and Ideology," 102, citing John Pechey's *The Compleat Midwife's Practice Enlarged*, 5th ed. (London: H. Rhodes, 1698). Two who firmly rejected the maternal feelings theory were James Blondel and Daniel Turner, physician-surgeons consulted by Queen Anne. Blondel, present at Anne's autopsy and a licentiate of the College of Physicians, wrote a pamphlet, *The Power of Mother's Imagination over the Fetus* (London: J. Brotherton, 1729), which refuted the widely held delusion that infant marks and deformities were attributable to maternal dreams.

24. Michael K. Eshleman, "Diet during Pregnancy in the Sixteenth and Seventeenth Centuries," 29–36; F. H. Champneys, "Midwives in England," *St. Bartholomew's Hospital Journal* 15 (1908): 45; and Thomas R. Forbes, "The Regulation of English Midwives in the Sixteenth and Seventeenth Centuries," *Medical History* 8 (1964): 235–44.

25. Crawford, "Attitudes to Menstruation," 52.

26. James Kemble, *Idols and Invalids* (Garden City, N.J.: Doubleday, 1936), 155.

27. Moore, *The History of the Study of Medicine*, 125. Floyer also constructed an instrument that could be used to measure the pulse rate. Nevertheless, he was among those physicians who still recommended the curative powers of the monarch, and advised the mother of young Samuel Johnson to take her tubercular child to be touched by Queen Anne in 1712.

28. T. R. Forbes has calculated fetal deaths, stillbirths, and miscarriages, in the Aldgate (London) parish of St. Botolph: from 1584 to 1598 there were 124.2 stillbirths for every thousand christenings; between 1609 to 1623 the ratio had fallen to 44.6: 1000. See Forbes, *The Midwife and the Witch* (New Haven, Conn.: Yale University Press, 1966).

29. One historian who offers the Rh factor solution is Maurice Anderson, " Queen Anne's Children," *British Medical Journal* (1963) 2: 684.

30. Kemble, *Idols and Invalids*, 171; Hester Chapman, *Queen Anne's Son* (London: Deutsch, 1954), 30; R. Scott Stevenson, *Famous Illnesses in History* (London: Eyre and Spottiswoode, 1962), 213–27. Stevenson says that Gloucester's hydrocephalus was due to syphilitic meningitis.

31. Dewhurst, *Royal Confinements*, 45–46. Dewhurst spurns the diagnosis of diabetes as a cause of Anne's reproductive woes, noting that diabetics produce larger babies; Anne's were small.

32. Ida Macalpine and Richard Hunter, *George III and the Mad Business* (New York: Pantheon, 1969), 195–222.

33. See "Syphilis," in *Clinical Symposia* 23/3 (1971): 7; and "Gastric Involvement in Syphilis," *Family Physician* 46/2 (1992): 552.

34. Brown, *Letters of Queen Anne*, 120, 127. The authors of *George III and the Mad Business* call this no "ordinary gout" but classic symptoms of porphyria: Macalpine and Hunter, *George III and the Mad Business*, 221.

35. From Elizabeth's Tilbury speech, August 9, 1588, quoted in Erickson, *The First Elizabeth*, 374–75.

36. Gideon Harvey, *The Vanities of Philosophy and the Physick*, (London: A. Roper, 1699), 34. Gideon Harvey the Elder was educated in the Low Countries, joined the College of Physicians in The Hague, and served Charles II. An opponent of elite medicine, he was Physician of the Tower under William and Mary, a lucrative sinecure, and was succeeded by his son in 1715. For the elder Harvey, see Munk, *Roll* 2: 11; *DNB*; and for the son's appointment see Add. MSS 38889, f. 164, British Library.

37. Since Anne was already corpulent, some wondered publicly how she could swell any more: Porter and Rousseau, *Gout*, 239, 246.

38. Philip Roberts, ed., *The Diary of Sir David Hamilton* (Oxford: Oxford University Press, 1975), 106.

39. For the black cat cure, see Daniel Turner, *De Morbis Cutaneis*, (London: R. Bonwicke, 1714), 24. See also Turner's *Syphilis* (London: R. Wilkin, 1737), and his *Discourse concerning Gleets* (London: n.p., 1729).

40. William Read, *A Short But Exact Account of All the Diseases Incident to the Eyes*, 2nd ed. (London: n.p., 1710); for the Swift comment, see *DNB*.

41. *The Oculist* (1705) ridiculed Read and another mocking verse read as follows:

> Her majesty sure was in a surprise
> Or else was very short-sighted
> When a tinker was sworn to look after her eyes
> And the mountebank tailor was knighted.

Quoted in Maple, *Magic, Medicine and Quackery*, 111; For Read, Grant, and Rugeley, see *DNB*; Munk, *Roll* 1: 267–68; Chapman, *Queen Anne's Son*, 122; and M. R. Hopkinson, *Anne of England* (New York: Macmillan, 1934), 148.

42. For a discussion of quinine's toxicity, see *Goodman and Gilman's The Pharmaceutical Basis of Therapeutics*, 9th ed., ed. Joel G. Hardman (New York: McGraw-Hill, 1996), 978–81.

43. Talbor, *English Remedy*, 44.

44. Ibid., 40, 63.

45. Dorothy McLaren, "Fertility, Infant Mortality, and Breast Feeding in the Seventeenth Century," *Medical History* 22 (1978): 380; Jane B. Donegan, *Women and Men Midwives* (Westport, Conn.: Greenwood Press, 1978). William Harvey, Jane Sharp, and Baldwin Hamey thought the better record of poor women in childbirth was due to less interference by midwives: see Harvey's *Anatomical Exercitations* (London: James Young, 1653), 488; and John Keevil, *Hamey the Stranger* (London: G. Bles, 1952), 48–49.

46. See Elizabeth Lane Furdell, "Medical Personnel at the Court of Queen Anne," *The Historian* 68 (1986): 412–29.

47. Given Lower's well-known anti-Catholic sentiments and later service to William as inspector of battlefield drugs, his advice to Anne may have been politically motivated, but she wrote to her sister that her doctors told her to go to Bath for the benefits to her health: Bathurst, *Letters of Two Queens*, 211. See also Luttrell, *Brief Historical Relation* 2: 161; Andrew J. Larner, "Portrait of Richard Lower," *Endeavor*, new series 11 (1987): 205–8; and for Lower's (and Dr. Millington's) scrutiny of rhubarb for wartime usage in 1690, see Moore, *History of St. Bartholomew's Hospital*, 2: 518.

48. The *DNB* spells it "Scarburgh," but spellings were still not standardized at the end of the seventeenth century, even for surnames.

49. Hone, *Life of Radcliffe*, 51; Porter and Rousseau, *Gout*, 241. Sainty and Bucholz found no royal warrant for Radcliffe during Anne's reign, but he was often consulted by the court and paid large sums for his prescriptions. Munk, *Roll* 1: 455.

50. Brown, *Letters of Queen Anne*, 51.

51. Annals of the College of Physicians, vol. 5, f. 94b, LRCP. Alex Sakula errs in asserting that Radcliffe "insisted on writing his directions in Latin"; just the opposite was true of this anti-Dispensarian. See Alex Sakula, "Dr. John Radcliffe, Court Physician, and the Death of Queen Anne," *Journal of the Royal College of Physicians of London* 19/4 (1985): 255.

52. Allen, "Medical Education in Seventeenth Century England," 127.

53. For the cough syrup, see Add. MSS 39289, f. 21, British Library; see also his *Pharmacopoeia Radcliffeanae*, 2nd ed., 2 vols., ed. Edward Strother (London: n.p., 1716) 2: 419.

54. All practitioners in the seventeenth century treated children as well as adults, and usually only quacks specialized; Samuel X. Radbill, "Pediatrics," in Debus, *Medicine in Seventeenth-Century England*, 241. Jack Dewhurst submits that Gloucester's troubles were not a consequence of his birth, but the result of an acute infection at six weeks: J. Dewhurst, *Royal Confinements*, 39.

55. Green, *Queen Anne*, 55–56, 64; J. B. Nias, *Dr. John Radcliffe* (Oxford: Oxford University Press, 1918), 15; Chapman, *Queen Anne's Son*, 42, 72.

56. See Turk and Allen, "Bleeding and Cupping," 128. Nonetheless, Radcliffe insisted that all cures are caused by "contraries," and he quoted Hippocrates' axiom that a physician should subtract from what abounds and add what is wanting.

57. Chapman, *Queen Anne's Son*, 138. Jack Dewhurst denies a genetic cause of Gloucester's hydrocephalus, a condition confirmed according to the autopsy report, instead attributing the excessive fluid in his cerebral ventricles to meningitis or a middle-ear infection: J. Dewhurst, *Royal Confinements*, 42. See also Jenkin Lewis, *Memoirs of Prince William Henry, Duke of Gloucester* (London: Payne, 1789).

58. Clemens, "Notes," 308.

59. Munk, *Roll* 1: 455.

60. Gregg, *Queen Anne*, 121; Maurice Ashley, *The Stuarts in Love* (New York: Macmillan, 1963), 229.

61. John M. Gray, ed., *Memoirs of Sir John Clerk* (Edinburgh: Edinburgh University Press, 1892), 79.

62. Anne's 1708 speech to Parliament, quoted in Hopkinson, *Anne of England*, 271. The Electress Sophia dropped dead in Hanover after running for shelter from a sudden rain at age eighty-four in 1714, two months before Queen Anne died: William Morgan, *English Political Parties and Leaders in the Reign of Queen Anne* (New Haven, Conn.: Yale University Press, 1920), 140–41.

63. *Clerk's Memoirs*, 62. Queen Anne called the Union with Scotland "the happiness of my reign": Hopkinson, *Anne of England*, 258.

64. Matthews, *Royal Apothecaries*, 135.

65. See Clippingdale, Medical Court Roll, 1: 153–54, LRCS. The *DNB* states that his father was a herbalist. Another critic accused Hannes of using a coat of arms for which he was not certified. For the exchange of letters between Hannes and Hans Sloane, then President of the College, see SL MSS 4059, folios 117–119, British Library.

66. Luttrell, *Brief Historical Relation* 4: 672.

67. A.H.T. Robb, "Cambridge Medicine," in *Medicine in Seventeenth Century England*, ed. Allen G. Debus (Berkeley: University of California Press, 1974), 329.

68. Perhaps because Portland, a Dutchman, was unpopular with English politicians, Lister dedicated his 1699 book, *A Journey to Paris*, to Baron Somers, Lord Chancellor of England. In it he reviewed medical discussions and experiments that he observed at the "Academie Royalle des Sciences."

69. Munk, *Roll* 1: 442; see also Benjamin Allen, *The Natural History of the Mineral Waters of Great Britain* (London: William Innys, 1711); Abel Boyer, *History of the Reign of Queen Anne Digested into Annals* (London: A. Roper, 1713), 345. For more works on Lister, consult Geoffrey

Keynes, *Dr. Martin Lister: A Bibliography* (London: St. Paul's Bibliographies, 1981); and G. P. Jefcoate, "Addendum to Keynes' Bibliography," *Book Collector* 33 (1984): 527.

70. Hamilton, *Diary*, xxxi, 3, 46, 55.

71. Ibid., xxiii.

72. Ibid., 71, 88.

73. Ibid., xxv, 6, 67.

74. Munk, *Roll* 2: 12. Philip Roberts has found no evidence either to support or to refute this widely accepted story; see Hamilton, *Diary*, xxii-xxiii. See also David Hamilton, *Treatise of a Miliary Fever* (London: A. Bettesworth, 1737), 60.

75. Maurice Ashley contends that Prince George may have had syphilis: see *Stuarts in Love*, 229. Shortly after Anne was crowned, she named Prince George Generalissimo of the armed forces and Lord High Admiral of England, a position he held until his death.

76. Sarah Jennings Churchill, Duchess of Marlborough, *The Letters of Sarah, Duchess of Marlborough* (London: Murray, 1875), 416; Agnes Strickland, *Queen Anne*, vol. 5 of *Lives of the Queens of England*, 8 vols. (London: H. Colborn, 1851), 593. Gregg reports that the Duchess was unsympathetic and callous, precipitating a final break between the two old friends: Gregg, *Queen Anne*, 282–83.

77. I thank Anita Guerrini for correcting Munk's record of the institution from which Arbuthnot received his medical degree.

78. Jonathan Swift, *Journal to Stella*, 2 vols. (London: Oxford University Press, 1948), 1: 239.

79. For more on Arbuthnot's satire, see Dennis Todd, "New Evidence for Dr. Arbuthnot's Authorship of 'Rabbit Man-Midwife,' " *Studies in Bibliography* 41 (1988): 257–67.

80. Shadwell's comments on Anne's health can be found in SL MSS 4034, f. 44, 46–50, British Library. To facilitate bleeding, physicians used the seton, a horsehair inserted beneath the skin to keep open a passage, and the moxa, Chinese wormwood burned on the skin as a counter-irritant or cauterizing agent.

81. W. E. Buckley, ed., *Memoirs of Thomas, Earl of Ailsbury* (London: n.p., 1890), 222–24.

82. Sloane wrote about his Caribbean adventure in *Voyage to Madeira, Barbados, Nieves, St. Christopher's and Jamaica*, 2 vols. (London: B. M., 1705–25). See also Richard Sheridan, "The Doctor and the Buccaneer: Hans Sloane's Case History of Henry Morgan," *Journal of the History of Medicine* 41 (1986): 76–87.

83. L. Jessop, "The Club at the Temple Coffee House," *Archives of Natural History* 16 (1989): 263–74.

84. Thomas, "Sir Hans Sloane and the Russian Academy of Sciences," 21–37.

85. Sloane may have been motivated to provide for his manuscripts after two arsonists set fire to his house in 1700; his collection is a keystone of the British Library and a necessity for medical historians. See M.A.E. Nickson, "Hans Sloane, Book Collector and Cataloguer," *British Library Journal* 14 (1988): 52–69; and Hans Sloane, *A Concise Narrative of His Life* (London: n.p., 1755).

86. Munk, *Roll* 2: 35. See Turner's pamphlet, *Short Review of the Quicksilver Controversy* (London: n.p., 1733); John Woodward, *State of Physick and of Diseases* (London: T. Horne, 1718). See also Levine, *Dr. Woodward's Shield*, 84–92.

87. See, for instance, SL MSS 4062, f. 3, (from James Welwood) and 4059, f. 24 (from a Mr. Eumbaring), British Library.

88. Munk, *Roll* 2: 40; Young, *Annals*, 375; and the posthumously published *Medical Works of Richard Mead* (London: C. Hitch 1762). See also Theodore M. Brown, "Medicine in the Shadow of the 'Principia,' " *Journal of the History of Ideas* 48 (1987): 629–48.

89. The cane subsequently passed to three more London doctors—William Pitcairne, Anthony Askew and Matthew Baillie—was then "retired in 1823," donated to the Royal College of Physicians by Baillie's widow. See MacMichael, *Gold-Headed Cane*.

90. Garrison, *Introduction to the History of Medicine*, 322. The ongoing feud between Mead and Woodward is well described in Levine, *Dr. Woodward's Shield*, 13–17. Other episodes of physical confrontation between medical men have been noted by historians, including the 1704 assault on

Radcliffe by the apothecary Cotsworth and the wounding by Foot Onslow of Dr. Shadwell in a 1705 duel in St. James's Park. Luttrell, *Brief Historical Relation*, 5: 572.

91. C. C. Booth, "Sir Samuel Garth, F.R.S.: The Dispensary Poet," *Notes and Records of the Royal Society of London* 40 (1986): 133.

92. For more of his verse, see *The Works of the Most Celebrated Minor Poets*, 2 vols. (London: F. Cogan, 1749).

93. "For thee she sheathed the terrors of her sword
For thee she broke her general and her word."

The Works of Sir Samuel Garth (Dublin: T. Ewing, 1769), 105–6. The statue referred to in the title had been erected in 1712, but the poem was not published during Anne's reign.

94. Munk, *Roll* 1: 498.

95. Garrison, *Introduction to the History of Medicine*, 389; SL 4046, f. 159, British Library. The letter mentions a man named Power, clerk of the Treasury, who would like to run the lottery and asks Sloane to put in a good word with chief minister Robert Walpole.

96. Munk, *Roll* 1: 467; Moore, *History of St. Bartholomew's*, 2: 351. Geoffrey Holmes argues that Blackmore's reputation was "barely reputable," but that might have been because of his support for the Apothecaries: Holmes, *Augustan England*, 190, 208.

97. Charles Bernard observed and recorded the reappearance of cancer in a patient at St. Bartholomew's; Moore, *History of St. Bartholomew's* 2: 629. Francis Bernard's recipes are preserved in SL MSS 2290, British Library.

98. Evidently, such dissections helped improve his own expertise. According to the *DNB*, Charles Bernard was acclaimed for saving the leg of a Mr. Hoadly, tutor at Catherine Hall.

99. Young, *Annals*, 563; Bloom and James, *Medical Practitioners*, 39; Dobson and Walker, *Barbers and Barber-Surgeons*, 123. Another Charles Bernard was clerk of the Barber-Surgeons in 1715.

100. Young, *Annals*, 570.

101. Add. MSS 38852, folios 1–8, British Library. Watkins was deputy judge advocate in Flanders.

102. Matthews, *Royal Apothecaries*, 133.

103. Ibid., 138. The Treasury paid him for his efforts. For Jones' appointment see *Calendar of Treasury Books*, 1702: 52, and for his travels, *Calendar of Treasury Books*, 1706: 452.

104. Munk, *Roll* 2: 6.

105. This story has been told extensively, but may be apocryphal. It is mentioned by Hone, *Life of Radcliffe*, 101; Strickland, *Queen Anne*, 410; Munk, *Roll* 1: 455; and Sakula, "Radcliffe and the Death of Queen Anne," 259.

106. Nias, *Dr. John Radcliffe*, 18–19.

107. The following is an excerpt from "Shepherd's Week":

A skilful leech (so God him speed)
They say had wrought this blessed deed.
This leech Arbuthnot was yclept,
Who many a night not once had slept;
But watch'd our gracious Sovereign still:
For who could rest while she was ill?
Oh! may'st though henceforth sweetly sleep,
Sheer swains! oh sheer your softest sheep
To swell his couch; for well I ween
He saved the realm, who saved the Queen.
Quoth I, please God, I'll high with glee
To court, this Arbuthnot to see.

From Lewis Melville, *Life and Letters of John Gay* (London: O'Connor, 1921), 24. Dr. Arbuthnot's career survived the queen's demise, and he enjoyed a lucrative practice in London.

108. Turk and Allen, "Bleeding and Cupping," 129. The patients of Richard Mead and Hans Sloane were routinely bled for fevers and apoplexy, often up to 35 ounces in the initial venesection, then up to 210 ounces within six days.

109. "Some Royal Deathbeds: Queen Anne," *British Medical Journal*, (1910) 2: 1530; and Henry L. Snyder, "The Last Days of Queen Anne: The Account of Sir John Evelyn Examined," *Huntington Library Quarterly* 34 (May 1971): 261–76.

110. Quoted in Gregg, *Queen Anne*, 394.

111. SL MSS 4034, f. 44, British Library; Morgan, *English Political Parties*, 122. James Kemble insists that Anne had varicose veins, and that a pulmonary embolism resulted from thrombophlebitis of the varicose saphenous vein: Kemble, *Idols and Invalids*, 170.

112. Sakula, "Radcliffe and the Death of Queen Anne," 259.

113. See Anthony Quinton, "Dr. John Radcliffe, the Benefactor and His Benefactions," *Journal of the Royal Society of Medicine* 79 (1986): 380–86.

114. Garth quoted in Otto Beckman, *A Pictorial History of Medicine* (Springfield, Ill.: Thomas, 1956), 192; Moore, *History of St. Bartholomew's*, 356. Radcliffe's prescriptions and observations were published posthumously in a two-volume tome intended as "of general use to all physicians, apothecaries and surgeons." The first volume sold sixteen hundred copies in less than six months. The second, nearly six hundred pages long, contains recipes for diuretic wine, nephritic pills, cephalic snuff, and hysteric electuary. More Radcliffe recipes can be found in Add. MSS 29568, f. 27, British Library.

115. Matthews, *Royal Apothecaries*, 140–41. Louis XIV exclaimed that the Stuarts were "an unlucky family" and that he "wished to hear no more of them." Quoted in Green, *Queen Anne*, 48.

116. Annals of the College of Physicians, 8: 100, LRCP.

117. Tessier moved up under George II to the post of extra physician in 1734 and physician to the person in 1739; Steigherthal, never on the regular medical staff, left England at George I's death. Munk, *Roll* 1: 69; 2: 38.

Epilogue

THE COLLECTIVE PROFILE AND LEGACY OF THE TUDOR AND STUART ROYAL DOCTORS

The Tudor-Stuart era of English history affords a convenient and instructive framework for examining the royal medical staff, the complex schism in the health-care profession, and the role of the sovereign in English medicine during a time of political and religious tumult. Of chief importance to our inquiry has been investigating the care that the royal doctors provided to the kings and queens of Great Britain and their families, care that affected every citizen. Reliable medical information is hard to come by in the biographies of monarchs and some of the most conscientious scholars have been forced to construct medical interpretations from questionable anecdotes. Amateur medical writing can be misleading even when based on the opinions of professionals contemporary to the patient; the king's doctors might understandably be reticent about the illnesses and deaths of their deceased sovereign. Moreover, medical description and its precise explication become even more difficult to verify in evidence hundreds of years old. Inaccurate and cavalier usage of psychological terms by laymen spawned many biographical mistakes in twentieth-century tomes. Nonetheless, pathography, the presentation of medical facts in biography, remains valuable for the student of a monarch's life.[1] The best sources from which to cull this sort of information about kings and queens are the unpublished notes and the arcane, albeit occasionally printed, accounts of the royal doctors.

Additionally, the archives yield much about the individual physicians, surgeons, and apothecaries who served the Tudor-Stuart households. Yet surprisingly, given the varied activities of aulic doctors as propagandists, diplomats, and medical politicians, medicine within the patrician setting of the royal court has been largely neglected.[2] Some of the illustrious professionals of the sixteenth and seventeenth centuries have received academic attention, but the past prominence of the aulic medical corps has faded except in the estimate of occupational antiquarians or genealogically minded descendants of the near-great. In recent years, medical and social historians have focused on ordinary practitioners and their patients, eschewing the study of acclaimed, elite doctors for political or publishing reasons.[3] Scholarly lack of interest coupled with partisan disdain edged the distinctive leaders of professional organizations off center-stage before their stories were written. Besides their individual import, the doctors at court are too consequential collectively and their multifaceted impact on medicine too great to be ignored. They correctly envisioned their function as pivotal in the protection of harmony throughout the kingdom through their attention to the ruler's health. Whatever their posthumous scientific reputation among historians, the royal doctors indisputably enjoyed positions of power and influence at court, among their colleagues, and in medical science.

The Tudor and Stuart generations witnessed a remarkable transformation in English medicine, some of which was directly precipitated by royal concerns. The healing arts were recast during the sixteenth and seventeenth centuries, galvanized by the scientific revolution and a growth in the professionalism produced by training, experimentation, and specialization.[4] At the beginning of the Tudor regime, physicians were classically educated gentlemen enamored with Galenic precepts; apothecaries and surgeons were merely craftsmen. By the end of Queen Anne's reign, Galenism was dead, apothecaries had evolved into practicing doctors, many British physicians had middle-class origins and degrees from Leiden or Reims, and surgeons were ready to split from the barbers, a move they finally effected in 1745. From the involvement of Henry VII and VIII in enabling the College of Physicians and the Barber-Surgeons' Company to regulate the practice of medicine in London to the cooperation of Queen Anne's government in legally leveling the professional playing field, monarchs interacted decisively with leaders in medicine. Princely intercession came sometimes at the behest of the royal medical personnel and sometimes in spite of their advice. Regardless of the monarch's medical politics, the iatric predilection of the royal family inevitably set the style for society inside and outside the court. The large majority of courtiers, nobles, clergy, affluent merchants, even prosperous artisans, all mimicked the monarch and patronized similar if not the same members of the medical community. The hoi polloi followed suit, buying medical publications written in the vernacular for the general public by physicians, surgeons, and apothecaries affiliated with the crown.

An analysis of the individual lives of these royal doctors reveals patterns that pertain to the group and further illustrates the transitional state of European medicine. Some commonalities are apparent in each of the aulic categories, even if the same caveat concerning untrustworthy evidence about ancient royalty applies to the royal doctors, all of them dead for at least 300 years and less notable than their imperial patients. Despite the sketchy nature of their recorded biographies, key details emerge about the medical corps of the Tudors and the Stuarts. They had their associations: most of the physicians to the crown and a handful of the surgeons and apothecaries held membership in the College of Physicians of London, and a significant number were Fellows of the Royal Society.[5] Approximately half of the physicians to the crown whose universities are known attended Oxford or Cambridge for their medical doctorates. Forty royal physicians had medical degrees from Oxford, thirty-eight from Cambridge. Over fifty royal doctors hailed from continental universities; the institutions of twenty-five, many of them with foreign M.D.s, are unknown, and approximately a dozen physician appointees lacked an earned doctoral degree in medicine. The dominance of the English sister universities reflects the lack of competition for medical degrees in Britain; prior to the end of the seventeenth century, no doctorates in medicine were awarded elsewhere in the British Isles.[6] On matriculating at Oxford or Cambridge for a medical diploma, students were first compelled to complete their undergraduate program of studies for a total of fourteen years, seven in the arts course (bachelor's and master's) and seven in medicine (bachelor's and doctorate). Continental universities expected their students to matriculate at several institutions.

Although many continental universities pursued the more experimental medical theories of Paracelsus and his followers, Oxford and Cambridge still deemed appropriate a Galenic curriculum in medicine until the mid-to-late seventeenth century when empiricism became the fashion in London.[7] Prompted by an enthusiastic Charles II and by a changed Royal College of Physicians in London, Oxbridge medical degrees began to reflect a new emphasis on finding specific cures for specific diseases. Since the Royal College of Physicians licensed men to practice in the London metropolitan area, and since nearly half of its membership by 1670 was continentally trained, it is not surprising that the English universities started to reshape their curricula to reflect the new medicine. Moreover, Oxford and Cambridge often incorporated foreign credentials and licensed unincorporated foreign degree holders, perhaps one-eighth of their total graduates. During the last half of the seventeenth century, when politics rather than letters necessitated overseas study, seventy-eight foreign medical degrees were incorporated at Oxford at the same time that 223 medical degrees were awarded to resident Oxonians. Nearly one-third of the Oxford and Cambridge Fellows of the College of Physicians were actually foreign degree holders, their licenses to practice medicine awarded by the Oxbridge faculties.[8] Among the royal doctors of the Tudor-Stuart period, eleven holders of foreign degrees had theirs incorporated at Oxford, ten at Cambridge.

As many as sixty doctors to the Tudors and the Stuarts received their medical degrees on the continent. Two universities that trained many British royal physicians were Padua and Leiden, among the foremost medical schools of the sixteenth and seventeenth centuries.[9] All Italian universities with the exception of Padua were closed to British students, as Reformation-era popes excluded non-Catholics from Italian institutions. The Venetian Republic controlled Padua and circumvented the papal order by creating a separate university for non-Catholics; as a result, many English and Scottish students enrolled there, especially in the sixteenth century. As a result of its policy of openness, Padua developed into the largest community of medical students and professors in Europe. Besides the size of its international faculty and the excellence of its curriculum, Padua could boast the first botanical garden in Europe.[10] Twenty of the Tudor-Stuart royal doctors held medical degrees from Padua, including Thomas Linacre, founder of the College of Physicians; William Harvey, discoverer of the circulation of the blood (and recipient of a later Cambridge M.D.); Laurence Wright, Cromwell's physician-in-ordinary; and William Stokeham, physician-in-ordinary to Charles II.

Considerable numbers of Oxford and Cambridge students in the seventeenth century went to Leiden for medical studies, as did graduates of Scottish universities. Among them were fourteen royal doctors, beginning with Elizabeth I's physician John James and including William Paddy, a Jacobean court appointee and advocate of public dissection. Though situated in Protestant territory, Leiden appealed to English-speaking students of various denominations, especially during times of domestic upheaval in Britain.[11] There were surely academic advantages to the medical student at Leiden, benefits born of the sophisticated teaching offered there. Clinical and chemical training, carried out by the professors themselves, added to orthodox lecturing and debating, made for an outstanding integrated curriculum. The medical faculty at Leiden was among the most innovative and distinguished in late seventeenth-century Europe, famed for stressing familiarity with human anatomy and observation of patient symptoms; public anatomical demonstrations in the anatomy theater complemented skeletal studies. Medical teaching was integrated into one of the city hospitals, giving students like Charles I's physician-in-ordinary Samuel Bispham and Thomas Burnet, physician in Scotland to the later Stuarts, the opportunity to observe sickness and its relief. Leiden's emphasis on anatomy, botany, chemistry, and the clinic differed substantially from the emphasis on medical philosophy still pursued at more traditional universities.

A number of British royal doctors received their medical certification at French universities including ten from Paris, Reims, and Montpellier. Many of the Scottish aulic physicians in particular obtained their credentials in France because of the Auld Alliance, the special relationship between the two countries; historically, Scottish Protestants had access to legal and medical studies at universities anywhere in France. Besides, there were no medical schools in Scotland until the end of the seventeenth century, and even then John Arbuthnot, physician to Queen Anne, obtained a medical degree from Aberdeen after being examined by a group of doctors, rather than by taking classes.[12] The University of Paris may have offered the dedicated student from Great Britain better medical facilities, and language presented no problem to English-speakers, since Latin functioned as the *lingua franca* in Europe well into the eighteenth century, encouraging the possibility of a cosmopolitan realm of learning in which national identities were obscured.

But, unlike the Italian or Dutch universities, French colleges, especially those in the provinces, had not made much progress in the study of medicine. Instead, the French were still devoted to a slavish reading of texts and to the medical wisdom of bleeding and purging; even the University of Paris manifested an unswerving Galenic bias until well into the 1600s.[13] However, Paris was one of only two French institutions demanding that its graduates have some experience observing and treating patients, and it had an amphitheater for dissections to augment its course in practical medicine. By the middle of the seventeenth century, a student would have been exposed to a faculty enamored of iatrochemistry and no longer completely acquiescing to the Galenic rationale behind phlebotomy. George Wakeman, Catherine of Braganza's harassed Roman Catholic doctor, had a medical diploma from Paris. A Protestant student like Samuel Haworth, physician to James, Duke of York, might have preferred to enroll in one of the lay and independent extra-university institutions in Paris, such as the Collège Royal, where research and teaching were promoted. This college had chairs of medicine, botany, surgery, and pharmacy; teaching was free and consisted of seventy to eighty lectures a year by each professor.

French provincial schools were easier to get into than Paris and had fewer prerequisites for matriculation, but they were not in general as rigorous in their pursuit of educational excellence. At Reims, one would have found a faculty and a course of study tardy in its awareness of the new medicine. Moreover, of the "eighty-seven doctors, officers, members, and their henchmen of the four faculties" at the University in the middle of the seventeenth century, most were priests.[14] Although the Roman Catholic church had become less directly influential in seventeenth-century Gallic education, the teaching of conventional medical doctrines predominated in the *ancien régime* for another century and a half. A few faculty mavericks, often Huguenot as well as Paracelsian, preferred the new metallic drugs like mercury and antimony over historic methods of bleeding and purging. For the most part, however, there is little novelty evident in the extant medical theses of English-speaking students who studied in France and in none of the theses of those who studied at Reims.[15] Contrary to contemporary opinion, however, Reims was no diploma factory in the Tudor-Stuart period; it required serious examinations and theses, never granting a degree *in absentia*. Historian Charles Coury suggests that the Reims medical faculty was reputable, if inferior to Paris and Montpellier. Based on the numbers of students and degrees awarded, the activity of the medical school at Reims placed it among the three or four most important of the old French faculties.[16] Among the Reims-trained royal doctors were James Welwood and Archibald Pitcairne, founding member of the Royal College of Physicians of Edinburgh. After the revocation of the Edict of Nantes in 1685, Reims became a less attractive collegiate destination for Britons.

The Faculty of Medicine at Montpellier is the oldest in France, its statutes dating from 1220 and, owing to its location in southern France, intellectually independent of Paris. Though under Galenic influence, its more liberal political climate persuaded the faculty from 1550 to teach anatomy and surgery despite the corporate separation between physicians and surgeons in France comparable to that in England; a chair in botany was established in 1593. Montpellier's example became contagious, as after 1600 Paris and other French institutions adopted regular courses in anatomy and botany. As early as 1650 some professors at Montpellier had abandoned the outmoded format of reading their own classical textual commentaries to students in favor of using more personal medical treatises; Montpellier was the first French institutional champion of Harvey's circulation of the blood.[17] Obtaining a doctorate at Montpellier was intended to be difficult, the severity of its medical examination reflecting the prestige of its faculty, among them Lazare Riverius, one of the foremost medical pedagogues, whose course of study encompassed physiology, pathology, semeiotics, hygiene, and therapy.[18] Montpellier produced royal doctors for England like physician Theodore Mayerne and serjeant-surgeon Gilbert Primrose, both on James I's aulic staff, and Alexander Fraizer, first physician to Charles I and Charles II. Various other European institutions like Basel, Bourges, Angers, and Nantes provided medical degrees to individual British royal doctors.

The continental medical educations of Englishmen during the Tudor and Stuart era created circles of discourse among scientists and doctors that significantly aided progress in health care both at home and abroad. Old school ties or new fraternities born of the intense and complex nature of scientific inquiry burgeoned into vigorous friendships nourished by frequent written discussions. Travel and personal visits further facilitated the strengthening of these communicative attachments across international borders. However, the ease of information exchange among physicians and scientists ceased once these men were drawn into the closed league of aulic service. Royal doctors simply could not disclose all that they knew to their counterparts in rival countries; their loyalties lay with the monarch and the nation.[19]

Like the physicians, the royal surgeons and apothecaries usually affiliated with occupational organizations in the capital. Most came from the London guilds, although foreign monarchs often brought their own personnel from their home soil. At least forty of the monarch's surgeons wore the livery of the London Barber Surgeons' Company, more than double the number of those who, by virtue of their alien status, did not. That means they had gone through the rigors of long apprenticeship, sometimes under their father's supervision, and trained under the watchful eye of the Company. By custom, the king's Serjeant- Surgeon became Master of the guild, although the foreign-born surgeons who served the Stuart queens and William of Orange did not even join the institution. A majority (twenty-three) of the royal apothecaries affiliated with the Grocers' Company of London until the Society of Apothecaries split off in the early seventeenth century. However, a sizable minority of the royal apothecaries, nineteen, either did not join these guilds or their affiliations are unknown.

Taken as a whole, the royal doctors are a varied group including quacks and geniuses, charlatans and scholars; generalizing about their role at court ignores that diversity. Their sheer numbers testify to the importance of the household staff for the Tudor-Stuart medical world. By examining their individual lives and activities, professional and personal, one can gain a better understanding of the diseases and ailments from which the Tudor-Stuart rulers and their courts suffered, and the medical personnel whom they summoned to attend them.

Appointees clearly used their influence with the monarch to foster careers and concepts. Some promoted Paracelsianism and in the post-Restoration age of empiricism, some advocated a sort of alternative medicine. Royal doctors published extensively, perhaps at first writing for those who served in subordinate positions within the profession, but ultimately they educated the general public. Their use of the press further undermined Galenic orthodoxy and the medical establishment. Several of the seventeenth-century royal doctors candidly championed the popularization of medical knowledge as an act of charity or as a political deed comparable to the printing of the Bible in the vernacular. Ironically, these publications also contributed to the development a medical entrepreneurship that changed the locus of intellectual and cultural reform from the court to the academies.[20] However, it is the intimate relationship between physician and princely patient, not politics or publications, that still intrigues us about the sovereign's medical personnel. Whatever a royal doctor's qualifications or competence, the destiny of the whole empire might ultimately depend on his therapies.

Notes

1. Milo Keynes, "Medical Sense and Nonsense in Biography," *Cambridge Review* 105 (January 30, 1984): 9–14.

2. Vivian Nutton, "Introduction," *Medicine at the Courts of Europe 1500–1837* (London: Routledge, 1990), 2–5.

3. See, for instance, Margaret Pelling, *The Common Lot: Sickness, Medical Occupations, and the Urban Poor in Early Modern England* (London: Longman, 1998); Beier, *Sufferers and Healers*; and Porter and Porter, *Patient's Progress*.

4. Robert G. Frank, Jr., "The Physician as Virtuoso in Seventeenth-Century England," in *English Scientific Virtuosi in the Sixteenth and Seventeenth Centuries*, ed. Barbara Shapiro and Robert G. Frank, Jr. (Los Angeles: University of California Press, 1979), 65; Bernice Hamilton, "The Medical Profession in the Eighteenth Century," *Economic History Review* 2nd series, 4/2 (1951): 141.

5. Of the regular and extraordinary appointees, 127 were Fellows of the College during the Tudor-Stuart period; twenty-seven royal doctors joined the Royal Society, some as founding members in 1662. James II's Scottish doctors figured prominently in the founding of the Royal College of Physicians of Edinburgh.

6. Moreover, religious qualifications barred native Nonconformists from study at either university. A.H.T. Robb-Smith, "Medical Education at Oxford and Cambridge Prior to 1850," in *The Evolution of Medical Education in Britain*, ed. F.N.L. Poynter (London: Pitman Medical Publishing, 1966), 19, 40.

7. For more on the medical course at Oxford and Cambridge, see Robert G. Frank, Jr., "Science, Medicine and the Universities of Early Modern England: Background and Sources, Part I," *History of Science* 11 (1973): 194–216.

8. Robb-Smith, "Medical Education at Oxford and Cambridge," 19, 39. For purposes of analysis, I have not counted incorporated foreign degrees as true Oxbridge M.D.s.

9. The universities of several of the royal doctors cannot be traced but, in addition to Padua and Leiden, the following continental institutions could claim alumni serving the Tudors and the Stuarts: Montpellier (5), Basel (4), Paris (3), Reims (2), and one each for Angers, Bourges, Caen, Ferrara, Franeker, Nantes, Orange, Pavia, and Sedan. A few royal physicians had degrees conferred by mandate or through unusual circumstances at universities, like St. Andrews in Scotland, without a graduate medical faculty.

10. Nancy G. Siraisi, *Medieval and Early Renaissance Medicine* (Chicago: University of Chicago Press, 1990), 64; Thomas A. Christopher, "The Seeds of Botany," *Natural History* 90 (1981): 50–58.

11. Smith, *English-Speaking Students at Leyden*, xvii-xviii.

12. John Durkan, "The French Connection in the Sixteenth and Early Seventeenth Centuries," in *Scotland and Europe, 1200–1850*, ed. T. C. Smout (Edinburgh: John Donald, 1986), 24.

13. Laurence Brockliss and Colin Jones, *The Medical World of Early Modern France* (Oxford: Clarendon Press, 1997), 107.

14. Pierre Desportes, ed., *Histoire de Reims* (Toulouse: Univers de la France et des Pays Francophone, 1983), 216.

15. For a critical analysis of Reims, see Laurence Brockliss, *French Higher Education in the Seventeenth and Eighteenth Centuries* (Oxford: Clarendon Press, 1987), 391–443.

16. Charles Coury, "The Teaching of Medicine in France from the Beginning of the Seventeenth Century," in *The History of Medical Education*, ed. Charles D. O'Malley (Berkeley: University of California Press, 1970), 122. Coury calls the medical programs at Orange, Avignon, Nancy, Nantes, and Angers discredited or marginal.

17. Coury, "Teaching of Medicine," 124, 133, 143; Brockliss, *French Higher Education*, 392–93, 402.

18. Brockliss, *French Higher Education*, 74–75, 392.

19. See David S. Lux and Harold J. Cook, "Closed Circles or Open Networks? Communicating at a Distance during the Scientific Revolution," *History of Science* 36 (1998): 179–212.

20. Brockliss and Jones, *Medical World of Early Modern France*, 280.

Bibliography

Primary Sources: Unpublished

Additional Manuscripts. British Library. London.
Annals of the Royal College of Physicians of London. Library of the Royal College of Physicians. London.
Calendar of Letter Books. Record Office. Corporation of London.
Egerton Manuscripts. British Library. London.
Establishment Books. Royal Archives. Windsor Castle.
Harleian Miscellany. British Library. London.
Journals of the Court of Common Council. Record Office. Corporation of London.
Lansdowne Manuscripts. British Library. London.
Registered Copy Wills, Prerogative Court of Canterbury. Family Records Centre. Public Record Office. London.
Repertories of the Court of Aldermen. Record Office. Corporation of London.
Royal Rolls. British Library. London.
Sloane Manuscripts. British Library. London.

Primary Sources: Published

Arbuthnot, John. *Essay Concerning the Effects of Air on Human Bodies*. London: J. Tonson, 1733.
_____. *Essay Concerning the Nature of Aliments*. 2 vols. London: J. Tonson, 1731.
Archer, John. *Every Man His Own Doctor*. London: Peter Lillicrap, 1671.
_____. *Secrets Disclosed of Consumptions*. London: The Author, 1684.
Baber, John. *A Poem upon the Coronation*. London: R. Everingham, 1685.
_____. *To the King, upon the Queen's Being Deliver'd of a Son*. London: Mary Thompson, 1688.
_____. *To the Poet Bavius*. London: Printed for the Author, 1688.
Bacon, Francis. *Sylva Sylvarum*. London: n.p., 1627.
Baker, George. *The Nature and Property of Quicksilver*. London: T. Cadman, 1585.
_____. *New Jewell of Health*. London: Henrie Denham. 1576.
Balfour, Andrew. *Letters Write [sic] to a Friend*. Edinburgh: n.p., 1700.
Bate, George. *Elenchus Motuum Nuperorum in Anglia: A Short Historical Account of the Rise and Progress of the Late Troubles in England*. London: A. Swalle, 1685.

Behn, Aphra. *To the Poet Bavius*. London: Printed for the Author, 1688.
Blackmore, Richard. *Medical Tracts*. London: n.p., 1725.
_____. *Report on William III's Autopsy*. London: n.p., 1702.
_____. *Treatise on Rheumatism and the King's Evil*. London: J. Pemberton, 1727.
_____. *Treatise upon Small Pox and Gout*. London: J. Clark, 1723.
_____. *A True and Impartial History of the Conspiracy against the Person and Government of King William III of Glorious Memory, in the Year 1695*. London: J. Knapton, 1723.
Blochwich, Martin. *Anatomie of the Elder*. Trans. Christopher Irvine. London: n.p., 1655.
Blondel, James. *The Power of Mother's Imagination over the Fetus*. London: J. Brotherton, 1729.
Boorde, Andrew. *The Book of Berdes*. London: n.p., 1547.
_____. *Breviarie of Health*. London: n.p., 1575.
_____. *Introduction and Dyetary with Barnes in the Defence of the Berde*. Edited F. J. Furnivall. London: Trubner, 1870.
_____. *First Book of the Introduction of Knowledge*. London: n. p., 1550.
_____. *Merry Tales of the Mad Men of Gotham*. London: Thomas Colwell, 1565.
Brewer, J.S., R. H. Brodie, and J. Gairdner, eds. *Letters and Papers, Foreign and Domestic, of the Reign of Henry VIII*. 2nd ed. 21 vols. London: HMSO, 1862–1920.
Brown, Beatrice C., ed. *The Letters and Diplomatic Instructions of Queen Anne*. London: Cassell, 1935.
Browne, Edward. *Journal of a Visit to Paris 1664*. London: John Murray, 1923.
Browne, John. *Adenochoiradelogia: Treatise on the King's Evil*. London: T. Newcomb, 1684.
_____. *Charisma Basilicon*. London: Thomas Newcomb, 1684.
_____. *Preternatural Tumours*. London: R. Clavel, 1678.
Buckley, W. E., ed. *Memoirs of Thomas, Earl of Ailsbury*. London, n.p., 1890.
Bullein, William. *Bulwarke of Defence against All Sicknes, Sorenes and Woundes*. London: John Kyngston, 1579.
Burnet, Gilbert. *History of His Own Time*. 2nd ed. 6 vols. Oxford: Oxford University Press, 1833.
Burnet, Thomas. *Thesaurus Medicinae Practicae*. London: Robert Boulter, 1683.
Caius, John. *Book of Sweats*. London: n.p., 1552.
_____. *Works of John Caius*. Ed. E. S. Roberts. Cambridge: Cambridge University Press, 1912.
Calendar of the Close Rolls Preserved in the Public Record Office (1485–1500). London: HMSO, 1955.
Calendar of the Patent Rolls Preserved in the Public Record Office: Henry VII (1485–1509). 2 vols. London: HMSO, 1914–16.Calendar of State Papers, Domestic Series, for the Commonwealth. 13 vols. London: Longmans, 1875–86.
Calendar of State Papers, Domestic Series, of the Reign of Anne. 2 vols. London: HMSO, 1916.

Calendar of State Papers, Domestic Series, of the Reign of Charles I, 1625–1649. 23 vols. London: Longman, Brown, Green, Longman, and Roberts, 1858–97.Calendar of State Papers, Domestic Series, of the Reign of Charles II, 1660–1685. 28 vols. London: Longman, Green, Longman, and Roberts, 1860–1939.

Calendar of State Papers, Domestic Series, for the Reign of James II. 3 vols. London: HMSO, 1960–72.

Calendar of State Papers, Domestic Series, for the Reign of William III. 6 vols. London: HMSO, 1908–37.

Calendar of State Papers, Domestic Series, for the Reign of William and Mary. 5 vols. London: Eyre and Spottiswoode, 1895–1906.Calendar of State Papers, Domestic Series, for the Reigns of Edward VI, Mary, Elizabeth, and James I. 12 vols. London: Longman, Green, Longman, and Roberts, 1853–72.

Calendar of Treasury Books (1660–1714). 32 vols. London: HMSO, 1904.

Calendar of Treasury Papers (1556–1728). 6 vols. London: Longmans, Green, Reader, and Dyer, 1868–89.

Catalogue of the Entire Library of Thomas Goodman, Physician. London: n.p., 1739.

Catalogue of the Library of Dr. Francis Bernard. London, n.p., 1698.

Chamberlen, Hugh. *Proposal for Better Securing of Health.* London: n.p., 1689.

_____. *Vomits in Fevers.* Edinburgh: n.p., 1700.

Chamberlen, Peter. *Public Baths.* London: n.p., 1648.

_____. *A Voice in Rhama.* London: William Bentley, 1646.

Charlton, Walter. *Dissertation on the Vindication of the Antiquity of Stonehenge.* London: J. Browne, 1730.

_____. *Immortality of the Human Soul.* London: W. Wilson, 1657.

Clowes, William. *Treatise for the Artificiall Cure of Struma.* Amsterdam: Da Capo Reprints, 1970.

_____. *Treatise on the King's Evil.* London: n.p., 1602.

Coxe, Daniel. *Discourse (about) Physick and Physicians.* London: n.p., 1669.

Culpeper, Nicholas. *Catastrophe Magnatum or the Fall of Monarchie.* London: Vere and Brooke, 1652.

_____. *Complete Herbal.* New ed. London: Thomas Kelly, 1835.

_____. *Directory for Midwives: A Guide for Women in Their Conception, Bearing, and Suckling Their Children.* London: Peter Cole, 1651.

_____. *Galen's Art of Physick.* London: Peter Cole, 1652.

_____. *Semiotica Uranica or An Strological Judgment of Diseases.* 4th ed. London: N. Brooke, 1671.

de Beer, E. S., ed. *The Diary of John Evelyn.* 6 vols. Oxford: Clarendon Press, 1955.

de Blegny, Nicolas. *The English Remedy or Talbor's Wonderful Secret.* London: J. Wallis, 1682.

Denton, William. *The Burnt Child Dreads the Fire.* London: J. Magnes, 1675.

Dickinson, Edmund. *Physica vetus et vera.* London: n.p., 1702.

Doebner, Richard, ed. *Memoirs of Mary, Queen of England*. London: David Nutt, 1886.
Elyot, Thomas. *The Castel of Helth*. London: Thomas Bertheleti, 1534.
Fanshawe, Anne Harrison. *Memoirs of Lady Fanshawe*. Ed. N. H. Nicolas. London: Henry Colburn, 1829.
Foxe, John. *Acts and Monuments of These Latter and Perilous Days*. 8th ed., 3 vols. London: Company of Stationers, 1641.
Freind, John. *Chemical Lectures*. London: J. Bowyer, 1712.
Fuller, William. *A Brief Discovery of the True Mother of the Pretended Prince of Wales*. London: n.p., 1696.
Gale, Thomas. *Certain Works of Chirurgery*. London: T. East, 1586.
Garth, Samuel. *The Dispensatory: A Poem*. London: John Nutt, 1699.
_____. *The Works of Sir Samuel Garth*. Dublin: T. Ewing, 1769.
Gerard, John. *The Herball or General History of Plants*. London: John Norton, 1597.
Gibson, Thomas. *Anatomy of Human Bodies*. London: Flesher, 1682.
Goddard, Jonathan. *A Discourse Setting Forth the Unhappy Condition of the Practice of Physick in London*. London: John Martyn, 1670.
Grafton, Richard. *A Chronicle at Large*. 2 vols. London: H. Denham, 1569.
Grant, Roger. *Full Account of a Miraculous Cure*. London: T. Childe, 1709.
Gray, John M., ed. *Memoirs of Sir John Clerk*. Edinburgh: Edinburgh University Press, 1892.
Greaves, Edward. *Morbus Epidemius*. Oxford: L. Lichfield, 1643.
Grey, Elizabeth, Countess of Kent. *Choice Manuall of Rare and Select Secrets in Physick and Chirurgerie*. London: W(illiam) J(arvis), 1653.
Halliwell, J. O., ed. *The Private Diary of Dr. John Dee*. London: Camden Society, xix, 1842.
Hamilton, David. *Diary of Sir David Hamilton*. Ed. Philip Roberts. Oxford: Oxford University Press, 1975.
_____. *Treatise of a Miliary Fever*. London: A. Bettesworth, 1737.
Harel, Adam. *Album Amicorum*. London: n.p., 1914.
Harris, Walter. *De Morbis Acutis Infantum*. London: Samuel Smith, 1689.
_____. *A Description of the King's Royal Palace and Gardens at Loo*. London: R. Roberts, 1699.
_____. *Farewell to Popery*. London: Walter Kettilby, 1679.
_____. *Pharmacologia Anti-Empirica, or A Rational Discourse of Remedies both Chymical and Galenical*. London: Richard Chiswell, 1683.
Hartman, George. *The Family Physitian*. London: R. Wellington, 1696.
Harvey, Gideon. *The Conclave of Physicians*. London: James Partridge, 1683.
_____. *The Family Physician and the House Apothecary*. 2nd ed. London: M. R., 1678.
_____. *The Vanities of Philosophy and the Physick*. London: A. Roper, 1700.
Harvey, William. *Anatomical Exercitation*. London: James Young, 1653.
Haworth, Samuel. *True Method of Curing Consumptions*. London: Samuel Smith, 1683.

Hinton, John. *Memoires of Sir John Hinton, Physitian in Ordinary*. London: n.p., 1679.

Historical Manuscripts Commission. *Manuscripts of His Grace, the Duke of Rutland*. 4 vols. London: HMSO, 1888–1905.

_____. *12th Report*. App. VII. London: HMSO, 1890.

Irvine, Christopher. *Medicina Magnetica*. Edinburgh: n.p., 1656.

James I, King of England. *A Counterblast to Tobacco*. London: R. B., 1604.

Jones, Inigo. *The Most Notable Antiquity of Great Britain*. Farnborough, England: Gregg, 1971.

King, William, ed. *Memoirs of Sarah, Duchess of Marlborough*. London: Dutton, 1930.

Latham, Robert, and William Matthews, eds. *The Diary of Samuel Pepys*. 10 vols. Berkeley: University of California Press, 1971.

LeFevre, Nicolas. *Discourse upon Sir Walter Rawleigh's Great Cordial*. London: J. F., 1664.

Lister, Martin. *The Art of Cooking*. London: B. Lintott, 1709.

_____. *A Journey to Paris*. London: A. Baldwin, 1699.

Lower, Martin. *De catarrhis*. Translated by Richard Hunter and Ida Macalpine. London: Dawson's, 1963.

_____. *Dr. Lower's Receipts*. London: John Nutt, 1700.

Luttrell, Narcissus. *A Brief Historical Relation of State Affairs, 1678–1714*. 6 vols. Oxford: Oxford University Press, 1857.

Marbecke, Roger. *A Defense of Tobacco*. London: Richard Field, 1602.

Marlborough, Sarah Jennings Churchill. *Letters of Sarah, Duchess of Marlborough*. London: Murray, 1875.

Mayerne, Theodore. *The Compleat Midwife's Practice Enlarged*. 5th ed. Ed. John Pechey. London: H. Rhodes, 1698.

_____. *Medicinal Counsels or Advices*. London: N. Ponder, 1677.

Mayerne, Theodore and Thomas Cadyman. *The Distiller of London*. London: Richard Bishop, 1639.

Mead, Richard. *The Medical Works of Richard Mead*. London: C. Hitch, 1762.

Meads, Dorothy, ed. *Diary of Lady Margaret Hoby*. London: Routledge, 1930.

_____. *Pharmacopoeia Pauperum*. London: T. Warner, 1718.

Memorial to Dr. William Briggs. London: n.p., 1702.

Newcome, Henry. *The Compeat Mother*. London: J. Wyat, 1695.

Nichols, John, ed. *The Progresses, Processions, and Magnificent Festivities of King James the First*. 4 vols. London: J. B. Nichols, 1828.

_____. *The Progresses and Public Processions of Queen Elizabeth*. 3 vols. London: Printed by the editor, 1788–1805.

Nichols, John Gough, ed. *The Diary of Henry Machyn*. New York: AMS Press, 1968.

Otten, Charlotte F., ed. *English Women's Voices 1540–1800*. Miami: Florida International University Press, 1992.

Parkinson, John. *Garden of Pleasant Flowers*. Ed. Alfred Hyatt. London: T. N. Foulis, 1904.

Pechey, John. *The Compleat Herbal of Physical Plants*. London: n.p., 1694.

_____. *The Compleat Midwife's Practice Enlarged*. 5th ed. London: H. Rhodes, 1698.

Peter, Charles. *Syphilis*. London: J. Bowyer, 1720.

Primrose, Gilbert. *Jacob's Vow*. London: F. Kingston, 1617.

Pyke, J. P. *A Hundred Notable Things*. London: n.p., 1686.

Radcliffe, John. *Memoirs of the Life of Radcliffe*. Ed. William Pittis. London: E. Curll, 1715.

_____. *Pharmacopoeia Radcliffeanae*. Ed. Edward Strother. London: n.p., 1716.

Ramesey, William. *Gentleman's Companion*. London: Rowland Reynolds, 1672.

Read, William. *A Short But Exact Account of All Diseases Incident to the Eyes*. 2nd ed. London: n.p., 1710.

Ronjat, Etienne. *Lettre Écrite de Londres à un Médecin*. London: n.p., 1703.

Royal College of Physicians of London. *London Pharmacopoeia of 1618 (Pharmacopoeia Londinensis)*, reproduced in facsimile. Madison: State Historical Society of Wisconsin, 1944.

Salmon, William. *Pharmacopoeia Bateana*. Translated by James Shipton. London: S. Smith, 1694.

_____. *Pharmacopoeia Londinensis or New London Dispensatory*. 5th ed. London: J. Dawk, 1696.

Scott-Moncrieff, Robert, ed. *The Household Book of Lady Grisell Baillie*. Edinburgh: Scottish History Society, 1911.

Sibbald, Robert. *The Autobiography of Sir Robert Sibbald*. Edinburgh: n.p., 1833.

_____. *The Memoirs of Robert Sibbald*. Ed. Francis Paget Hett. London: H. Milford, 1932.

Skeyne, Gilbert. *Tracts by Dr. Gilbert Skeyne, Mediciner to His Majesty*. Edinburgh: Bannatyne Club, 1860.

Sloane, Hans. *A Concise Narrative of His Life*. London: n.p., 1755.

_____. *Discourse on the State of Health in Jamaica*. London: n. p., 1679.

_____. *Voyage to Madeira, Barbados, Nieves, St. Christopher'sand Jamaica*. 2 vols. London: B. M., 1705–25.

Swift, Jonathan. *Journal to Stella*. 2 vols. London: Oxford University Press, 1948.

Talbor, Robert. *Pyretologia: A Rational Account of the Causes and Cures of Agues*. London: R. Clavel, 1672.

Thompson, E. M., ed. *Correspondence of the Family of Hatton*. 2 vols. New York: Johnson Reprints, 1965.

To That Most Incorrigible Scribbler Bavius. London: "Printed for the Coffee-Houses," 1688.

The Tryals of George Wakeman. London: H. Hills, 1679.

Turner, Daniel. *De Morbid Cutaneis*. London: R. Bonwicke, 1714.

_____. *Discourse concerning Gleets*. London: n.p., 1729.
_____. *The Drop and Pill of Mr. Ward Considered*. London: n.p., 1735.
_____. *Present State of Surgery*. London: n.p., 1703.
_____. *A Short Review of the Quicksilver Controvery*. London: n.p., 1733.
_____. *Syphilis*. London: R. Wilkin, 1737.Vicary, John. *Anatomie of the Bodie of Man*. Ed. F. J. Furnivall and Percy Furnivall. London: Trubner, 1888.
_____. *The English-Man's Treasure*. 7th ed. London: B. Alsop, 1626.
Welwood, James. *Memoirs of the Most Material Transactions in England*. London: T. Goodwin, 1700.
_____. *A True Relation of the Wonderful Cure of M. Maillard to which is added a letter from Dr. Welwood upon that subject*. London: R. Baldwin, 1694.
Whitaker, Tobias. *An Elenchus of Opinions concerning the Cure of the Small Pox*. London: n.p., 1661.
_____. *The Tree of Human Life*. London: n.p., 1638.
Wild, Robert. *The Grateful Non-Conformist*. London: n.p., 1665.
Willis, Robert., ed. *The Works of William Harvey*. London: Sydenham Society, 1847.
Willis, Thomas. *Cerebri anatome*. London: Thomas Roycroft, 1664.
_____. *The Remaining Medical Works*. Translated by S. Pordage. London: T. Dring, 1681.
Wiseman, Richard. *Charisma Basilicon*. London: Thomas Newcomb, 1684.
_____. *Severall Chirurgical Treatises*. London: Flesher and Macock, 1676.
Woodward, John. *The State of Physick and of Diseases*. London: T. Horne, 1718.

Secondary Sources: Books

Akrigg, G.P.V. *Jacobean Pageant or the Court of James I*. London: Hamish Hamilton, 1962.
Allen, Benjamin. *Natural History of the Mineral Waters of Great Britain*. London: William Innys, 1711.
Arber, Agnes. *Herbals, Their Origins and Evolution*. (Cambridge: Cambridge University Press, 1912.
Arrizabalaga, Jon, John Henderson, and Roger French. *The Great Pox: The French Disease in Renaissance Europe*. New Haven, Conn.: Yale University Press, 1997.
Ashley, Maurice. *Charles II*. New York: Praeger, 1971.
_____. *James II*. Minneapolis: University of Minnesota Press, 1977.
_____. *The Stuarts in Love*. New York: Macmillan, 1963.
Aveling, J. H. *The Chamberlens and the Midwifery Forceps*. London: Churchill, 1882.
_____. *English Midwives*. London: Churchill, 1872.
Aylmer, G. E. *The State's Servants: The Civil Service of the English Republic 1649–1660*. London: Routledge and Kegan Paul, 1973.
Badger, John. *Exact Alphabetical Catalogue of All that Have Their Degree in Physick, 1659–1695*. London: n.p., 1695.

Barrett, C.R.B. *History of the Society of Apothecaries of London*. London: E. Stock, 1905.

Barwick, Peter. *Life of Dr. John Barwick*. London: J. Bettenham, 1724.

Bathurst, Bejamin, ed. *Letters of Two Queens*. London: R. Holden, 1924.

Beaven, Alfred. *Aldermen of the City of London*. 2 vols. London: Eden Fisher, 1913.

Beck, R. Theodore. *The Cutting Edge: The Early History of theSurgeons of London*. London: Lund Humphries, 1974.

Beckman, Otto. *A Pictorial History of Medicine*. Springfield, Ill.: Thomas, 1956.

Beer, Barrett L. *Northumberland*. Kent, Ohio: Kent State University Press, 1973.

_____. *Rebellion and Riot: Popular Disorder during the Reign of Edward VI*. Kent, Ohio: Kent State University Press, 1985.

_____. *Tudor England Observed*. Stroud, England: Sutton, 1998.

Beier, Lucinda McCray. *Sufferers and Healers: The Experience of Illness in Seventeenth Century England*. London: Routledge and Kegan Paul, 1987.

Beresford, John. *Gossip of the Seventeenth and Eighteenth Centuries*. 2 vols. London: R. Cobden-Sanderson, 1923.

Bergeron, David M. *Royal Family, Royal Lovers: King James of England and Scotland*. Columbia: University of Missouri Press, 1991.

Berlant, Jeffrey L. *Profession and Monopoly*. Berkeley: University of California Press, 1975.

Bingham, Caroline. *James V of Scotland*. London: Collins, 1971.

_____. *The Stewart Kings of Scotland*. New York: St. Martin's Press, 1974.

Bloch, Marc. *The Royal Touch*. London: Routledge, 1973.

Blomberg, William N. *An Account of the Life of Edmund Dickinson, M.D*. London: R. Montague, 1737.

Bloom, J. H., and R. R. James. *Medical Practitioners 1529–1725*. Cambridge: Cambridge University Press, 1935.

Bond, Edward A. *Russia at the Close of the Sixteenth Century*. London: Hakluyt Society, 1856.

Bowers, Toni. *The Politics of Motherhood: British Writing and Culture, 1680–1760*. New York: Cambridge University Press, 1996.

Bradford, C. A. *Hugh Morgan, Queen Elizabeth's Apothecary*. London, E. T. Heron, 1939.

Brockliss, L.W.B. *French Higher Education in the Seventeenth and Eighteenth Centuries*. Oxford: Clarendon Press, 1987.

Brockliss, Laurence, and Colin Jones. *The Medical World of Early Modern France*. Oxford: Clarendon Press, 1997.

Brown, Keith. *Bloodfeud in Scotland, 1573–1625*. Edinburgh: J. Donald, 1986.

Bucholz, R. O. *The Augustan Court: Queen Anne and the Decline of Court Culture*. Stanford, Calif.: Stanford University Press, 1993.

Buchanan, Patricia Hill. *Margaret Tudor, Queen of Scots*. Edinburgh: Scottish Academic Press, 1985.

Bush, M. L. *The Government Policy of Protector Somerset*. Montreal: McGill-Queen's University Press, 1975.

Butler, Iris. *Rule of Three*. London: Hodder and Stoughton, 1967.

Calvert, E. M., and R.T.C. Calvert. *Serjeant Surgeon John Knight*. London: W. Heinemann, 1939.

Cannon, John, and Ralph Griffiths. *Oxford Illustrated History of the British Monarchy*. Oxford: Oxford University Press, 1988.

Carlton, Charles. *Charles I: The Personal Monarch*. 2nd ed. London: Routledge, 1995.

_____. *Royal Childhoods*. London: Routledge and Kegan Paul, 1986.

Carr, John Dickinson. *The Murder of Sir Edmund Godfrey*. New York: International Polygontics, 1989.

Carrier, Irene. *James VI and I, King of Great Britain*. Cambridge: Cambridge University Press, 1998.

Carruthers, Robert, ed. *The Poetical Works of Alexander Pope*. 4 vols. London: Ingraham, 1953.

Carswell, John. *The Descent on England*. New York: John Day, 1969.

Chamberlin, Frederick. *The Private Character of Henry the Eighth*. New York: Washburne, 1931.

Chapman, Hester. *Lady Jane Grey*. London: Jonathan Cape, 1962.

_____. *Mary II, Queen of England*. Westport, Conn.: Greenwood Press, 1976.

_____. *The Last Tudor King*. London: Jonathan Cape: 1958.

_____. *Queen Anne's Son*. London: Deutsch, 1954.

_____. *The Thistle and the Rose*. New York: Coward, McCann and Geoghegan, 1969.

Chauvois, Louis. *William Harvey: Life and Times*. London: Philosophical Library, 1957.

Chrimes, S. B. *Henry VII*. Berkeley: University of California Press, 1972.

Clark, George. *History of the Royal College of Physicians of London*. 2 vols. Oxford: Clarendon Press, 1964.

Claydon, Tony. *William III and the Godly Revolution*. Cambridge: Cambridge University Press, 1996.

Clippingdale, Samuel Dodd. Medical Court Roll, 2 vols. (unpublished). Royal College of Surgeons Library, London.

Comrie, John D. *History of Scottish Medicine*. 2nd ed. 2 Vols. London: Bailliere, Tindall and Cox, 1932.

Cook, Harold J. *The Decline of the Old Medical Regime in Stuart London*. Ithaca, N.Y.: Cornell University Press, 1986.

_____. *Trials of an Ordinary Doctor*. Baltimore: Johns Hopkins University Press, 1994.

Cook, Richard I. *Sir Samuel Garth*. Boston: Twayne, 1980.

Copeman, W. S. C. *The Apothecaries of London 1617–1967*. London: Pergamon, 1967.

_____. *Doctors and Disease in Tudor Times*. London: Dawson's, 1960.

Coward, Barry. *Oliver Cromwell*. London: Longman, 1991.

Craig, W. S. *History of the Royal College of Physicians of Edinburgh*. Oxford: Basil Blackwell, 1976.

Crawfurd, Raymond. *The King's Evil*. Oxford: Oxford University Press, 1911.

_____. *The Last Days of Charles II*. Oxford: Clarendon Press, 1909.

Creighton, Charles. *A History of Epidemics in Britain*. 2nd ed. 2 vols. Cambridge: Cambridge University Press, 1891.

Cutter, I. S., and Harry R. Viets. *A Short History of Midwifery*. Philadelphia: Saunders, 1964.

Daniel, Thomas M. *Captain of Death: The Story of Tuberculosis*. Rochester, N.Y.: University of Rochester Press, 1997.

deBeer, G. R. *Sir Hans Sloane and the British Museum*. London: Oxford University Press, 1953.

Debus, Allen G. *The Chemical Philosophy: Paracelsian Science and Medicine in the Sixteenth and Seventeenth Centuries*. 2 vols. New York: Science History Publications, 1977.

_____. *The English Paracelsians*. London: Oldbourne, 1965.

_____, ed. *Medicine in Seventeenth-Century England*. Berkeley: University of California Press, 1974.

Desportes, Pierre, ed. *Histoire de Reims*. Toulouse: Univers de la France et des Pays Francophone, 1983.

Dewhurst, Jack. *Royal Confinements: A Gynaecological History of Britain's Royal Family*. New York: St. Martin's Press, 1980.

Dewhurst, Kenneth. *Dr. Thomas Syndenham*. Berkeley: University of California Press, 1966.

_____. *The Quicksilver Doctor*. Bristol, England: Wright, 1957.

_____. *Thomas Willis's Oxford Lectures*. Oxford: Sandford Publications, 1980.

Dickens, A. G. *The English Reformation*. 2nd ed. University Park: University of Pennsylvania Press, 1991.

Dictionary of National Biography. 22 vols. New York: Macmillan, 1908; first published 1885–1901 in 66 vols.

Dictionary of National Biography Supplement: Corrections and Additions. Boston: G. K. Hall, 1966.

Digby, Anne. *Making a Medical Living*. Cambridge: Cambridge University Press, 1994.

Dobson, Jessie, and R. Milnes Walker. *Barbers and Barber-Surgeons of London*. London: Blackwell, 1979.

Donald, Peter. *An Uncounselled King: Charles I and the Scottish Troubles, 1637–1641*. Cambridge: Cambridge University Press, 1990.

Donaldson, Gordon. *All the Queen's Men: Power and Politics in Mary Stewart's Scotland*. New York: St. Martin's Press, 1983.

Donegan, Jane B. *Women and Men Midwives*. Westport, Conn.: Greenwood Press, 1978.

Donnison, Jean. *Midwives and Medical Men*. New York: Schocken, 1977.

Duran-Reynals, M. L. *The Fever-Bark Tree*. Garden City NY: Doubleday, 1946.
Durston, Christopher. *James I*. New York: Routledge, 1993.
Dutton, Ralph. *English Court Life from Henry VII to George II*. London: Batsford, 1963.
Eccles, Audrey. *Obstetrics and Gynaecology in Tudor and Stuart England*. London: Croom Helm, 1982.
Elton, G. R. *England under the Tudors*. London: Methuen, 1956.
Reform and Reformation England. London: Arnold, 1977.
Emmison, F. G. *Tudor Secretary: Sir William Petre at Court and Home*. Cambridge: Cambridge University Press, 1961.
Erickson, Carolly. *Bloody Mary*. Garden City, N. Y.: Doubleday, 1978.
_____. *The First Elizabeth*. New York: Summit Books, 1983.
Feiling, Keith. *A History of the Tory Party 1640–1714*. Oxford: Clarendon Press, 1924.
Fines, John. *Biographical Register of Early English Protestants*. Oxford: Sutton Courtenay, 1981.
Fluckiger, Friedrich A. *The Cinchona Barks*. Philadelphia: Blakiston, 1884.
Forbes, T. R. *The Midwife and the Witch*. New Haven, Conn.: Yale University Press, 1966.
Foster, Joseph. *Alumnae Oxonienses, 1500–1714*. 4 vols. Oxford: Parker, 1891–92.
Fox, Frank L. A *Distant Storm: The Four Days' Battle of 1666*. Rotherfield, England: Press of Sail Publications, 1996.
Fraser, Antonia. *Cromwell*. New York: Dell, 1973.
_____. *Mary, Queen of Scots*. London: Weidenfeld and Nicolson, 1969.
_____. *Royal Charles*. New York: Delta, 1979.
_____. *The Weaker Vessel*. New York: Vintage, 1985.
_____. *The Wives of Henry VIII*. New York: Alfred A. Knopf, 1992.
French, Peter. *John Dee*. London: Ark, 1987.
French, Roger, and Andrew Wear, eds. *The Medical Revolution of the Seventeenth Century*. Cambridge: Cambridge University Press, 1989.
Froude, J.A. *The Reign of Mary Tudor*. London: J.M. Dent, 1924.
Furdell, Elizabeth Lane. *James Welwood: Physician to the Glorious Revolution*. Conshohocken, Penn.: Combined Publishing, 1998.
Gairdner, James. *Henry the Seventh*. London: Macmillan, 1902.
Garrett, C. H. *The Marian Exiles*. Cambridge: Cambridge University Press, 1938.
Garrison, Fielding. *Introduction to the History of Medicine*. 4th ed. Philadelphia: W. B. Saunders Co., 1929.
Getz, Faye. *Healing and Society in Medieval England: A Middle English Translation of the Pharmaceutical Writings of Gilbertus Anglicus*. Madison: University of Wisconsin Press, 1991.
_____. *Medicine in the English Middle Ages*. Princeton, N.J.: Princeton University Press, 1998.

Gillingham, John. *The Wars of the Roses*. Baton Rouge: Louisiana State University Press, 1981.

Gottfried, Richard S. *Doctors and Medicine in Medieval England, 1340–1530*. Princeton, N.J.: Princeton University Press, 1986.

Grant, Alexander. *Henry VII*. London: Methuen, 1985.

Gray, Robert. *The King's Wife*. London: Secker and Warburg, 1990.

Green, David. *Queen Anne*. London: Collins, 1970.

Gregg, Edward. *Queen Anne*. London: Routledge and Kegan Paul, 1980.

Gregg, Pauline. *King Charles I*. Berkeley: University of California Press, 1981.

Hackett, L. W. *Malaria in Europe*. London: Oxford University Press, 1937.

Haigh, Christopher. *Elizabeth I*. London: Longman, 1988.

Hainsworth, D. R., and Christine Churches. *The Anglo-Dutch Naval Wars 1652–1674*. Stroud, England: Sutton, 1998.

Hamel, J. *England and Russia*. Trans. John S. Leigh. New York: DaCapo, 1968.

Hardman, Joel G., ed. *Goodman and Gilman's The Pharmaceutical Basis of Therapeutics*. 9th ed. New York: McGraw-Hill, 1996.

Harris, Tim. *Politics under the Later Stuarts: Party Conflict in a Divided Society, 1660–1715*. London: Longman, 1993.

Haswell, Jock. *James II: Soldier and Sailor*. London: Hamilton, 1972.

Hayward, John. *The Life and Raigne of King Edward the Sixth*. Ed. Barrett L. Beer. Kent, Ohio: Kent State University Press, 1993.

Hembry, Phyllis. *The English Spa, 1560–1815*. London: Athlone Press, 1990.

Hill, Christopher. *Change and Continuity in Seventeenth-Century England*. Rev. ed. New Haven, Conn.: Yale University Press, 1991.

_____. *God's Englishman*. New York: Harper, 1972.

Hogrefe, Pearl. *The Life and Times of Sir Thomas Elyot, Englishman*. Ames: Iowa State University Press, 1967.

Hole, Christina. *The English Housewife in the Seventeenth Century*. London: Chatto and Windus, 1953.

Holmes, Geoffrey. *Augustan England: Professions, State and Society 1680–1730*. London: George Allen and Unwin, 1982.

_____. *British Politics in the Age of Anne*. London: Melbourne, 1967.

Hone, Campbell R. *The Life of Dr. John Radcliffe*. London: Faber and Faber, 1950.

Hopkinson, M. R. *Anne of England*. New York: Macmillan, 1934.

Horton-Smith, L. G. *Dr. Walter Bailey*. St. Alban's, England: Campfield Press, 1952.

Hunter, Lynette, and Sarah Hutton, eds. *Women, Science and Medicine 1500–1700*. Stroud, England: Sutton, 1997.

Hunter, Michael. *The Royal Society and Its Fellows 1660–1700*. Chalfont St. Giles, England: British Society for the History of Science, 1982.

_____. *Science and Society in Restoration England*. Cambridge: Cambridge University Press, 1981.

Hunting, Penelope. *A History of the Society of Apothecaries*. London: Society of Apothecaries, 1998.

Isler, Hansruedi. *Thomas Willis, 1621–1675: Doctor and Scientist*. New York: Hafner, 1968.

Jameson, Eric. *The Natural History of Quackery*. London: C. C. Thomas, 1961.

Jaramillo-Arango, Jaime. *The Conquest of Malaria*. London: Heinemann, 1950.

Jenkins, Elizabeth. *Elizabeth and Leicester*. New York: Coward-McCann, 1962.

Jesse, John H. *Memoirs of the Court of England during the Reign of the Stuarts*. 4 vols. London: R. Bentley, 1840.

Johnston, William. *Bibliography and Portraits of Arthur Johnston, M.D., Physician to James I and Charles I*. Aberdeen: privately printed, 1896.

Jones, J. R. *The First Whigs*. Rev. ed. London: Oxford University Press, 1970.

_____. *The Revolution of 1688 in England*. New York: Norton, 1973.

Jones, Whitney. *William Turner*. London: Routledge, 1988.

Jordan, W. K. *Edward VI: The Threshold of Power*. Cambridge, Mass.: Harvard University Press, 1970.

_____. *Edward VI: The Young King*. London: George Allen and Unwin, 1968.

Katz, David S. *The Jews in the History of England, 1485–1850*. Oxford: Clarendon Press, 1994.

Kearney, Hugh. *Scholars and Gentlemen: Universities and Society in Pre-Industrial Britain 1500–1700*. Ithaca, N.Y.: Cornell University Press, 1970.

Keele, Kenneth. *William Harvey*. London: Nelson, 1965.

Keevil, John. *Hamey the Stranger*. London: G. Bles, 1952.

Kemble, James. *Idols and Invalids*. Garden City, N.J.: Doubleday, 1936.

Kenyon, John P. *The Popish Plot*. New York: Penguin, 1974.

Keynes, Geoffrey. *Dr. Martin Lister: A Bibliography*. London: St. Paul's Bibliographies, 1981.

_____. *The Life of William Harvey*. Oxford: Clarendon Press, 1966.

King, Lester S. *The Medical World of the Eighteenth Century*. Chicago: University of Chicago Press, 1958.

_____. *The Road to Medical Enlightenment, 1650–1695*. New York: American Elsevier, 1970.

Knachel, Philip A., ed. *Eikon Basilikon: The Portraiture of His Sacred Majesty in His Solitude and Sufferings*. Ithaca, N.Y.: Cornell University Press, 1966.

Kolin, Philip C. *Elizabethan Stage Doctor*. Salzburg: Institut fur Englische Sprache und Literatur, 1975.

Larkey, Sanford V. *Medical Knowledge in Tudor England*. San Marino, Calif.: Huntington Library, 1932.

_____. *Vesalian Compendium of Geminus and Nicholas Udall's Translation*. London: n.p., 1933.

Lawson-Dick, Oliver, ed. *Aubrey's Brief Lives*. London: Mandarin, 1992.

Lee, Maurice. *Great Britain's Solomon: James VI and I in His Three Kingdoms*. Urbana: University of Illinois Press, 1990.

Lehmberg, S. E. *Sir Thomas Elyot: Tudor Humanist*. Austin: University of Texas Press, 1960.

LeNeve, J. *Lives and Characters of the Most Illustrious Persons Who Died in the Year*. London: S. Holt, 1712.

Leti, Gregorio. *La vie d'Elisabeth reine d'Angleterre*. Amsterdam: Chez Henri Desbordes, 1714.

Levin, Carole. *The Heart and Stomach of a King*. Philadelphia: University of Pennsylvania Press, 1994.

Levine, Joseph M. *The Battle of the Books*. Ithaca, N.Y.: Cornell University Press, 1991.

_____. *Dr. Woodward's Shield: History, Science, and Satire in Augustan England*. Ithaca, N.Y.: Cornell University Press, 1991.

Lewis, Jenkin. *Memoirs of Prince William Henry, Duke of Gloucester*. London: Payne, 1789.

Lindeboom, G. A. *Dutch Medical Biography*. Amsterdam: Rodopi, 1984.

Loach, Jennifer. *Parliament and Crown in the Reign of Mary Tudor*. Oxford: Oxford University Press, 1986.

Loades, David. *John Dudley, Duke of Northumberland*. Oxford: Clarendon Press, 1996.

_____. *Mary Tudor*. Oxford: Blackwell, 1989.

Lockyer, Roger. *Buckingham*. London: Longman, 1981.

_____. *James VI and I*. London: Longman, 1998.

Longmore, T. *Richard Wiseman*. London: Longmans, Green and Co., 1891.

Macalpine, Ida, and Richard Hunter. *George III and the Mad Business*. New York: Pantheon, 1969.

MacCaffrey, Wallace. *Elizabeth I*. London: Edward Arnold, 1993.

Mackie, R. L. *King James IV of Scotland*. Edinburgh: Oliver and Boyd, 1958.

Macmichael, William. *The Gold-Headed Cane*. London: Longmans, 1884.

_____. *Lives of British Physicians*. London: J. Murray, 1830.

MacNalty, Arthur. *The Doctor in Politics and Diplomacy*. London: Privately printed, 1937.

_____. *Elizabeth Tudor: The Lonely Queen*. New York: Frederick Ungar, 1961.

_____. *Henry VIII: A Difficult Patient*. London: C. Johnson, 1952.

Madden, Frederic, ed. *Privy Purse Expenses of the Princess Mary*. London: W. Pickering, 1831.

Maddison, Francis, Margaret Pelling, and Charles Webster. *Essays on the Life and Work of Thomas Linacre*. Oxford: Clarendon Press, 1977.

Maple, Eric. *Magic, Medicine and Quackery*. S. Brunswick, N.J.: A. S. Barnes, 1968.

Marshall, J. D. *Lancashire*. London: David and Charles, 1974.

Matthews, Leslie G. *The Royal Apothecaries*. London: Wellcome Medical Library, 1967.

McMains, H. F. *The Death of Oliver Cromwell*. Lexington: University Press of Kentucky, 2000.

Melville, Lewis. *Life and Letters of John Gay*. London: O'Connor, 1921.

Merkel, Ingrid, and Allen G. Debus, eds. *Hermeticism and the Renaissance*. Washington, D.C.: Folger Library, 1988.

Merton, R. K. *Science, Technology and Society in Seventeenth Century England*. New York: H. Fertig, 1970.

Miller, John. *James II*. Hove, England: Wayland, 1978.

_____. *Popery and Politics in England 1660–88*. Cambridge: Cambridge University Press, 1973.

_____. *William and Mary*. London: Weidenfeld and Nicolson, 1974.

Milne, Gustav. *The Great Fire of London*. New Barnet, England: Historical Publications, 1986.

Morgan, Bruce T., ed. *Patronage and Institutions: Science, Technology and Medicine at the European Court 1500–1750*. Rochester, N.Y.: Boydell Press, 1991.

Morgan, William. *English Political Parties and Leaders in the Reign of Queen Anne*. New Haven, Conn.: Yale University Press, 1920.

Moore, Norman. *History of St. Bartholomew's Hospital*. 2 vols. London: C. A. Pearson, 1918.

_____. *History of the Study of Medicine in the British Isles*. Oxford: Clarendon Press, 1908.

Mullett, Michael. *James II and the English Revolution*. New York: Routledge, 1994.

Munk, William. *Roll of the Royal College of Physicians*. 2 vols. London: Longman, Green and Roberts, 1861.

Myers, J. Arthur. *Captain of All These Men of Death*. St. Louis, Mo.: Warren Green, 1977.

Naylor, Kate. *Richard Smith, M.D.* Lincoln, England: Governors of the Foundation of Christ's Hospital, 1951.

Nias, J. B. *Dr. John Radcliffe*. Oxford: Oxford University Press, 1918.

Nicolas, N. H. *The Life and Times of Sir Christopher Hatton*. London: Richard Bentley, 1847.

_____, ed. *The Privy Purse Expenses of Elizabeth of York*. New York: Barnes and Noble Reprint, 1972.

Nutton, Vivian. *John Caius and the Manuscripts of Galen*. Cambridge: Cambridge Philological Society, 1987.

_____, ed. *Medicine at the Courts of Europe, 1500–1837*. London: Routledge, 1990.

O'Day, Rosemary. *The Tudor Age*. London: Longman, 1995.

O'Malley, Charles D. *English Medical Humanists*. Lawrence: University of Kansas Press, 1965.

_____, ed. *The History of Medical Education*. Berkeley: University of California Press, 1970.

Ore, Oystein. *Cardano*. New York: Dover, 1953.

Orme, Nicholas, and Margaret Webster. *The English Hospital 1070–1570*. New Haven, Conn.: Yale University Press, 1995.

Osler, William. *Thomas Linacre*. Cambridge: Cambridge University Press, 1908.

Pagel, Walter. *From Paracelsus to Van Helmont*. Ed. Marianne Winder. London: Variorum Reprints, 1986.

_____. *Jean Baptista van Helmont*. Cambridge: Cambridge University Press, 1982.

_____. *Paracelsus*. New York: S. Karger, 1958.

Parks, G. B. *Richard Hakluyt and the English Voyages*. 2nd ed. Ed. James A. Williamson. New York: Ungar, 1961.

Peck, D. C., ed. *Leicester's Commonwealth*. Athens: Ohio University Press, 1985.

Peck, Linda Levy. *Court Patronage and Court Corruption in Early Stuart England*. London: Routledge, 1990.

_____. *Northampton: Patronage and Policy at the Court of James I*. London: Allen and Unwin, 1982.

Pollard, A. F. *History of England from the Accession of Edward VI to the Death of Elizabeth*. London: Longmans, Green, and Co., 1929.

Poole, H. Edmund. *The Wisdom of Andrew Boorde*. Leicester, England: E. Backus, 1936.

Porter, Dorothy, and Roy Porter. *Patient's Progress: Doctors and Doctoring in Eighteenth-Century England*. Stanford, Calif.: Stanford University Press, 1989.

_____, eds. *Doctors, Politics and Society*. Amsterdam: Rodopi, 1993.

Porter, Roy. *Disease, Medicine and Society in England 1550–1860*. London: Macmillan, 1987.

_____. *Health for Sale: Quackery in England 1660–1850*. Manchester: Manchester University Press, 1989.

_____. *London*. Cambridge, Mass.: Harvard University Press, 1996.

_____, ed. *Medicine: A History of Healing*. New York: Marlowe, 1997.

_____, ed. *Patients and Practitioners*. Cambridge: Cambridge University Press, 1985.

_____, ed. *The Popularization of Medicine 1650–1850*. New York: Routledge, 1992.

Porter, Roy, and G. S. Rousseau. *Gout: The Patrician Malady*. New Haven, Conn.: Yale University Press, 1998.

Porter, Roy, and Mikulas Teich, eds. *The Scientific Revolution in National Context*. Cambridge: Cambridge University Press, 1992.

Potterton, David, ed. *Culpeper's Color Herbal*. New York: Sterling Publishing, 1983.

Power, D'Arcy. *Dr. Walter Bayley and His Works 1529–1592*. London: Royal Medical and Chirurgical Society of London, 1907.

_____. *The Education of A Surgeon under Vicary*. Bristol, England: Wright, 1921.

_____. *Epoch-Making Books in British Surgery*. Bristol,England: n.p., 1928.

_____, ed. *Plarr's Lives of the Fellows of the Royal College of Surgeons*. London: John Wright, 1930.

Poynter, F. N. L. *The Evolution of Medical Education in Britain*. London: Pitman, 1966.

_____. *The Evolution of Medical Practice in Britain*. London: Pitman, 1961.

_____, ed. *The Evolution of Pharmacy in Britain*. Springfield, Ill.: C. C. Thomas, 1965.

_____, ed. *Selected Writings of William Clowes*. London: Harvey and Blythe, 1948.

Prescott, H.F.M. *A Spanish Tudor*. New York: AMS Press, 1970.

Prest, Wilfred, ed. *The Professions in Early Modern England*. London: Croom Helm, 1987.

Purver, Margery. *The Royal Society*. London: Routledge and Kegan Paul, 1967.

Pye, John Patrick. *Thomas Linacre: Scholar, Physician, Priest*. London: Catholic Truth Society, 1912.

Rae, James. *Deaths of the Kings of England*. London: Sherratt and Hughes, 1913.

Raven, Charles E. *English Naturalists from Neckam to Ray*. New York: Cambridge University Press, 1968.

Reeves, L. J. *Charles I and the Road to Personal Rule*. Cambridge: Cambridge University Press, 1989.

Ridley, Jasper. *Elizabeth I*. New York: Viking, 1987.

Roberts, E. S., ed. *The Works of John Caius, M.D.* Cambridge: Cambridge University Press, 1912.

Rohde, Eleanour Sinclair. *The Old English Herbals*. New York: Dover, 1971.

Rosenberg, Eleanor. *Leicester: Patron of Letters*. New York: Columbia University Press, 1955.

Rosenthal, M. B., and D. H. Smith, eds. *Psychosomatic Obstetrics and Gynecology*. New York: Karger, 1985.

Rowse, A. L. *The Elizabethan Renaissance*. 2 vols. New York: Scribner, 1971–72.

Royal College of Physicians of London. *Mutual Admiration: An Exhibition Catalogue*. London: RCP, 1989.

Russell, Conrad. *Parliaments and English Politics 1621–1629*. Oxford: Oxford University Press, 1979.

Russell, Andrew W., ed. *The Town and State Physician in Europe from the Middle Ages to the Enlightenment*. Wolfenbuttel, Germany: Herzog August Bibliothek, 1981.

Sainty, J. C., and R. O. Bucholz. *Officials of the Royal Household 1660–1837. Part I: Department of the Lord Chamberlain and Associated Offices*. London: Institute of Historical Research, 1997.

Saxl, Fritz, and Rudolf Wittkower. *British Art and the Mediterranean*. New York: Oxford University Press, 1948.

Scarisbrick, J. J. *Henry VIII*. Berkeley: University of California Press, 1970.

Seaward, Paul. *The Restoration, 1660–1688*. New York: St. Martin's Press, 1991.

Sena, John F. *The Best-Natured Man*. New York: AMS Press, 1986.

Shapiro, Barbara, and Robert G. Frank, Jr. *English Scientific Virtuosi in the Sixteenth and Seventeenth Centuries*. Los Angeles: University of California Press, 1979.

Sharpe, Kevin. *The Personal Rule of Charles I*. New Haven, Conn.: Yale University Press, 1992.

Sherwood, Roy. *The Court of Oliver Cromwell*. London: Croom Helm, 1977.

Shumaker, Wayne. *Renaissance Curiosa*. Binghamton: State University of New York Press, 1982.

Sigerist, Henry E. *The Great Doctors*. New York: Norton, 1933.

Simon, John. *English Sanitary Institutions*. 2nd ed. London: John Murray, 1897.

Simons, Eric N. *Henry VII: The First Tudor King*. London: Frederick Muller, 1968.

Siraisi, Nancy. *Medieval and Early Renaissance Medicine*. Chicago: University of Chicago Press, 1990.

Skinner, Henry A. *The Origin of Medical Terms*. Baltimore: Johns Hopkins University Press, 1961.

Slack, Paul. *The Impact of Plague in Tudor and Stuart England*. Boston: Routledge and Kegan Paul, 1985.

Smith, Lacey Baldwin. *Henry VIII: Mask of Royalty*. Boston: Houghton Mifflin, 1973.

Smith, R. W. Innes. *English-Speaking Students of Medicine at the University of Leyden*. Edinburgh: Oliver and Boyd, 1932.

Solomon, Harry M. *Sir Richard Blackmore*. Boston: Twayne, 1980.

Somerset, Anne. *Elizabeth I*. New York: Knopf, 1991.

_____. *Unnatural Murder: Poison at the Court of James I*. London: Weidenfeld and Nicolson, 1997.

Somerville, Johann P., ed. *King James VI and I: The Political Writings*. Cambridge: Cambridge University Press, 1994.

Spencer, Herbert R. *History of British Midwifery 1650–1800*. London: Bale, 1927.

_____. *William Harvey, Obstetric Physician and Gynecologist*. London: Harrison and Sons, 1921.

Starkey, David, et al, eds. *The English Court from the Wars of the Roses to the Civil War*. London: Longman, 1987.

Statt, Daniel. *Foreigners and Englishmen*. Newark DE: University of Delaware Press, 1995.

Steensma, Robert. *Dr. John Arbuthnot*. New York: Twayne, 1979.

Stevenson, David. *King's College, Aberdeen*. Aberdeen: University of Aberdeen Press, 1990.

Stevenson, R. Scott. *Famous Illnesses in History*. London: Eyre and Spottiswoode, 1962.

Stow, John. *Survey of London*. New York: Dutton, 1912.

Strickland, Agnes. *Queen Anne*. Vol. 5 of *Lives of the Queens of England*. 8 vols. London: H. Colborn, 1851.

Strong, Roy. *Henry, Prince of Wales, and England's Lost Renaissance*. New York: Thames and Hudson, 1986.

Strype, John. *Ecclesiastical Memorials*. 3 vols. London: B. Aylmer, 1721.

_____. *A Survey of London and Westminster Brought down from 1633 to the Present*. 2 vols. London: A. Churchill, 1720.

Talbot, C. H., and E. A. Hammond. *The Medical Practitioners in Medieval England: A Biographical Register*. London: Wellcome Medical Library, 1965.

Temkin, Owsei. *Galenism*. Ithaca, N.Y.: Cornell University Press, 1973.

Thomas, Keith. *Religion and the Decline of Magic*. London: Weidenfeld and Nicolson, 1971.

Thompson, C.J.S. *Quacks of Old London*. Philadelphia: Lippincott, 1929.

Thompson, Silvanus P. *William Gilbert, Physician*. London: C. Whittingham, 1903.

Thulesius, Olav. *Nicholas Culpeper*. New York: St. Martin's Press, 1992.

Trease, George Edward. *Pharmacy in History*. London: Bailliere, Tindall and Cox, 1964.

Treue, Wilhelm. *Doctor at Court*. Translated by Frances Fawcett. London: Weidenfeld and Nicolson, 1958.

Trevor-Roper, Hugh. *Renaissance Essays*.. Chicago: University of Chicago Press, 1985.

Turner, F. C. *James II*. London: Eyre and Spottiswoode, 1948.

Underwood, E. A. *Boerhaave's Men at Leyden and After*. Edinburgh: Edinburgh University Press, 1977.

van der Zee, Henri, and Barbara van der Zee. *William and Mary*. New York: Knopf, 1973

Venn, John, and J. A. Venn. *Alumni Cantabrigienses*. 2 vols. Cambridge: Cambridge University Press, 1924–1927.

Vines, S. H., and G. Claridge Druce. *Account of the Morisonian Herbarium*. Oxford: Clarendon Press, 1914.

Waldman, Milton. *Elizabeth and Leicester*. Boston: Houghton-Mifflin, 1945.

Wall, Cecil. *History of the Surgeons Company*. London: Oxford University Press, 1937.

_____. *The London Apothecaries*. London: Apothecaries' Hall, 1955.

Wall, Cecil, H. Charles Cameron, and E. Ashworth Underwood. *History of the Worshipful Society of Apothecaries of London: Vol. 1 1617–1815*. (London: Oxford University Press, 1963.

Warnicke, Retha. *The Marrying of Anne of Cleves*. Cambridge: Cambridge University Press, 2000.

_____. *The Rise and Fall of Anne Boleyn*. Cambridge: Cambridge University Press, 1989.

Weatherill, Lorna. *Consumer Behaviour and Material Culture in Britain, 1660–1760*. London: Routledge, 1988.

Webster, Charles S. *From Paracelsus to Newton*. Cambridge: Cambridge University Press, 1982.

_____. *The Great Instauration: Science, Medicine and Reform in England 1626–1660*. New York: Holmes and Meier, 1976.

_____, ed. *Health, Medicine and Mortality in the Sixteenth Century*. Cambridge: Cambridge University Press, 1979.

Weir, Alison. *The Children of Henry VIII*. New York: Ballantine Books, 1996.

Westfall, Richard. *Science and Religion in Seventeenth-Century England*. New Haven, Conn.: Yale University Press, 1958.

Whittet, T. D. *Clerks, Bedels, and Chemical Operators of the Society of Apothecaries*. London: Apothecaries' Hall, 1977.

Whitteridge, Gweneth. *William Harvey and the Circulation of the Blood*. London: Macdonald, 1971.

Williams, E. C. *Anne of Denmark*. Harlow, England: Longmans, 1970.

Williams, Neville. *Henry VIII and His Court*. New York: Macmillan, 1971.

Williamson, James A. *The Tudor Age*. London: Longman, 1979.

Willson, D. Harris. *King James VI and I*. New York: Henry Holt, 1956.

Wood, Anthony. *Athenae Oxonienses*. 5 vols. London: Rivington, 1813–20.

Woolfson, Jonathan. *Padua and the Tudors: English Students in Italy, 1485–1603*. Cambridge: Cambridge University Press, 1999.

Yates, Frances. *Giordano Bruno and the Hermetic Tradition*. Chicago: University of Chicago Press, 1964.

Youings, Joyce. *Sixteenth-Century England*. New York: Penguin Books, 1984.

Young, Sidney. *Annals of the Barber-Surgeons of London*. London: Blades, East and Blades, 1890.

Zimmerman, L. M., and I. Veith. *Great Ideas in the History of Surgery*. Baltimore: William and Wilkins, 1961.

Secondary Sources: Articles and Chapters

Allen, Phyllis. "Medical Education in Seventeenth-Century England." *Journal of the History of Medicine and Allied Sciences* 1 (1946): 115–43.

Anderson, Maurice. "Queen Anne's Children." *British Medical Journal* (1963) 2: 684.

Andrews, Jonathan. "In Her Vapours . . . or Indeed in Her Madness?" *History of Psychiatry* 1 (1990): 125–43.

Appleby, John H. "Some of Arthur Dee's Associations before Visiting Russia Clarified, including Two Letters from Sir Theodore Mayerne." *Ambix* 26 (1979): 1–15.

Arthure, Humphrey. "The Midwife." *Journal of Obstetrics and Gynecology of the British Commonwealth* 80 (1973): 1–9.

Axtell, J. L. "Education and Status in Stuart England: The London Physicians." *History of Education Quarterly* 10 (1970): 141–59.

Bakay, Louis. "Richard Wiseman, a Royalist Surgeon of the English Civil War." *Surgical Neurology* 27 (1987): 415–18.

Baker, George. "Observations on the Late Intermittent Fevers." *Medical Transactions* 3 (1785): 141–216.

Bates, Donald G. "Thomas Sydenham and the Medical Meaning of 'Method.' " *Bulletin of the History of Medicine* 51 (1977): 324–38.
Bayles, Howard. "The Rose Case." *Chemist and Druggist* 132 (1940): 473–74.
Beasley, A. W. "The Disability of James VI and I." *Seventeenth Century* 10 (1995): 151–62.
Beer, Barrett L. "Northumberland: The Myth of the Wicked Duke and the Historical John Dudley." *Albion* 11 (1979): 1–14.
Beier, Lucinda. "The Creation of the Medical Fringe." *Society for the Social History of Medicine Bulletin* 29 (1981): 29–32.
Benedek, Thomas G. "The Changing Relationship between Midwives and Physicians during the Renaissance." *Bulletin of the History of Medicine* 51 (1977): 550–64.
Bindoff, S. T. "A Kingdom at Stake, 1553." *History Today* 3 (1953): 642–48.
Birken, William J. "The Royal College of Physicians of London and Its Support of the Parliamentary Cause in the English Civil War." *Journal of British Studies* 23 (1983): 47–62.
Boehrer, Bruce Thomas. "Early Modern Syphilis." *Journal of the History of Sexuality* 1 (1990): 197–214.
Booth, C. C. "Sir Samuel Garth, F.R.S.: The Dispensary Poet." *Notes and Records of the Royal Society of London* 40 (1986): 125–45.
Brinch, Ove. "The Medical Problems of Henry VIII." *Centaurus* 5/3–4 (1958): 339–69.
Brockliss, L. W. B. "The Literary Image of the *Médicins du Roi* in the Literature of the Grand Siècle." In *Medicine at the Courts of Europe 1500–1838*, ed. Vivian Nutton. London: Routledge, 1990.
_____. "Medical Teaching at the University of Paris, 1600–1720." *Annals of Science* 35 (1978): 221–51.
Brown, James. "Historical Cards." *Gentleman's Magazine* 84/1 (1814): 128–29.
Brown, Theodore M. "The College of Physicians and the Acceptance of Iatromechanism in England 1665–1695." *Bulletin of the History of Medicine* 44 (1970): 12–30.
_____. "Medicine in the Shadow of the 'Principia.' " *Journal of the History of Ideas* 48 (1987): 629–48.
Bruce-Chwatt, L. J. "George Bate—Cromwell's Devious Physician." *Journal of the Royal College of Physicians of London* 17/2 (1983): 144–46.
Bucholz, R. O. " 'Nothing But Ceremony': Queen Anne and the Limitations on Royal Ritual." *Journal of British Studies* 30 (1991): 288–323.
Buckman, Robert F., Jr., and J. William Futrell. "William Cowper." *Surgery* 99/5 (1986): 582–90.
Bynum, W. F. "Medicine at the English Court, 1688–1837." In *Medicine at the Courts of Europe, 1500–1838*, ed. Vivian Nutton. London: Routledge, 1990.
Champneys, F. H. "Midwives in England." *St. Bartholomew's Hospital Journal* 15 (1908): 45.
Chaplin, A. "A History of Medical Education in the Universities of Oxford

and Cambridge 1500–1850." *Proceedings of the Royal Society of Medicine* 13 (1920): 83–107.

Christopher, Thomas A. "The Seeds of Botany." *Natural History* 90 (1981): 50–58.

Clemens, J. R. "Notes on English Medicine." *Annals of Medical History*. New Series, 3 (January 1931): 308–16.

Clericuzio, Antonio. "From van Helmont to Boyle: A Study of the Transmission of Helmontian Chemical and Medical Theories in Seventeenth-Century England." *British Journal for the History of Science* 26 (1993): 303–35.

Clippingdale, Samuel Dodd. "Sir William Butt, M.D.: A Local Link with Shakespeare." *West London Medical Journal* (July 1916).

Cook, Harold J. "Good Advice and Little Medicine: The Professional Authority of Early Modern English Physicians." *Journal of British Studies* 33 (1994): 1–31.

_____. "Living in Revolutionary Times: Medical Change under William and Mary." In *Patronage and Institutions: Science, Technology and Medicine at the European Court 1500–1750*, ed. Bruce T. Moran. Rochester, N.Y.: Boydell Press, 1991.

_____. "Policing the Health of London: The College of Physicians and the Early Stuart Monarchy." *Social History of Medicine* 2 (1989): 1–33.

_____. "Practical Medicine and the British Armed Forces after the 'Glorious Revolution.' " *Medical History* 34 (1990: 1–26.

_____. "The Rose Case Reconsidered: Physicians, Apothecaries, and the Law in Augustan England." *Journal of the History of Medicine and Allied Sciences* 45 (1990): 527–55.

_____. "Sir John Colbatch and Augustan Medicine." *Annals of Science* 47 (1990): 475–505.

Cornwallis, Charles. "The Life and Death of Our Late Most Incomparable and Heroique Prince Henry, Prince of Wales," in *Somers Tracts*. Revised edition. Ed. Walter Scott. 13 vols. New York: AMS, 1965. 2: 225–52.

Coury, Charles. "The Teaching of Medicine in France from the Beginning of the Seventeenth Century." In *The History of Medical Education*, ed. Charles D. O'Malley. Berkeley: University of California Press, 1970.

Crawford, Patricia. "Attitudes to Menstruation in 17th-Century England." *Past and Present* 91 (1981): 47–73.

Cuddy, Neil. "The Revival of the Entourage: The Bedchamber of James I." In *The English Court from the Wars of the Roses to the Civil War*, ed. David Starkey et al. London: Longman, 1987.

Cunningham, Andrew. "Sir Robert Sibbald and Medical Education, Edinburgh." *Clio Medica* 13/2 (1978): 135–61.

Currie, A. S. "Notes on the Obstetrical History of Catherine of Aragon and Anne Boleyn." *Edinburgh Medical Journal* 38 (1888): 1–34.

de Beer, E. S. "Earliest Fellows of the Royal Society." *Bulletin of the Institute of Historical Research* 15 (1937–38): 79–93.

Debus, Allen G. "The Paracelsian Compromise in Elizabethan England." *Ambix* 8 (1960): 71–97.

DeKrey, Gary S. "Political Radicalism in London after the Glorious Revolution." *Journal of Modern History* 55 (1983): 585–617.

Dewhurst, Kenneth. "The Death of Queen Mary II: A Mistaken Diagnosis by Dr. Radcliffe." *Oxford Medical School Gazette* 14 (1962): 104–6.

Dimock, Arthur. "The Conspiracy of Dr. Lopez." *English Historical Review* 9 (1894): 440–72.

Dobson, J. "The Royal Dentists." *Annals of the Royal College of Surgeons* 46 (1970): 277–91.

Dobson, M. "Marsh Fever." *Journal of Historical Geography* 6 (1980): 357–89.

"Doctors at Court: The Medical Household." *British Medical Journal* (1953) 1: 1217–18.

Dowling, Maria. "Anne Boleyn as Patron." In *Henry VIII: A European Court in England,* ed. David Starkey. London: Collins and Brown, 1991.

Durkan, John. "The French Connection in the Sixteenth and Seventeenth Centuries." In *Scotland and Europe, 1200–1850,* ed. T. Smout. Edinburgh: John Donald, 1984.

Ellis, Frank. "The Background of the London Dispensary." *Journal of the History of Medicine* 20 (1965): 197–212.

Emerson, Roger L. "Sir Robert Sibbald, Kt., the Royal Society of Scotland, and the Origins of the Scottish Enlightenment." *Annals of Science* 45 (1988): 41–72.

Emslie-Smith, D. "Great Doctors and Medical Worthies." *Scottish Medical Journal* 33 (1988): 280–84.

Eshleman, Michael K. "Diet during Pregnancy in the Sixteenth and Seventeenth Centuries." *Journal of the History of Medicine* 30 (1975): 29–36.

'Espinasse, Margaret. "The Decline and Fall of Restoration Science." *Past and Present* 14 (July 1958): 74–89.

Fischer, Irving. "Hypothalamic Amenorrhea: Pseudocyesis." In *Psychosomatic Obstetrics, Gynecology and Endochrinology,* ed. William S. Kroger. Springfield, Ill.: Thomas, 1962.

Forbes, Thomas R. "The Case of the Casual Chirurgeon." *Yale Journal of Biology and Medicine* 51 (1978): 583–88.

_____. "The Regulation of English Midwives in the Sixteenth and Seventeenth Centuries." *Medical History* 8 (1964): 235–44.

_____. "The Regulation of English Midwives in the Eighteenth and Nineteenth Centuries." *Medical History* 15 (1971): 352–62.

Frank, Robert G., Jr. "The Physician as Virtuoso in Seventeenth-Century England." In *English Scientific Virtuosi in the Sixteenth and Seventeenth Centuries,* ed. Barbara Shapiro and Robert G. Frank, Jr. Los Angeles: University of California Press, 1979.

_____. "Science, Medicine and the Universities of Early Modern England:

Background and Sources, Part 1." *History of Science* 11 (1973): 194–216; "Part 2," 239–69.

Franklin, Alfred White. "Clinical Medicine." In *Medicine inSeventeenth-Century England*, ed. Allen G. Debus. Berkeley: University of California Press, 1974.

Furdell, Elizabeth Lane. "At the King's Arms in the Poultrey': The Bookshop Emporium of Dorman Newman." *London Journal* 23 (1998): 1–20.

_____. " 'Every Man His Own Doctor': Medical Publishers and Booksellers in the Augustan Age." Unpublished paper read at the DeBartolo Conference on "Revolutions in Print." Tampa, Fla., 1999.

_____. "The Life and Work of Samuel Dodd Clippingdale, Physician and Antiquarian." *Journal of the Royal Society of Medicine* 82 (1989): 758–60.

_____. "Medical Personnel at the Court of Queen Anne." *The Historian* 68 (1986): 412–29.

Futrell, J. W. "William Cowper." *Surgery* 99 (1986): 582–90.

Garrison, Fielding H. "The Medical and Scientific Periodicals of the Seventeenth and Eighteenth Centuries." *Bulletin of the Institute of the History of Medicine* 2/8 (October 1934): 285–343.

_____. "Medicine in *The Tatler, The Spectator*, and *The Guardian*.." *Bulletin of the Institute for the History of Medicine* 2 (1934): 477–503.

"Gastric Involvement in Syphilis." *Family Physician* 46/2 (1992): 552.

Gelbart, Nina Rattner. "The Intellectual Development of Walter Charlton." *Ambix* 18/3 (1971): 149–68.

Geshwind, Max. "Gerard's Herbal Revisited." *Bulletin of the History of Dentistry* 36 (1988): 54–56.

Goldie, Mark. "The Revolution of 1689 and the Structure of Political Argument." *Bulletin of Research in the Humanities* 83 (1980): 473–564.

Guy, John. "Tudor Monarchy and Political Culture." In *Tudor and Stuart Britain*, ed. John Morrill. Oxford: Oxford University Press, 1996.

Gysel, C. "Dental Aspects of Bidloo's 'Anatomy.' " *Medical Hygiene* 44 (1986): 2213–14.

Haggis, A. W. "Fundamental Errors in the Early History of Cinchona." *Bulletin of the History of Medicine* 11 (1942): 568–87.

Hall, A. Rupert and Marie Boas Hall. "The First Human Blood Transfusion: Priority Disputes." *Medical History* 24 (1980): 461–65.

Hambridge, Roger A. "Epiricomany or an Infatuation in Favour of Empiricism or Quackery." In *Literature, Science and Medicine*, ed. Serge Soupel and Roger A. Hambridge. Los Angeles: University of California Press, 1982.

Hamilton, Bernice. "The Medical Professions in the Eighteenth Century." *Economic History Review*, 2nd Series, 4/2 (1951): 141–63.

Henry, John. "Medicine and Pneumatology." *Medical History* 31 (1987): 15–40.

Hill, Christopher. "William Harvey and the Idea of Monarchy." *Past and Present* 27 (1964): 55–72.

Hoak, Dale. "Two Revolutions in Tudor Government." In *Revolutions Reassessed*, ed. Christopher Coleman and David Starkey. Oxford: Oxford University Press, 1986.

Hotine, Margaret. "The Politics of Anti-Semitism: 'The Jew of Malta' and 'The Merchant of Venice.' " *Notes and Queries* 38 (1991): 35–39.

Huffman, William H. and Robert A. Seelinger, Jr. "Robert Fludd's Brevis to James I." *Ambix* 24 (1978): 69–92.

"A Huguenot Surgeon." *Proceedings of the Huguenot Society of London* 17 (1942–43): 70–71.

Hunter, Lynette. "Women and Domestic Medicine." In *Women, Science and Medicine 1500–1700*, ed. Lynette Hunter and Sarah Hutton. Stroud, England: Sutton, 1997.

Jackson, Stanley W. "Melancholia and the Waning of the Humoral Theory." *Journal of the History of Medicine* (1978): 367–76.

James, R. R. "Earliest List of Surgeons to Be Licensed by the Bishop of London." *Janus* 41 (1937): 255–60.

Jaramillo-Arango, Jaime. "A Critical Review of the Basic Facts in the History of Cinchona." *Journal of the Linnaeus Society* 53/351 (March 1949): 272–309.

Jefcoate, G. P. "Addendum to Keynes' Bibliography." *Book Collector* 33 (1984): 527.

Jessup, L. "The Club at the Temple Coffee House." *Archives of Natural History* 16 (1989): 263–74.

Jewson, N. D. "Medical Knowledge and the Patronage System." *Sociology* 8/3 (1974): 369–85.

"John Baber." *Notes and Queries*, 12th Series, 12 (1922): 516.

Kerwin, William. "Where Have You Gone, Margaret Kennix?" In *Women Healers and Physicians*, ed. Lilian R. Furst. Lexington: University Press of Kentucky, 1997.

Keynes, Milo. "Medical Sense and Nonsense in Biography." *Cambridge Review* 105 (January 30, 1984): 9–14.

Kocher, Paul H. "Paracelsian Medicine in England: The First Thirty Years." *Journal of the History of Medicine* 2 (1947): 451–80.

Krivatsy, Nati H. "Walsingham's Copy of Bailey's *Brief Discourse*." *Library*, Series 6, 1 (1979): 166–68.

Kybett, Susan Maclean. "Henry VIII—A Malnourished King?" *History Today* 39 (September 1989): 19–25.

Lane, Joan. "The Household of a Stuart Physician." *Medical History* 17 (1973): 82–86.

Larkin, Edward. "Biographies and Doctors." *Times Literary Supplement* 22 (1974): 289.

Larner, Andrew J. "Portrait of Richard Lower." *Endeavor*, New Series, 11 (1987): 205–8.

Lawler, John. "Dr. Bernard's Library." *Book Auctions in England in the Seventeenth Century*. London: E. Stock, 1898.

Lawrence, James Henry. "History of the Antient Family of Lawrence." *Gentleman's Magazine* 85/2 (1815): 12–17.

Lenman, Bruce. "Physicians and Politics in the Jacobite Era." *The Jacobite Challenge*, ed. Eveline Cruickshanks and Jeremy Black. Edinburgh: John Donald, 1988.

Lindeboom, G. A. "Cowper's Brutale 'Plagiaat' van Bidloo's Anatomische Atlas." *Nederlands Tijdschrift voor Geneeskund* 126/41 (1982): 1878–82.

"Literary Notes." *British Medical Journal* (1912) 1: 688.

Lux, David S. and Harold J. Cook. "Closed Circles or Open Networks?: Communicating at a Distance during the Scientific Revolution." *History of Science* 36 (1998): 179–212.

MacLennan, Hector. "A Gynaecologist Looks at the Tudors." *Medical History* 11 (1967): 66–74.

MacNalty, Arthur. "Medicine in the Time of Queen Elizabeth I." *British Medical Journal* (1953) 1: 1179–84.

Marin, Louis. "Le Corps Pathétique du Roi." *Revue des Sciences Humaines* 69/198 (1985): 31–49.

Martin, Graham. "Prince Rupert and the Surgeons." *History Today* 40 (December 1990): 38–43.

Matthews, Leslie G. "The Day Book of the Court Apothecary 1691–93." *Medical History* 22 (1978): 161–73.

_____. "Italian Charlatans in England." *Pharmaceutical Historian* 9/2 (1979): 2–5.

_____. "Licensed Mountebanks in Britain." *Journal of the History of Medicine* 19 (1964): 30–45.

_____. "Royal Apothecaries of the Tudor Period." *Medical History* 8 (1964): 170–80.

McLaren, Dorothy. "Fertility, Infant Mortality, and Breast Feeding in the Seventeenth Century." *Medical History* 22 (1978): 378–96.

Meyers, William. "Shakespeare, Shylock, and the Jews." *Commentary* 101 (April 1996): 32–38.

Mitchell, R. G. "William Harvey and Celtic Medicine." *Scottish Medical Journal* 29 (1984): 247–56.

Morgan, D.A.L. "The House of Policy." In *The English Court from the Wars of the Roses to the Civil War*, ed. David Starkey et al. London: Longman, 1987.

Morris, G.C.R. "A Portrait of Thomas Hollier, Pepys' Surgeon." *Annals of the Royal College of Surgeons of England* 61 (1979): 224–29.

_____. "Which Molins Treated Cromwell for the Stone and Did Not Prescribe for Pepys?" *Medical History* 26 (1982): 429–35.

"Mr. Serjeant Surgeon John Knight." *British Medical Journal* (1940) 2: 129.

Mullett, Charles F. "Physician vs. Apothecary, 1669–1671." *Scientific Monthly* 49 (1930): 558–65.

Murphy, John. "The Illusion of Decline: the Privy Chamber." In *The English Court from the Wars of the Roses to the Civil War*, ed. David Starkey et al. London: Longman, 1987.

Newman, George. "Thomas Sydenham, Reformer of English Medicine." *Interpreters of Nature: Essays*. Freeport, N.Y.: Books for Libraries, 1968.

Nickson, M.A.E. "Hans Sloane, Book Collector and Cataloguer." *British Library Journal* 14 (1988): 52–69.

Nutton, Vivian. "Conrad Gesner and the English Naturalists." *Medical History* 29 (1985): 93–97.

_____. "Dr. Butler Revisited." *Medical History* 22 (1978): 417–30.

_____. "John Caius and the Linacre Tradition." *Medical History* 23 (1979): 373–91.

_____. "Medicine, Diplomacy and Finance: The Prefaces to a Hippocratic Commentary of 1541." In *New Perspectives on Renaissance Thought*, ed. John Henry and Sarah Hutton. London: Duckworth, 1990.

Nutton, Vivian, and Jeffrey Boss. "Dr. Butler Revisited." *Medical History* 22 (1978): 417–30.

Osler, Margaret. "Descartes and Charlton on Nature and God." *Journal of the History of Ideas* 40 (1979): 445–56.

Pagel, Walter. "Religious Motives in the Medical Biology of the Seventeenth Century." *Bulletin of the History of Medicine* 3 (1935): 97–128, 213–31, 265–312.

Payne, Leonard. "A Plagiarist Plagiarised." *Journal of the Royal College of Physicians of London* 19/1 (1985): 44–47.

Peachey, George C. "Thomas Trapham—Cromwell's Surgeon—and Others." *Proceedings of the Royal Society of Medicine* 24 (1931): 1441–49.

Pelling, Margaret. "Medical Practice in Early Modern England: Trade or Profession?" In *The Professions in Early Modern England*, ed. Wilfrid Prest. London: Croom Helm, 1987.

_____. "Thoroughly Resented? Older Women and the Medical Role in Early Modern London." In *Women, Science and Medicine 1500–1700*, ed. Lynette Hunter and Sarah Hutton. Stroud, England: Sutton, 1997.

Pelling, Margaret and Charles S.Webster. "Medical Practitioners." In *Health, Medicine and Mortality in the Sixteenth Century*, ed. Charles S. Webster. Cambridge: Cambridge University Press, 1979.

Perry, Norma. "Anglo-Jewry, the Law, Religious Conviction, and Self-Interest (1655–1753)." *Journal of European Studies* 14 (1984): 1–23.

Petrelli, R. L. "The Regulation of French Midwifery during the Ancien Régime." *Journal of the History of Medicine* 25 (1971): 276–92.

Phelps, Wayne E. "John Gerard the Herbalist." *Library*, Series 6, 2 (1980): 76–80.

Pocock, J. G. A. "Robert Brady." *Cambridge Historical Journal* 10 (1950–52): 186.

Power, D'Arcy. "Serjeant Surgeons of England and Their Office." *St. Bartholomew's Hospital Journal* 8 (March 1901): 81–84.

_____. "Some Notes on Edmund Harman, King's Barber." *Proceedings of the Royal Society of Medicine* 9 (1916): 67–88.

Poynter, F.N.L. "Gideon de Laune and His Family Circle." *The Wellcome History of Medicine Library Publications Lecture Series*. No. 2. London: Wellcome Medical Library, 1965.

_____. "Nicholas Culpeper and His Books." *Journal of the History of Medicine* 17 (1962): 152–67.

_____. "Nicholas Culpeper and the Paracelsians." *Science, Medicine and Society in the Renaissance*, ed. Allen G. Debus. 2 vols. New York: Science History Publications, 1972.

Proust, Jacqueline. "Le Dialogue de William Bullein." In *Le Dialogue au Temps de la Renaissance*, ed. M. T. Jones-Davies, 59–73. Paris: J. Touzot, 1984.

Quinton, Anthony. "Dr. John Radcliffe, the Benefactor and His Benefactions." *Journal of the Royal Society of Medicine* 79 (1986): 380–86.

Radbill, Samuel X. "Pediatrics." In *Medicine in Seventeenth-Century England*, ed. Allen G. Debus. Berkeley: University of California Press, 1974.

Rather, L. J. "Pathology at Mid-Century." In *Medicine in Seventeenth-Century England*, ed. Allen G. Debus. Los Angeles: University of California Press, 1974.

Rattansi, Pyarali M. "The Helmontian-Galenist Controversy in Restoration England." *Ambix* 12 (1964): 1–23.

_____. "Paracelsus and the Puritan Revolution." *Ambix* 11 (1963): 24–32.

Robb, A.H.T. "Cambridge Medicine." in *Medicine in Seventeenth- Century England*, ed. Allen G. Debus. Berkeley: University of California Press, 1974.

_____. "Medical Education at Oxford and Cambridge Prior to 1850." In *The Evolution of Medical Education in Britian*, ed. F.N.L. Poynter. London: Pitman Medical Publishing, 1966.

Roberts, K. B. "Bidloo, Cowper and Plagiarism of Anatomical Illustrations." *Canadian Social History of Medicine Newsletter*. September 1970: 7–10.

Roberts, R. S. "The Personnel and Practice of Medicine in Tudor and Stuart England. Part 1: The Provinces." *Medical History* 6 (1962): 363–82.

_____. "The Personnel and Practice of Medicine in Tudor and Stuart England. Part 2: London." *Medical History* 8 (1964): 217–34.

Ronalds, Francis S. "Sir William Scroggs and Sir George Wakeman." In *The Attempted Whig Revolution of 1678–1681*. Urbana: University of Illinois Press, 1937.

Roush, Robert E. "The Development of Midwifery." *Journal of the Nurse Midwife* 24/3 (May-June 1979): 27–37.

Russell, K. F. "John Browne 1642–1702." *Bulletin of the History of Medicine* 33/5 (1959): 393–414; 33/6 (1959): 503–22.

Sakula, Alex. "Dr. John Radcliffe, Court Physician, and the Death of Queen Anne." *Journal of the Royal College of Physicians of London* 19/4 (1985): 255–60.

Saxbe, W. B. "Listeria monocytogenes and Queen Anne." *Paediatrics* 49 (1972): 97.

Schaffer, Simon. "The Glorious Revolution and Medicine in Britain and the Netherlands." *Notes and Records of the Royal Society* 43 (1989): 167–90.

Schofield, Roger, and E. A. Wrigley. "Infant and Child Mortality in England in the Late Tudor and Early Stuart Period." In *Health, Medicine and Mortality in the Sixteenth Century*, ed. Charles Webster. Cambridge: Cambridge University Press, 1979.

"Serjeant-Surgeons of England and Their Office." *British Medical Journal* (1900) 1: 583.

"The Serjeant-Surgeons to the King." *British Medical Journal* (1925) 1: 224.

Sharp, Lindsay. "The Royal College of Physicians and Interregnum Politics." *Medical History* 19 (1975): 107–28.

Sharpe, Kevin. "Faction at the Early Stuart Court." *History Today* 33 (October 1983): 39–47.

_____. "The Image of Virtue: The Court and Household of Charles I." In *The English Court from the Wars of the Roses to the Civil War*, ed. David Starkey et al. London: Longman, 1987.

Shepard, Alan. " 'O seditious citizen of the physicall Common-Wealth!': Harvey's Royalism and His Autopsy of Old Parr." *University of Toronto Quarterly* 65 (1996): 482–506.

Sheridan, Richard. "The Doctor and the Buccaneer: Hans Sloane's Case History of Henry Morgan." *Journal of the History of Medicine* 41 (1986): 76–87.

Siegel, Rudolph E., and F.N.L. Poynter. "Robert Talbor, Charles II and Cinchona." *Medical History* 6 (1962): 82–85.

Slack, Paul. "Mirrors of Health and the Treasures of Poor Men." In *Health, Medicine and Mortality in the Sixteenth Century*, ed. Charles Webster. Cambridge: Cambridge University Press, 1979.

Smith, Dale. "Quinine and Fever." *Journal of the History of Medicine* 31 (1976): 344–45.

Smith, Hilda. "Gynecology and Ideology in Seventeenth Century England." In *Liberating Women's History*, ed. Berenice A. Carroll. Urbana: University of Illinois Press, 1976.

Snyder, Henry L. "The Last Days of Queen Anne: The Account of Sir John Evelyn Examined." *Huntington Library Quarterly* (May 1971): 261–76.

"Some Royal Deathbeds: Queen Anne," *British Medical Journal* (1910) 2: 1530.

Starkey, David. "Intimacy and Innovation: The Use of the Privy Chamber." In *The English Court from the Wars of the Roses to the Civil War*, ed. David Starkey et al. London: Longman, 1987.

Stevenson, Lloyd G. "New Diseases of the Seventeenth Century." *Bulletin of the History of Medicine* 39 (1965): 1–21.

Stewart, Byron S. "The Cult of the Royal Martyr." *Church History* 38 (1969): 175–87.

Stubbs, Blaxland. "Royal Recipes for Plasters, Ointments and Other Medicaments." *Chemist and Druggist* 114 (1931): 792–94.

"Syphilis." *Clinical Symposia* 32/3 (1971): 7.

"Tabor's (or Talbor's) Cure of Ague." *Journal of the Royal College of Physicians of London*. 21/1 (1987): 66.

Thomas, Christine G. "Sir Hans Sloane and the Russian Academy of Sciences." *British Library Journal* 14 (1988): 21–37.

_____. "The Society of Chemical Physitians." In *Science, Medicine, and History*, ed. E. A. Underwood. London: Oxford University Press, 1953.

Thompson, Henry R. "Serjeant Surgeons to Their Majesties." *Annals of the Royal College of Surgeons* 26 (1960): 1–23.

Thorndike, Lynn. "Newness and Novelty in Seventeenth-Century Science and Medicine." In *Roots of Scientific Thought*, ed. P. P. Wiener and A. Noland. New York: Basic Books, 1957.

Thornton, J. L., and Patricia C. Want. "William Harvey, 'Father of British Obstetrics' and His Friend Percival Willughby." *British Journal of Obstetrics and Gynaecology* 85/4 (1978): 241–45.

Todd, Dennis. "New Evidence for Dr. Arbuthnot's Authorship of 'Rabbit Man-Midwife.' " *Studies in Bibliography* 41 (1988): 257–67.

Trevor-Roper, Hugh. "The Court Physician and Paracelsianism." In *Medicine at the Courts of Europe, 1500–1838*, ed. Vivian Nutton. London: Routledge, 1990.

_____. "Medicine in Politics." *American Scholar* 51 (Winter 1982): 23–42.

Turk, J. L., and Elizabeth Allen. "Bleeding and Cupping." *Annals of the Royal College of Surgeons* 65/2 (March 1983): 128–29.

Underwood, E. Ashworth. "Medicine and the Crown." *British Medical Journal* 1 (1953): 1185–87.

Ungerer, Gustav. "George Baker: Translator of Aparicio de Zubia's Pamphlet on the 'Oleum Magistrale.' " *Medical History* 30 (1986): 203–11.

Vigne, Randolph. "Mayerne and His Successors." *Journal of the Royal College of Physicians of London* 20/3 (1986): 222–26.

Wear, Andrew. "Interfaces: Perceptions of Health and Illness in Early Modern England." In *Problems and Methods in the History of Medicine*, ed. Roy Porter and Andrew Wear. London: Croom Helm, 1987.

_____. "Puritan Perceptions of Illness in Seventeenth-Century England." In *Patients and Practitioners*, ed. Roy Porter. Cambridge: Cambridge University Press, 1985

Webster, Charles. "The College of Physicians: 'Solomon's House' in Commonwealth England." *Bulletin of the History of Medicine* 41 (1967): 393–412.

_____. "English Medical Reformers of the Puritan Revolution: A Background to the 'Society of Chymical Physitians.' " *Ambix* 14 (1967): 16–41.

Weigall, Rachell. "An Elizabethan Gentlewoman: The Journal of Lady Mildmay." *Quarterly Review* 215 (1911): 119–36.

Whitfield, A.G.W. "Roger Marbeck—First Registrar." *Journal of the Royal College of Physicians of London* 15/1 (1981): 59–60.

Whittet, T. D. "Sir Thomas Clarges, Apothecary and Envoy." *Journal of the Royal Society of Medicine* 81 (1988): 464–67.

Wilson, Adrian. "Memorial of Eleanor Willughby." In *Women, Science and Medicine 1500–1700*, ed. Lynette Hunter and Sarah Hutton. Stroud, England: Sutton, 1997.

Wolf, Lucien. "Jews in Elizabethan England." *Transactions of the Jewish Historical Society of England* 11 (1928): 1–91.

Wyman, A. L. "Samuel Barrow, M.D., Physician to Charles II and Admirer of John Milton." *Medical History* 18 (1974): 335–48.

INDEX